Clinical Sports Psychiatry

Clinical Sports Psychiatry

An International Perspective

Edited by

David A. Baron

Claudia L. Reardon

Steven H. Baron

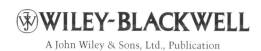

A John Wiley & Sons, Ltd., Publication

Registered Office
John Wiley & Sons, Ltd, The Atrium, Southern Gate, Chichester, West Sussex, PO19 8SQ, UK

Editorial Offices
9600 Garsington Road, Oxford, OX4 2DQ, UK
The Atrium, Southern Gate, Chichester, West Sussex, PO19 8SQ, UK
2121 State Avenue, Ames, Iowa 50014–8300, USA

For details of our global editorial offices, for customer services and for information about how to apply for permission to reuse the copyright material in this book please see our website at www.wiley.com/wiley-blackwell.

Library of Congress Cataloging-in-Publication Data

Clinical sports psychiatry : an international perspective / edited by David A. Baron, Claudia L. Reardon, Steven H. Baron.
       p. ; cm.
   Includes bibliographical references and index.
   ISBN 978-1-118-40488-1 (cloth)
I. Baron, David A.   II. Reardon, Claudia L.   III. Baron, Steven H.
[DNLM: 1. Athletes–psychology.   2. Mental Disorders–therapy.   3. Sports–psychology.   QT 260]
   616.89–dc23
                                      2012048022
A catalogue record for this book is available from the British Library.

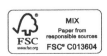

Contents

Contributors

Samir Abolmagd
Addiction Medicine Unit,
Cairo University, Cairo, Egypt

Ezzat Abdelazeem A. Awad
NTNU Norway, Hail,
Kingdom of Saudi Arabia

David A. Baron
International Relations, Keck School
of Medicine at the University of
Southern California, Los Angeles, CA, USA
Department of Psychiatry,
Keck School of Medicine at the
University of Southern California,
Los Angeles, CA, USA
Keck Medical Center at University of
Southern California, Los Angeles, CA, USA
Global Center for Exercise,
Psychiatry, and Sports at USC,
Health Sciences Campus, Los Angeles,
CA, USA

Steven H. Baron
Montgomery County Community
College, Blue Bell, PA, USA

Antonia L. Baum
Department of Psychiatry
and Behavioral Sciences,
George Washington University
School of Medicine and Health
Sciences, Washington, DC, USA

Krisztina Berczik
Doctoral School of Psychology,
Eötvös Loránd University,
Hungary
Institute of Psychology,
Eötvös Loránd University, Budapest,
Hungary

Ugur Cakir
Department of Psychiatry,
Derince Education and Research Hospital,
Kocaeli, Turkey

Brandon J. Cornejo
Northwest Permanente,
East Interstate Medical Office,
Mental Health, Portland, OR, USA

Bulent Coskun
Department of Psychiatry,
Community Mental Health Center,
Kocaeli University, Kocaeli, Turkey

Jeremy DeFranco
Department of Psychiatry,
Keck School of Medicine at the University
of Southern California,
Los Angeles, CA, USA

Zsolt Demetrovics
Institute of Psychology,
Eötvös Loránd University,
Budapest, Hungary

Robert M. Factor
Department of Psychiatry,
University of Wisconsin School of
Medicine and Public Health, Madison,
WI, USA

Heba M. Fakher M. Hendawy
Department of Neuropsychiatry,
Faculty of Medicine,
Institute of Psychiatry,
Ain Shams University, Cairo,
Egypt

Michael W. Fitzgerald
Warrior Behavioral Health,
U.S. Army Health Center,
Schofield Barracks,
HI, USA

Ira D. Glick
Psychiatry and Behavioral Sciences,
Stanford University School of
Medicine, Stanford, CA, USA

Mark D. Griffiths
International Gaming
Research Unit, Psychology
Division, Nottingham Trent
University, Nottingham, UK

Dora Kurimay
SPiN New York, New York, NY, USA

Tamás Kurimay
Department of Psychiatry
and Psychiatric Rehabilitation,
Saint John Hospital,
Budapest, Hungary

Michael T. Lardon
Department of Psychiatry,
School of Medicine,
University of California, San Diego,
San Diego, CA, USA

Saul I. Marks
FINA Sports Medicine Committee,
Toronto, ON, Canada
International Society for
Sport Psychiatry,
North York General Hospital, Toronto, ON,
Canada
Department of Health and Disease,
Department of Psychiatry,
University of Toronto,
Toronto, ON, Canada

Sally Mohamed
Kasr El Maadi Hospital, korniche El
Maadi, Maadi, Cairo, Egypt

Eric D. Morse
Carolina Performance,
North Carolina
State University, Raleigh, NC, USA

Thomas Newmark
Department of Psychiatry,
Robert Wood Johnson
Medical School, Cooper
University Hospital, Camden, NJ, USA

Aslihan Polat
Department of Psychiatry,
Kocaeli University Medical Faculty,
Kocaeli, Turkey
Women's Mental Health Unit,
Kocaeli University School of Medicine,
Kocaeli, Turkey

Pavel A. Ponizovskiy
Department of Mental Disorders
Complicated by Substance Abuse,
Moscow Research Institute of
Psychiatry, Moscow, Russia

Claudia L. Reardon
Department of Psychiatry,
University of Wisconsin
School of Medicine and
Public Health, Madison, WI, USA

Eva C. Ritvo
Department of Psychiatry
and Behavioral Sciences,
University of Miami School of
Medicine, Miami, FL, USA

Mark A. Stillman
Department of Psychology,
School of Liberal Arts,
Georgia Gwinnett College,
Lawsenceville, GA, USA

Joshua Tompkins
Keck School of Medicine
at the University of
Southern California, Los Angeles, CA,
USA

Kathy Toon
GlamSlam Tennis, El Cerrito, CA, USA

Thomas Wenzel
Division of Social Psychiatry,
Medical University of Vienna,
Vienna, Austria

Li Jing Zhu
Division of Social Psychiatry,
Medical University of Vienna,
Vienna, Austria
Physical Education College,
Zheng Zhou University,
Zheng Zhou, Henan, Peoples Republic
of China

Foreword by Steve Peters

I am very pleased and honored to have been invited to write a foreword for this groundbreaking book. I have been a consultant psychiatrist for over 20 years and have worked in the field of elite sport since 2001, going on to become the first full-time sports psychiatrist in the United Kingdom in 2005.

Forging new pathways can be fraught with danger, and it would have been very helpful when I first started working with athletes to have had some guidance on the more unfamiliar areas that I was about to encounter. A few examples would be abuse in sport, sexual harassment, substance use, and cultural issues. Although these topics have previously been considered independently, there has never been a concise volume that draws them together in a manner that offers the would-be sports psychiatrist or practicing clinician a comprehensive coverage of the work and research undertaken to date. Alongside the more familiar psychiatric areas of expertise such as eating disorders, these less familiar areas have been woven together to provide, within this book, a balanced and comprehensive coverage of the range of subjects the psychiatrist could possibly expect to encounter in sport. As psychiatry within sport is a relatively new discipline within medicine and arguably in its embryonic phase, attempting to draw together the spectrum of areas that psychiatry covers across various sports is a commendable endeavor. In addition, to coordinate international perspectives is ambitious. I believe that the editors and their authors have not only admirably succeeded in this venture but also established a foundation for future work in the field.

This book, therefore, has drawn together experts who have offered a comprehensive review of recent research in their specialist fields. The book does not claim to be authoritative but rather offers the reader the opportunity to survey the work of others with the addition of personal experience and interpretation. For example, in my own area of expertise, optimizing the functioning of the human mind, the reader is introduced to a selected number of psychological practices and techniques for consideration. These are not presented as superior illustrations or definitive models but rather as examples to consider. This approach is representative of the style of the book and I believe gives it its strength. It offers information as a forum for discussion, to be thought provoking and yet also offers practical advice. As such, the book is a very useful tool to all psychiatrists working in the field of sport or who have an interest in it.

The book is well balanced both in the range and depth of its contents. It could be viewed as having three major themes. The first theme deals with the more standard aspects of mental health and covers notoriously difficult areas within clinical practice such as addictions, suicidal ideation, and posttraumatic stress. The second major theme covers the general health of the athlete from both the physical and psychological perspectives, and within this does not shirk from tackling the more challenging subjects of potential abuse, sexual harassment, doping, and lifestyle choices encountered within various cultures in sport. The final theme looks at how the psychiatrist can contribute toward improving the athlete's performance. The information offered has a lot of practical advice and will be a great asset to the psychiatrist.

This book is very forward looking and will help provide a basis for the development of the specialism of sports psychiatry within medicine. It offers a future curriculum for training those who wish to specialize in this field, and I recommend it as extremely useful reading to both the trainee and the experienced specialist already engaged in sport.

ABOUT THE AUTHOR

Dr. Peters has worked with the Great Britain Cycling Team, the Professional Procycling Team SKY, and numerous other elite national sports, such as England Rugby, Track and Field, Taekwondo, and Canoeing. He holds positions with the UK anti-doping organization and has acted in a consultancy capacity to the World Anti-Doping Agency. He introduced his own mind management model for sport, encapsulated in the book *The Chimp Paradox*. He is a Senior Clinical Lecturer and Undergraduate Dean at Sheffield Medical School and a member of the examination panel for the Royal College of Psychiatrists.

Foreword by Thomas Newmark

My entire life, I have been a sports fan. As President of The International Society for Sports Psychiatry (ISSP) for the past 4 years and a member of the ISSP for 20 years, I have seen the evolution and growing interest in the field of sports psychiatry. The ISSP has held annual symposia at the American Psychiatric Association (APA) annual scientific meeting. Psychiatrist experts have presented, and athletes have enriched the programs by sharing their experiences. Traumatic brain injury and the impact of injury, doping, and addiction in athletes are among the topics presented and discussed in recent years. I have participated in and been very inspired by and impressed with these programs. The level of interest shown by members and nonmembers, both nationally and internationally, has continued to soar. Members have often inquired about how they can learn about the field and if there is a textbook for sports psychiatry. We now have this comprehensive volume *Clinical Sports Psychiatry: An International Perspective*. This textbook is written with scientific rigor and practical information to facilitate your sports psychiatry practice.

I have long known and worked with editors David Baron, D.O., MSEd, and Claudia Reardon, M.D. Both are extraordinarily dynamic individuals. Steven Baron, Ph.D., is a noted social scientist whose current research focuses on sports psychology and traumatic brain injury.

David Baron, D.O., is a giant in the field of sports psychiatry. He is one of the world experts on concussion, doping, and mood disorders in athletes and has written and presented extensively. Dr. Baron is an outstanding researcher and has always pushed to have sports psychiatry as a field based in scientific data. He has worked with Olympians and has been a consultant at the Olympic Games. Claudia Reardon, M.D., is an expert in the use of treatment modalities and medications in athletes. She is a dedicated researcher and educator. She has a broad, visionary perspective of the status and future of sports psychiatry.

I learned about the field of sports psychiatry by attending and presenting sports psychiatry-related topics at the APA and by developing a sports psychiatry program for local high-school athletes. In addition, I read articles written by many of the authors and editors featured in *Clinical Sports Psychiatry: An International Perspective*. In treating athletes and in 20 years of educating medical students and training psychiatry residents, I have seen few comprehensive resources for sports psychiatry practice, the only other notable one being *Sports Psychiatry: Theory and Practice* (Eds. Begel and Burton, 2000). Having treated athletes for performance anxiety, issues related to recovery from injury, and postconcussion syndrome, I felt the need for a resource current with the evolving science, research, and knowledge. *Clinical Sports Psychiatry: An International Perspective* fulfills that need. We at the ISSP have also encouraged the increased interest, participation, and contributions of international psychiatrists in the field. Their contributions are included in this new textbook.

Indeed, the editors have recruited an outstanding team of experts for the book. In reading this volume, psychiatrists will develop greater competence in working with athletes and teams. The global perspective is unique. Through the ISSP, I know and work with many of the authors. All are nationally and internationally known psychiatrists in their areas of expertise. Eric Morse, M.D., has developed behavioral and addiction service programs for college athletes and teams. Saul Marks, M.D., from Canada, has studied, consulted with, and treated athletes who have been sexually harassed or abused. Antonia Baum, M.D., has expertise in eating disorders in athletes and has extensively researched suicide risk in athletes. Ira Glick, M.D., has written and spoken throughout the world on psychotherapy treatments for athletes and their families and collaborates routinely with Eva Ritvo, M.D. Michael Lardon, M.D., has worked extensively with golfers on performance enhancement. Finally, other authors and I speak to the current status and challenges of sports psychiatry.

Be enriched and enjoy.

ABOUT THE AUTHOR

Thomas Newmark, M.D., is President of the International Society for Sports Psychiatry. Presently, he is Professor of Psychiatry at Cooper Medical School of Rowan University (CMSRU) in Camden, New Jersey. Previously, Dr. Newmark was Professor at Robert Wood Johnson Medical School (RWJMS) and Chief of Psychiatry at Cooper University Hospital (CUH), serving from 1997 to 2011. He served as President of the Cooper Medical Staff from 2002 to 2007. Dr. Newmark is President-Elect of the American Association of Psychiatric Administrators. He is a past president of the New Jersey Psychiatric Association and South Jersey Psychiatric Association and continues to serve as the head of the Ethics Committee for NJPA. In his 25 years of service at CUH and RWJMS, Dr. Newmark has served on numerous committees for RWJMS, including those for Admissions, Appointment and Promotions, Curriculum, CME, and the Executive Committee.

Dr. Newmark earned his medical degree from Hahnemann University Medical School (now Drexel University School of Medicine). He completed his internship at Albert Einstein Medical Center in Philadelphia and his residency at the Medical University of South Carolina. He is board certified in adult, psychosomatic medicine, and administrative psychiatry. Dr. Newmark has been recognized consistently by his colleagues, being named a Top Doc many times. He serves on the Editorial Board of Academic Psychiatry. Dr. Newmark has made numerous presentations and has published on sports psychiatry. Very interested in psychiatric education, Dr. Newmark has received several teaching awards, including seven Golden Apple Teaching Awards from the RWJMS and the Sol Sherry M.D. Award from CUH. He is a Distinguished Life Fellow of the American Psychiatric Association.

Acknowledgments

The coeditors are very grateful to the International Society for Sports Psychiatry and to the World Psychiatric Association Section on Exercise and Sports Psychiatry. Both organizations endorsed this work and supported its development by providing as chapter authors many of the world's leading experts in sports psychiatry. We would also like to acknowledge the athletes across the globe who give so much of themselves in order to pursue and model excellence.

Preface

*Spanning the globe to bring you the
constant variety of sport...the thrill of
victory...and the agony of defeat...the
human drama of athletic competition
...this is ABC's Wide World of Sports!*

This was the weekly opening of the first television broadcast to showcase sports from around the globe. It first aired on 29 April 1961 on the American Broadcasting Company, but became an international phenomenon, focusing on sports not commonly covered by international networks. It introduced viewers from around the world to sports rarely seen by the average sports fan. The editors of this text were inspired by this approach. This book is one of the first to address current issues in sports psychiatry from a global perspective (the chapter authors represent over half a dozen countries). It does not concentrate on any individual sport, but rather provides analysis of the most important, contemporary issues in sports psychiatry, including concussion in sports, suicide in athletes, doping, and sexual harassment and abuse in sport. Our goal is to span the globe to bring the reader the full variety of sports psychiatry topics in one text, from an international perspective.

Much of the lay public and many members of the sporting world do not understand the differences between sports psychologists and sports psychiatrists. As behavioral health providers, both disciplines offer valuable contributions in providing for the well-being of athletes, on and off the field of competition. Sports psychology, an older and more established field, tends to focus on performance enhancement strategies and techniques, whereas sports psychiatry addresses the etiology and treatment of psychiatric symptoms and syndromes presenting in athletes. Importantly, overlap between the fields does exist. For example, sports psychiatrists may discuss performance enhancement strategies such as goal setting and mental imagery in the context of addressing an athlete's depression or anxiety. Not only is this holistic approach helpful for the overall functioning of the athlete, but it also helps to achieve "buy in" from the athlete who may otherwise be reluctant to seek psychiatric treatment solely for the purpose of treating a psychiatric disorder.

We believe athletes, especially elite competitors, should be viewed as a unique patient population with diagnostic and treatment interventions sensitive to their needs. Just as child or geriatric psychiatrists are knowledgeable about different clinical presentations of and treatments for their patient population, psychiatrists evaluating and treating athletes should be aware of issues impacting their clinical cohort. After reading this book, we believe the learner will have a better appreciation of these unique concepts.

Athletic competition has been an integral component of culture worldwide for thousands of years. Successful athletes are treated like royalty, with the most accomplished becoming national icons. Few events can match the impact of a world champion national team on the collective psyche of an entire country. Olympic champions in marquee sports are given rock star status after their victory. Youth athletes dream of someday attaining the fame and financial rewards given to elite competitors. As all athletes know, success does not come without paying the price. Years of dedication and self-sacrifice are the universal blueprint for victory. Only recently has the impact of emotional stress and physical injury been acknowledged as important factors to consider. The potential long-term adverse consequences of multiple head trauma are changing the culture of contact sports around the globe. We have learned that nonelite athletes may suffer from sport-related psychiatric conditions such as exercise addiction. Moreover, even after retirement, athletes may be at risk for sport-related psychiatric conditions including depression and substance abuse.

Through the topics mentioned and several others, we have introduced the reader to the most important contemporary issues in sports psychiatry. Our goal is to inspire the reader to engage in the education and research needed to better address the mental health needs of athletes around the world. The "game" is just beginning, and everyone wins if we do it right. Sport has many known mental health benefits, and it is the hope of sports psychiatrists to optimize the benefits while successfully preventing and treating psychiatric symptoms and disorders that may arise.

We hope you feel encouraged to contribute to the emerging field of sports psychiatry. This book is endorsed by the two major sports psychiatry organizations, the International Society for Sports Psychiatry (ISSP) and the World Psychiatric Association Section on Exercise and Sports Psychiatry. We thank their leadership for the endorsement and encourage all qualified readers to consider joining both of these excellent groups.

David A. Baron
Claudia L. Reardon
Steven H. Baron

Part One

Mental Health Challenges Faced by Athletes

1 Substance Use in Athletes

Eric D. Morse

Carolina Performance, North Carolina State University, USA

KEY POINTS

- A strong, clear, enforceable drug testing policy with frequent, random drug tests would reduce substance use in athletes.
- Assessment of positive drug tests and treatment of substance use disorders and co-occurring mental illness by sports psychiatrists would help athletes continue to perform at a high level.
- The higher the stakes, the more the risk of doping and the use of performance-enhancing drugs, and the greater the need for sports psychiatrists working with athletes.

BACKGROUND AND SCOPE OF PROBLEM

Despite the risk of negative consequences of loss of performance, pay, and scholarships, elite athletes seem to use most substances at higher rates than age-matched nonathletes in the general population [1–10]. The rates may be lower in some sports, ethnicities, and nationalities [7, 11]. Comparing the National Collegiate Athletic Association (NCAA) survey data from 2005 to 2009, there was a drop in reported use of amphetamines (3.7% of U.S. college athletes reported use), ephedrine (0.9%), and anabolic steroids (0.6%), and increases in cannabis (22.6% reported use), cocaine (1.8%), opioids (3.3%), alcohol (83.1%), and alcohol binges (38.8%) [12]. While sometimes used initially for performance-enhancing reasons, many of these substances can represent gateways to other drug use. There are certainly risks of "stimulant stacking" (energy drinks, excitatory amino acids, caffeine, nicotine, ephedrine, and amphetamines) that can lead to "upper–downer" pairings (adding cannabis, alcohol, or prescription sleeping medications to stimulants) [4]. Sports psychiatrists must be aware of these pairings and patterns of use among their athletes to avoid enabling. Sports psychiatrists must be able to urine drug test their athletes for diagnostic purposes, in a way that would not lead to negative consequences and that would encourage treatment and assistance over penalties. Our elite athletes are role models for our youth; thus, creating prevention and intervention programs to reduce substance use in athletes may have a significant impact on substance use in general.

Clinical Sports Psychiatry: An International Perspective, First Edition. Edited by David A. Baron,
Claudia L. Reardon and Steven H. Baron.
© 2013 John Wiley & Sons, Ltd. Published 2013 by John Wiley & Sons, Ltd.

REASONS FOR USE

Athletes often use substances to objectively or subjectively assist performance. McDuff lists the most common reasons for elite athletes to initially use substances: to fit in, boost self-confidence, produce pleasure, escape problems, and have fun. Reasons for continued use may include: stress relief, psychological dependence, negative emotions reduction, and tolerance/withdrawal [4]. In this author's and others' experiences, a leading reason for athletes to use substances is to get high. Looking at the reasons for an individual athlete can help in the development of a treatment plan. Developing new coping mechanisms other than substance use is vital.

Enhancing performance with substances may involve getting bigger, stronger, or faster. For some athletes, substances are used to get thinner or to pay better attention. Relieving pain with opioids may lead to an iatrogenic addiction. Some athletes compete using opioids. A recent study by the National Institute on Drug Abuse and the National Football League (NFL) of 644 former NFL players found that 52% used pain medication while playing. Of those players, 63% received medication from a nonmedical source; 15% of the retired players are still misusing pain medications [5].

Substance use to celebrate wins or console losses may be done on an individual or team level. Particularly in individual sports, individual athletes may deal with the stress of winning (and higher expectations) or losing (and disappointment) with substances. It seems to be acceptable in many societies to celebrate a tough win with alcohol, as evident from many sports-related television commercials. Champion teams and athletes pop open and shower each other with champagne to celebrate. When substance use is part of the team culture through peer pressure, hazing rituals, or even as part of the team's recruiting process, it can be propagated from class to class or from old professional veterans to rookies.

Career termination

Of all the challenges with which athletes must contend, the termination of their athletic career certainly ranks among one of the most difficult [13]. When athletes recognize that professional sports participation is no longer an option, they may be reluctant to give up the identity of athlete. For many athletes whose identity has been drawn from athletic participation, anticipation of life after athletics can be scary. It is common for athletes experiencing the termination phase of their career to deal with the anxiety and fear by using substances [14]. Unexpected, early career termination due to injury, poor academic performance, or positive drug tests are even more challenging and may lead to more substance use. Unresolved physical pain may lead to substance use as well. The loss of identity and remaining stuck in the past may be seen in reunions, alumni functions, and frequent unexpected visits to the training room long after athletic careers are over. Substance use at these times may peak. Sports psychiatrists need to screen, warn, and treat their athletes of these common occurrences. Athletes often do not like to discuss what they would do if their athletic careers were over tomorrow, but discussing the subject and developing a Plan B may help prevent maladaptive behaviors in the future and should be part of the work of the sports psychiatrist.

Weight management

Most athletes are concerned with weight management at one time or another, to enhance performance, make specific weight classes, or appear attractive for judges [15]. For some, the focus on weight management becomes obsessive and eating disorder behaviors develop.

While misusing substances like diet pills, stimulants, or laxatives is expected with eating disorders, some athletes may develop a co-occurring substance use disorder [16]. Suspecting an eating disorder should be probable cause for a urine drug screen within athletic drug testing policies. While there is a sport-specific prevalence for eating disorders, no sport or individual should be considered exempt from developing an eating disorder. Anabolic steroids may be used to trim down and reduce body fat, or to bulk up and gain weight. Some athletes use cannabis to improve their appetites and gain weight for their sport.

Performance effects

Athletes may use substances for performance-enhancing effects. When sports psychiatrists refer to performance-enhancing drugs, we may think of anabolic steroids and stimulants. However, athletes may see some initial improvement in their game with alcohol, cannabis, or benzodiazepines if they are too energized or have difficulties with intensity regulation when competing. They may pair uppers (steroids, stimulants, or cocaine) with downers (alcohol, benzodiazepines, or cannabis) as they continue to use and require assistance with resulting insomnia or fatigue. Continued use or abuse may lead to dependence and/or a drop-off in performance. Tolerance develops and higher doses must be consumed to gain the same performance or euphoric effect. An athlete may have a difficult time deciding if continued use is for performance-enhancement reasons or for relaxation and coping with the deterioration in performance. Substance use usually increases during the off-season and on days off [5].

Athletes, coaches, trainers, or administrators may ask sports psychiatrists to prescribe performance-enhancing medications to athletes. Importantly, proper testing, diagnosing, treatment planning, and prescribing appropriate medication for mental illness should not be considered performance enhancing, but performance enabling [17]. Sports psychiatrists help athletes return to their previous level of functioning and performance with the use of psychiatric medications. However, sports psychiatrists must be aware of the psychiatric medications that are on the banned list of the sport in which their athlete-patient participates (particularly stimulants, modafinil, and beta-blockers) and, if a prescription of one of these medications is appropriate, submit the proper documentation for Therapeutic Use Exemptions (TUE) for most professional and Olympic sports [18]. The NCAA also has certain guidelines [19]. Medications to treat addictions, such as methadone or buprenorphine, may be on some banned lists as well.

TRAUMATIC BRAIN INJURY

Athletes with traumatic brain injury (TBI) are more susceptible to the intoxicating effects of substances and may get in trouble more easily due to the disinhibiting effects of the brain injury. Cognitive impairments may become more pronounced. Athletes with postconcussive symptoms or syndromes may rely on substances to help manage the headaches and frustrations of not being able to practice or compete. The risk of suicide may be magnified when TBI is complemented with substances. Athletes with TBI may become more impulsive, have more emotional dysregulation, have less cognitive reserve, and require more time to clear from substances, particularly from longer-acting benzodiazepines, which may be inappropriately prescribed for sleep by some physicians.

RECOGNIZING SUBSTANCE USE

Prior to or besides urine drug testing, how might sports psychiatrists recognize substance use in athletes? First and foremost, sports psychiatrists might not recognize substance use unless they ask. Other members of the sports medicine team might not feel comfortable or have much training in asking the questions. Asking yes/no questions such as "Do you drink alcohol?" often leads to a quick "no" from the athlete. On the other hand, asking "How much alcohol do you drink in a typical week?" usually results in a response of some number of drinks. When the answer is "zero," the sports psychiatrist should probe why the athlete does not drink. The same series of questions should continue for other commonly used substances – stimulants, cannabis, anabolic steroids, cocaine, and others depending on the location and what substances are popular in that region or campus. To find out what other substances are popular in your region or campus, the sports psychiatrist may simply ask, "What are your teammates usually using?"

Besides responses to direct questions, students having difficulty reporting to practice, study hall, or class on time might be a clue to substance use problems. There may be a drop-off in their academic or athletic performance. Other odd behaviors or changes in attitude or work ethic are common. Sometimes substance intoxication is more obvious than substance withdrawal. More specific signs and symptoms of substance use are listed in Table 1.1.

For universities and teams, a good substance use prevention or drug testing policy will allow drug testing for cause. Discovering some of the signs mentioned previously should prompt someone to order a drug test. A good substance use prevention or drug testing policy is not designed to punish the athlete, but rather to help the athlete get the assistance she may

Table 1.1 Signs and symptoms of substance use.

Substance	Signs and symptoms of use	Signs and symptoms of withdrawal
Stimulants	Dilated pupils, anxiety, jitteriness, increased heart rate/blood pressure, mood, somnolence, dry mouth, nasal problems, restlessness, insomnia, talkativeness, loss of appetite, tics	Fatigue, headaches, anxiety, depression
Cannabis	Smell on clothes, bloodshot eyes, memory problems, lack of motivation, paranoia, increased appetite, use of eyedrops, drowsiness, giggling, slowed responses, cough	Insomnia, cravings, irritability, anxiety, reduced appetite
Alcohol	Sedation, disinhibition, slurred speech, euphoria, ataxia, blackouts, memory problems, flushing, impulsiveness, vomiting, fights, legal problems, nystagmus	Increased heart rate/blood pressure, tremor, seizures, irritability, insomnia, fatigue, depressed mood, headache, sweating
Anabolic steroids	Acne, rapid weight gain, irritability, rage, gynecomastia or hair loss in males, deepening of voice and facial hair in females, injection sites, cysts, bloating, night sweats, joint pain, insomnia, mood swings	Depressed mood, weakness, fatigue, aches, insomnia, weight loss, restlessness

need. Treatment and education should be emphasized over suspensions. There should be a "treatment track" that may allow an athlete who tests positive to return to play sooner if the athlete is compliant with treatment recommendations.

TREATMENT

Individual treatment

Sports psychiatrists may be asked to assess and intervene when an athlete tests positive on a random urine drug test from a team, university, NCAA, or professional league. Teams, universities, or leagues must have a very clear, fair drug testing policy that allows for assessment, treatment, and enforceable consequences for positive drug tests with little wiggle room for exceptions for more talented athletes in money-generating sports or for influential coaches. The best deterrent for drug use in sports is frequent, accurate, very closely observed, truly random urine drug testing. Masking agents must be tested for as well. If athletes know they will be tested and suspended for testing positive, they are much less likely to use. If athletes know that their parents, agents, or coaches can argue and have the result thrown out, they are more likely to use.

It is not unusual for athletes to deny any use, despite mass spectroscopy confirmation of their urine drug tests. The athlete may be in the precontemplation stage of change and not interested in treatment of or intervention for their substance use. A good sports psychiatrist can use motivational interviewing techniques in these circumstances. He can agree to disagree with the athlete, roll with resistance, and make the most of the mandated treatment. Discussing some of the reasons the athlete uses his substance of choice can be helpful. Pointing out the pros and cons of the athlete's drug use and the discrepancies between where the athlete wants to go in life and the impact that continued use of that substance might have on that dream can move the athlete along the stages of change from precontemplation to contemplation, preparation, action, and then maintenance [20].

When an athlete is unable to cut down on use, has withdrawal symptoms when not using, develops tolerance, continues to use despite knowledge of the dangers, spends increasing time focused on using or finding drugs, uses drugs to escape responsibilities, or increases the amount used over time, then a serious substance use disorder should be considered [21]. Other substance use disorders should be ruled out, as athletes may use downers such as alcohol or benzodiazepines to counteract the effects of stimulants, as discussed earlier.

Besides motivational interviewing, 12-step facilitation, cognitive behavioral therapy/relapse prevention, and network therapy can be helpful treatment modalities. Concerns about confidentiality may make it more challenging to convince most athletes to go to a 12-step meeting (AA or NA). Because athletes have so much to lose by testing positive again, they tend to be willing to try pharmacologic interventions (disulfiram, acamprosate, naltrexone, buprenorphine, etc.). Co-occurrence of addiction together with mental illness is the rule rather than the exception. The co-occurring mental illness must also be treated.

Team treatment

Sports psychiatrists are consulted to do team interventions when administrators or coaches discover substance use problems that are widespread. When called in, sports psychiatrists need familiarity with which substances are being used, the drug testing policy, who the team leaders are, what attitudes the coaches have toward substance use, and what the expectations of their service are. Permissive attitudes must change. When substance use is part of the team culture through peer pressure, hazing rituals, or even as part of the team's recruiting process, interventions need to be made at the team level. Athletes, coaches, administrators, and sometimes athlete alumni need to be on the same page in terms of substance use policies and team expectations. Teammates tend to use together. The team itself may need to draft its own substance use policy to establish new norms. More sessions may be required to check the progress, and the work needs to be solidified at the beginning of each season to maintain the change to the team culture.

COLLEGE VERSUS PROFESSIONAL

Colleges vary in if they do drug testing above that conducted by the NCAA or other national college athletics organizations and in if they offer or mandate treatment. Different professional leagues have different rates of substance use and different substance use policies. Some mandate treatment, while others rely on suspensions and do not offer treatment. Some professional teams do additional testing beyond league testing to help identify their at-risk athletes and subsequently offer treatment to them. Some teams will trade athletes who test positive with the knowledge that their athletic performance will probably drop due to continued substance use. Most college and professional athletic careers are relatively short and are shortened further by substance use difficulties. The more money that is involved in a sport, the higher the stakes and sometimes the more the resources, for better or worse, made available to the athlete. The more money an athlete makes, the more the athlete can afford designer drugs, masking agents, and novel anabolic steroids that may go undetected on standard urine drug testing. These athletes may also be more likely to try to cheat with the use of doping in ways that are just beginning to be described, for example, with gene doping.

SPECIFIC SUBSTANCES

Cannabis

Cannabis (marijuana) has a relatively long half-life in the urine. A heavy, daily user may continue to test positive for up to 2 months. Cannabis is lipophilic, which means that its half-life can be shorter in elite athletes with low body fat. Some athletes use synthetic cannabinoids (e.g., K2 or Spice) to avoid detection in urine drug testing. The NCAA and some professional leagues have banned cannabis for legal and safety reasons. Some athletes, coaches, and administrators have permissive attitudes toward marijuana. The potency of today's cannabis is significantly higher than it was 20–30 years ago. Cannabis use has been associated with amotivational syndrome, panic, depression, and psychosis. Due to its long half-life and relatively frequent use, sports psychiatrists are more commonly consulted for positive urine drug tests for marijuana than for most other substances. A case study later in this chapter illustrates an athlete who struggled with cannabis.

Stimulants

Amphetamines have been used in sports for performance-enhancing reasons since the 1940s [22]. Athletes may recognize and seek the performance-enhancing effects of stimulants, which are first-line treatment for attention deficit hyperactivity disorder (ADHD). It is very easy to research and memorize the diagnostic criteria for ADHD in the hope of being prescribed stimulants for performance enhancement. When prescribed for well-documented ADHD, stimulants may be performance enabling, not performance enhancing. The prescription of stimulants strictly for performance enhancement must be considered a doping violation and unethical, and the sports psychiatrist should be reprimanded. Some of the external pressures to diagnose and aggressively treat ADHD may come from coaches, trainers, academic support, and/or athletic directors. The sports psychiatrist may want to feel like a team player and treat the athlete before proper testing is performed. The athlete may border on academic ineligibility and feel pressured by their support system to initiate stimulants as soon as possible. He may fear the loss of his scholarship or college career. Professional athletes may feel that if they do not perform at their best, they may lose games, contracts, or endorsement dollars. General managers, trainers, sports medicine physicians, and/or coaches may feel the need to get their athlete diagnosed and treated immediately for ADHD. A significant number of amphetamines prescribed to college students are illegally sold on college campuses by the people for whom the prescriptions were intended. Some athletes share their prescribed stimulants with teammates. When that teammate responds to the stimulant positively, that teammate may feel she must have ADHD too. Starting with extended-release formulations of stimulants for legitimate ADHD will reduce the likelihood of abuse for performance-enhancing purposes, addiction, and diversion.

Athletes are now using energy drinks in a similar pattern as amphetamines. Athletes may ingest ephedrine, pseudoephedrine, synephrine, phenylpropanolamine, nicotine, excitatory amino acids, ginseng, and high-dose caffeine. Athletes may ask for modafinil and armodafinil by name. These are easily obtainable via internet pharmacies and are not detected on standard urine drug screens. Sports psychiatrists may be unknowingly asked to treat these stimulants' common side effects, such as anxiety, insomnia, tremors, motor tics, irritability, overheating, and loss of appetite. Screening for all stimulant use is vital when encountering these complaints, and such screening is especially important during the season, when use increases. Prescribing good sleep hygiene prior to a sleep medication may be helpful.

Alcohol

Alcohol is the most commonly used substance by athletes. An NCAA 2001 study shows that college athletes drink overwhelmingly for social reasons (83.9%) compared to purposes of feeling good (12.9%), coping (3%), or performance (0.2%) [23]. It is a common part of hazing, team building, celebrating, and consoling. Binges lead to drop-offs in attending classes and practices, poor athletic performance, fights, injuries, legal problems, and public relation problems. Athletes who drink at least weekly have injury rates twice that of nondrinkers [24]. Alcohol consumption can reduce hand–eye coordination, muscle strength, muscle memory, and running and cycling times and lead to dehydration, insomnia, and myopathies [25]. Standard urine drug tests for alcohol will typically only pick up heavy alcohol users [4], unless testing for ethyl glucuronide (ETG). Sports psychiatrists have expertise in prescribing disulfiram, acamprosate, and naltrexone for cases of alcohol dependence.

Anabolic steroids

Anabolic steroid use seems to be on the decline. It has received more media coverage, and the NCAA and professional leagues are testing for it more. Sports psychiatrists may still be asked by athletes, coaches, and trainers about the half-lives of performance-enhancing drugs such as anabolic steroids for the purposes of preparing for urine drug testing and about masking agents. Some athletes may ask to be prescribed a low dose of an anabolic steroid while claiming that it would be a harm reduction as opposed to taking an internet steroid at a higher dose. Besides the 1990 Anabolic Steroid Act making such a practice illegal, such behavior is unethical, immoral, and violates the purpose of sport. A sports psychiatrist's special knowledge may (unbeknownst to him or not) be used for doping purposes, and educational information must be given with the proper ethical considerations. One exception to this rule may be an athlete who is addicted to anabolic steroids and requires a medical detoxification. Cutting an athlete off cold turkey has reportedly resulted in acute depression and suicide attempts, according to the work of the Taylor Hooten Foundation [26]. Estimates suggest that up to 30% of anabolic steroid users develop a dependence disorder, which can be complicated by other substance use disorders (particularly disorders involving alcohol, opiates, and sedatives) [27]. Development of a detoxification protocol for anabolic steroids is necessary and in the works under the leadership of the Taylor Hooten Foundation.

Case Study

A college sophomore tennis player is referred to the sports psychiatrist after testing positive for marijuana on a university random urine drug test. She had been highly recruited, and despite some injuries, competed at a high level her freshman year. Her trainer reported at the time of the referral that she had recently purposely lost her NCAA semifinal championship match at the end of the third set so as to avoid the urine drug test required of the champion and runner-up. She knew she would test positive for marijuana and would face suspension and public humiliation. The trainer believed she had the talent and ability to have won the championship had she been free of marijuana. Typically, per this student's athletic department's drug testing policy, the first positive urine drug test would result in an evaluation by a substance abuse counselor and a requirement to attend a few group classes on substance abuse prevention. After that initial evaluation, the substance abuse counselor suggested a referral to the sports psychiatrist for addiction treatment. Subsequent to that referral, and partly because she had that potential to win a national championship, the sports psychiatrist met with her regularly for the rest of her college career.

In treatment together, while using a combination of motivational interviewing, network therapy, and development of a relapse prevention plan, the athlete and sports psychiatrist were able to move her from precontemplation to the maintenance phase of her recovery. She admitted that everyone in her family and all of her childhood friends smoked marijuana. Some of her teammates did so as well. The athlete and psychiatrist worked to find and develop friendships with clean and sober people. She experienced significant protracted withdrawal, which required a low dose of a sleeping medication. She refused to attend 12-step facilitation or other support group meetings. The sports psychiatrist spoke to several of her family members regarding her relapse prevention plan and asked them not to smoke in front of or offer marijuana to the student athlete. She had several slips and relapses, particularly when visiting her hometown. The athlete and psychiatrist thoroughly examined every relapse, trying to identify her triggers and develop other coping mechanisms when facing those triggers and cravings. She used her phone network, which included her sports psychiatrist. She in fact called her sports psychiatrist twice while dealing with cravings. The athlete and psychiatrist met every other week for several months, until she was more confident in her recovery. Thereafter, meetings occurred once a month, with instant urine drug screens for marijuana.

The psychiatrist and athlete also discussed mental skills that involved shifting attention, reducing precompetitive anxiety, and improving positive self-talk. She won the national championship in her junior year. She continued to remain marijuana-free, and her academic performance also improved. She continued to pass random urine drug screens with the sports psychiatrist for treatment purposes only (off the books). In her senior year, she withdrew from her semifinal match due to a shoulder injury that later required a surgical repair. She denied any marijuana use around the time of that championship tournament and ultimately graduated from college with 14 months' sobriety.

CONCLUSIONS

Sports psychiatrists need to be well-trained in recognizing, preventing, and treating substance use disorders. Substance use is a common reason why professional teams, leagues, and university athletic departments hire sports psychiatrists. Substance use is easily tracked by urine drug tests, and the success or failure of treatment can be easily measured by decision makers. Medications can be helpful in treating addictions and co-occurring mental illness in athletes, and sports psychiatrists are the experts in these medical decisions. While helping athletes off substances, sports psychiatrists can help athletes perform at a high level. Sports psychiatrists are helpful in developing strong drug prevention and testing policies that emphasize education and treatment over sanctions. Sports psychiatrists should be aware of the common drugs used for performance enhancement and abuse on their teams and in their regions. The more elite the athlete and the more the financial gain that is involved, the greater the risk of doping and the use of performance-enhancing drugs, and the greater the need for sports psychiatrists working with athletes.

REFERENCES

1. Greene GA, Uryasz FD, Petr TA, *et al*. (2001). NCAA study of substance use and abuse habits of college student athletes. *Clinical Journal of Sports Medicine* 1, 51–56.
2. Millman RB, Ross EJ (2003). Steroid and nutritional supplement use in professional athletes. *American Journal of Addictions* 12(Suppl.), 48–54.
3. Ambrose PJ (2004). Drug use in sports: a veritable arena for pharmacists. *Journal of the American Pharmacists Association* 44, 501–514.
4. McDuff DR, Baron, DA (2005). Substance use in athletics: a sports psychiatry perspective. *Clinical Journal of Sports Medicine* 24, 885–897.
5. McDuff DR (2012). *Sports Psychiatry: Strategies for Life Balance and Peak Performance*. Washington, DC: American Psychiatric Publishing, 86.
6. Yusko DA, Buckman JF, White HR, *et al*. (2008). Alcohol, tobacco, illicit drugs, and performance enhancers: a comparison of use by college student athletes and nonathletes. *Journal of American College Health* 57, 281.

7. Hoberman J (2002). Sports physicians and the doping crisis in elite sports. *Clinical Journal of Sports Medicine* 12, 203–208.
8. Buckman JF, Yusko DA, Farris SG, *et al.* (2011). Risk of marijuana use in male and female college student athletes and nonathletes. *Journal of Studies on Alcohol and Drugs* 72, 586–591.
9. Ford JA (2007). Alcohol use among college students: a comparison of athletes and nonathletes. *Substance Use & Misuse* 42, 1367–1377.
10. Ford JA (2008). Nonmedical prescription drug use among college students: a comparison between athletes and nonathletes. *Journal of American College Health* 57, 211–220.
11. Dunn M, Thomas JO, Swift W, *et al.* (2011). Recreational substance use among elite Australian athletes. *Drug and Alcohol Review* 30, 63–68.
12. Hendrickson B. (2011) NCAA drug-use study shows large majority have not used banned drugs. http://www.ncaa.org/wps/wcm/connect/public/ncaa/resources/latest+news/2012/january/ncaa+drug-use+study+shows+large+majority+have+not+used+banned+drugs/. Accessed on 28 April 2012.
13. Pinkerton R, Hinz L, Barrow J (1989). The college student athlete: psychological considerations and interventions. *Journal of American College Health* 37, 218–226.
14. Parham W (1993). The intercollegiate athlete: a 1990's profile. *The Counseling Psychologist* 21, 411–429.
15. Swoap RA, Murphy SM (1995). Eating disorders and weight management in athletes. In: Murphy SM. *Sport Psychology Interventions*. Champaign: Human Kinetics, pp. 307–329.
16. Currie A, Morse ED (2005). Eating disorders in athletes: managing the risks. *Clinical Journal of Sports Medicine* 24, 871–883.
17. Morse ED (2011). Professional boundaries in sport psychiatry. *Journal of Clinical Sport Psychology* 4, 173–174.
18. World Anti-Doping Agency (2012). List of prohibited substances and methods, January 1. http://list.wada-ama.org. Accessed on 12 May 2012.
19. NCAA guidelines to document ADHD treatment with banned stimulant medications. Addendum to the January 2009 guidelines (July 20, 2010). http://www.ncaa.org/drugtesting (with a login and password). Accessed on 12 May 2012.
20. Miller WR, Rollnick S (2004). Talking oneself into change: motivational interviewing, stages of change, and therapeutic process. *Journal of Cognitive Psychotherapy: An International Quarterly* 18 (4), 299–308.
21. American Psychiatric Association (1994). *Diagnostic and Statistical Manual of Mental Disorders*, 4th edition. Washington, DC: American Psychiatric Association.
22. Jones AR, Pinchot JT (1998). Stimulant use in sports. *American Journal of Addictions* 7, 243–255.
23. NCAA study of substance abuse habits of college student-athletes (2001). http://www.ncaa.org/wps/wcm/connect/public/NCAA/Resources/Research/NCAA+Studies+of+Substance+Use+Habits+of+College+Student-Athletes. Accessed on 18 January 2013.
24. O'Brien CP, Lyons F (2000). Alcohol and the athlete. *Sports Medicine* 29, 295–300.
25. Nelson TF, Wechsler H (2001). Alcohol and college athletes. *Medicine and Science in Sports and Exercise* 33(1), 43–47.
26. What happens when you stop using anabolic steroids? http://taylorhooton.org/steroid-ed-faq/. Accessed on 12 May 2012.
27. Kanayama G, Brower KJ, Wood RJ, *et al.* (2009). Anabolic-androgenic steroid dependence: an emerging disorder. *Addiction* 104, 1966–1978.

2 Addiction in Retired Athletes

Pavel A. Ponizovskiy

Department of Mental Disorders Complicated by Substance Abuse, Moscow Research Institute of Psychiatry, Russia

KEY POINTS

- Athletic retirement is a challenge that results in healthy adjustment or a distressful response.
- Substance abuse in former athletes is one of the signs of career transition distress.
- Extensive studies investigating substance abuse in retired athletes are needed to improve preventive measures.

BACKGROUND

Changes in social roles occurring during the life course of every person are difficult transitional periods requiring adaptation. Successful coping with career termination is followed by effective adjustment to life after retirement. It is recommended that athletes prepare in advance for their athletic career termination.

Conceptual models of adaptation to career transition suggest that retirement planning, voluntary termination, multiple personal identity (see Chapter 6), availability of social and medical support, and active coping strategies facilitate athletes' adaptation to the postcareer.

Alternatively, failure in coping with a transition is often followed by negative consequences. Substance misuse can become a significant problem in retirement as athletes turn to alcohol and drugs in order to reduce residual injury-related pain, for emotional relief, or to exchange exercise dependence for substance addiction. Due to preserved high-level adaptive physiological potential, addiction in retired athletes has unique clinical features.

ATHLETIC RETIREMENT – ALWAYS TRAUMATIC?

Career termination is considered to be one of the most challenging and potentially traumatic transitions encountered by athletes [1, 2]. Athletes must adapt to the ordeal of career termination with a renewed sense of personal worthiness outside of the sport world [3–6].

Clinical Sports Psychiatry: An International Perspective, First Edition. Edited by David A. Baron, Claudia L. Reardon and Steven H. Baron.
© 2013 John Wiley & Sons, Ltd. Published 2013 by John Wiley & Sons, Ltd.

The summarized findings of 14 studies ($n = 2653$) conducted between 1982 and 1998 that evaluated psychological adjustment to career termination among athletes in amateur, collegiate, Olympic, and professional sports indicated that 20.1% of the athletes manifested psychological difficulties in response to athletic termination and had a need for psychological assistance [7].

Conversely, some studies have indicated that athletic retirement may not be traumatic, but rather an important event that influences the retiring athletes' well-being and development [8–11]. Though the initial response of many of the athlete-subjects to career termination was frustration and anxiety, overall they perceived it as an opportunity to reestablish more traditional social roles and lifestyles. The authors suggest that the issue of retirement from sport should be treated as "sport specific" rather than generalized across the broader sporting framework [10–12].

A MODEL OF ADAPTATION TO ATHLETIC RETIREMENT

According to Taylor and Ogilvie [13], career termination is not an event, but a process. Their conceptual model of adaptation to athletic retirement provides a thorough framework for examining the transition process. This multidimensional model involves psychosocial (emotional, social, financial, and occupational) factors that interact in response to the sport-career transition and account for the disposition of the athlete in transition. The model proposes five developmental stages:

- Stage 1 presents the causes of career termination (age, deselection, injury, free choice).
- Stage 2 enumerates the factors related to the adaptation (developmental experiences, self-identity, perception of control, social identity, tertiary contributors).
- Stage 3 describes available resources for adaptation (coping skills, social support, preretirement planning).
- Stage 4 addresses the overall quality of the career transition, resulting in either a healthy or distressful response to retirement. By this stage, the athlete's reaction to the transition will be evident, and the quality of the individual's transition is dependent upon the previous steps of the retirement process.
- Stage 5 lists intervention strategies for retirement difficulties (cognitive, emotional, behavioral, social, and organizational).

Positive and negative adjustment factors

It has been well described that voluntary/planned retirement under the athlete's own terms is a positive adjustment factor [14] associated with fewer difficulties and greater emotional and social adjustment after retirement [5, 15]. Conversely, involuntary/unplanned retirement in which the athlete has no other option is a negative adjustment factor [14] associated with difficulties such as emotional tension and increased feelings of anger, failure, and loss.

The main reasons for involuntary termination of an active sport career are age, injury, or deselection when the intense competition forces athletes to leave sports via a coach's decision. In these cases, many athletes are confronted by financial challenges and lack of purpose and significance and face the necessity of obtaining additional education or professional training. Many elite athletes who are accustomed to significant public recognition and personal perceptions of physical invulnerability turn out to be unprepared for life after sport and experience retirement distress. Lack of retirement planning, undeveloped personal lives, and an inability to build new social networks increase the transition crisis [14]. The bigger the difference between the social status in sport and after career termination, the more painful is the transition under otherwise equal conditions [6].

Some former athletes manage to remain involved in sport to different extents (playing, coaching, refereeing, managing national or local junior teams, working in sports administration), which is a positive factor that may contribute to healthy career transition. However, the level of such sport-related involvement fluctuates from 42% to 88%, depending on the country and specific kind of sport [11, 16].

A blended model of adaptation to career transition

Based on the results of a phenomenological exploration of the sport-career transition experiences that affect subjective well-being of former National Football League (NFL) players, the Conceptual Model of Adaptation to Career Transition [13] was modified into the Blended Model of Adaptation to Career Transition [17]. The model lists the signs of healthy career transition as follows:

- gainful employment
- financial security
- enrollment in undergraduate/postgraduate studies
- ≥ slightly satisfied subjective well-being score
- strong interpersonal relationships
- healthy management of pain/physical health

Signs of career transition distress include:

- adjustment difficulties
- occupational/financial problems
- family/social problems or social isolation
- psychopathology
- substance abuse/gambling

When trying to summarize the main international research results on career termination obtained by North American, West European, and Australian researchers, the following conclusions are made [18]:

- Career termination is caused by multiple sources and is often the result of a long process of reasoning and decision making.
- Though career termination may result in distress for many athletes (~20%), there are great individual differences in these reactions.
- Regardless of the particular causes of career termination, the athlete's subjective feeling about the decision as voluntary or involuntary is a crucial determinant of adaptation. Voluntary retirement contributes to a smoother transition process.
- The coping process depends not only on the causes, but also on the individual resources (e.g., education and goal-setting for the postcareer) and social resources (e.g., support from the family and postcareer services) of the athlete.

SUBSTANCE ABUSE AND ADDICTION IN RETIRED ATHLETES

Substance abuse as negative coping behavior is an often distressful response to retirement that can be observed in athletes [5, 13, 19]. While the rates of abuse or addiction may be lower during one's active athletic career, it may increase after retirement.

Case Study

Ivan was 37 years old when he was admitted to the hospital for detoxification with signs and symptoms of severe alcohol withdrawal: psychomotor agitation, hand tremor, sweating, a pulse of 106, insomnia, lack of appetite, and craving for alcohol. At the age of 7, he had started to play ice hockey. Being fond of playing and showing fast progress, he joined the local junior team. At the age of 17, he was invited to play for the professional national team. At the same time, he entered a university of physical training and sports, and after 5 years earned a specialization of coach. He continued to play ice hockey professionally until he suffered a trauma (complex left ankle joint fracture) during a match when he was 27 years old. He had undergone several surgeries, but still had to terminate his active professional career. After retirement, he described his emotions as "depression," "confusion," and "lack of understanding what to do next." He realized he "was not ready for such a quick turn" and was asking: "Why did it happen to me?" His rehabilitation course after the surgical treatment took 1 year. He intermittently experienced pain at the site of the former fracture. For the next 4 years, he worked as a coach for a local junior team but was not satisfied with the salary. Later he started to work as a sales manager in a sport fashion outlet. He got married at the age of 30 and had a son who is now 6 years old.

Before the termination of his active hockey career, Ivan was an infrequent drinker, having two vodka drinks once a month. After suffering the injury, he became a moderate drinker, having seven vodka drinks every week. Ivan recalled that at that point he had much spare time and "alcohol was making life brighter" and helped to reduce the occasional pain in his ankle. By the age of 32, he had become a heavier drinker, having up to 15 vodka drinks two to three times a week. By the age of 35, he developed physical dependence on alcohol, which manifested with withdrawal symptoms of headache, hand tremor, insomnia, lack of appetite, and anxiety. By then, hard drinking periods lasted up to 1 week, with daily consumption of 20–25 vodka drinks. Abstinence periods lasted up to 2 weeks, but alcohol consumption inevitably was resumed because of increased craving and dysphoria. In the hospital, Ivan was diagnosed with alcohol dependence and alcohol withdrawal.

In the described case, alcohol dependence developed after forced retirement from active sport due to injury incompatible with resumption of active professional ice hockey playing. During the initial stage of abuse, the analgesic and thymoleptic effects of alcohol were sought. Involuntary termination of sport career, lack of preretirement planning, and decrease of financial status, and thus a need to look for a new job, contributed to career transition distress and subsequent addiction.

PRERETIREMENT PREDISPOSITIONS TO ADDICTIONS

As described in Chapter 1 as well as in other references, cases of substance addiction are not common in active, preretirement professional athletes [20–22]. Moreover, estimates suggest that 15–20% of individuals with exercise addiction, as discussed in Chapter 4, may also have addictions to nicotine, alcohol, or illicit drugs [23]. Thus, preretirement professional athletes are at risk of developing chemical dependency, and specific preventive measures are ideally implemented at that stage, well before retirement [24].

Psychological examination of athletes who are about to finish or recently finished their athletic career revealed increased rates of predisposition to addictive behavior [25]. Low levels of predisposition were revealed in 30% of subjects, while 55% and 15% demonstrated moderate and high risk of developing addiction, respectively. Direct correlation between rates of predisposition to alcohol addiction, predisposition to drug abuse, and predisposition to cigarette smoking was revealed.

The analysis of cases of former high-level athletes has shown that after retirement, their excessive physical activity (exercise addiction in many cases) may be replaced by chemical dependency (l'addiction de remplacement) [26]. The possible neurobiological explanation may be that physical activity involves the synthesis and release of dopamine in the basal ganglia [27], while the dopaminergic mesocorticolimbic system is considered to be involved in reward-related associative learning [28], reinforcement [29], and incentive salience [30], playing a crucial role in the development of drug addiction. Therefore, the dopaminergic mesocorticolimbic brain system seems particularly involved in both the execution of physical activity and in some characteristics that may lead to the development of drug addiction. Based on that idea, some studies suggest that regular physical activity may help in the treatment of amphetamine addiction and may be used for relapse prevention [31].

PAINKILLERS MISUSE

Athletes with injury-related pain are at increased risk for opioid analgesic use and misuse, which may result in medical, psychiatric, and social problems [32]. Retired NFL players misuse painkillers at three times the rate of the general population. Those who misused during their active sport career are most likely to misuse after retirement compared to others. Current misuse is associated with more severe pain, undiagnosed concussions, and heavy drinking. Longitudinal studies are needed to determine the long-term effects of opioid analgesic misuse among athletes.

SMOKING

It is well known that athletes are less likely to smoke cigarettes than those who do not practice physical training, with "sedentary nonathletes" the heaviest smokers [33]. A shift away from sports participation can signal increased risk for smoking [19]. One study of high school students found that those whose participation level decreased over a 2-year period were nearly twice as likely to smoke as those with low participation overall and three times as likely to smoke as those with high participation overall [34]. Nevertheless, the study of former NFL players revealed that athlete retirees are much less likely to have ever smoked than are men in general, and also less likely to be current smokers. Less than 8% of NFL retirees smoke, compared with over 20% of the general population in the United States [35].

DRINKING

The recent exhaustive review of 34 peer-reviewed quantitative data-based studies completed on high school and college sports involvement and drug use has proven that sports participation is positively correlated with alcohol use, but inversely correlated with cigarette smoking and illicit drug use [36]. It has been identified that sport involvement among college students is related to high risk for excessive alcohol consumption and results in negative alcohol-related consequences [37, 38]. Highly active athletes drink more frequently than low-activity nonathletes and are more likely to binge drink [33, 39].

Intensive and systematic physical training during an athlete's sports career modifies her physiological status, for example, via increased muscle mass and pulmonary functional reserves. This allows athletes to consume alcohol in substantially higher rates than nonathletes. The study of former professional athletes addicted to alcohol [40] compared some of their physiological characteristics to those of alcohol-addicted nonathletes. Former athletes were found to have increased body mass index and reduced muscle mass, but compared to nonathletes, their muscle power was superior. The results suggest that functional adaptive potential of former athletes remains at a high level for some period of time even under the condition of chronic alcohol intoxication.

Perhaps related to these physiological differences, alcohol addiction in retired athletes has unique clinical features [41]. Although regular alcohol consumption starts in former athletes at an older age than in nonathletes, they demonstrate rapid development of tolerance with higher maximum daily intake of alcoholic beverages and longer drinking bouts.

The study of retired NFL players [35] revealed that compared to men in the general population, former athletes are less likely to be lifetime abstainers or current nondrinkers. They are slightly more likely to be light drinkers (fewer than 180 drinks per year or one every other day) and considerably more likely to be moderate drinkers (fewer than 730 drinks per year or two per day). The rates of heavy drinking (more than 730 drinks per year) and binge drinking (five or more drinks on a single occasion) are slightly higher among NFL retirees than the general population. Six percent of older retirees and less than 5% of younger ones reported that they had undergone treatment for alcohol problems.

All evidence combined, then, suggests that former professional athletes probably consume larger amounts of alcohol than nonathletes in the general population.

CONCLUSION

To date, most of the literature investigating the relationship between sports participation and substance use has focused upon active athletes, with little focus being given to retired athletes. Extensive studies are still required to investigate the use of cannabis, ecstasy, meth/amphetamine, cocaine, gamma-hydroxybutyrate and ketamine among former athletes. Nevertheless, the presented data suggest that:

- Substance abuse or addiction in retired athletes is often a sign of career transition distress.
- The rates of substance abuse or addiction may increase after retirement.
- Retired athletes may use some substances in substantially higher rates than nonathletes due to preserved high-level adaptive physiological potential.
- Former athletes often misuse substances to relieve residual pain from past sport injuries.

Further identifying why some athletes are at a greater risk for substance abuse and addiction after their career termination will help in the design and implementation of prevention initiatives.

REFERENCES

1. Taylor J, Ogilvie BC, Lavallee D. (2006) Career transition among athletes: Is there life after sports? In: Williams JM (ed.) *Applied Sport Psychology*. New York: McGraw Hill, pp. 595–615.
2. Chow BC. (2002) Support for elite athletes retiring from sport: The case in Hong Kong. *Journal of the International Council for Health, Physical Education, Sport and Dance* **38**, 37–42.
3. Ogilvie BC, Howe M. (1986) The trauma of termination from athletics. In: Williams JM (ed.) *Applied Sport Psychology: Personal Growth to Peak Performance*. Mountain View: Mayfield Publishing Co., pp. 365–382.
4. Ogilvie BC, Taylor J. (1993) Career termination issues among elite athletes. In: Singer RN, Murphy M, Tennant LK (eds.) *Handbook of Research in Sport Psychology*. New York: Macmillan, pp. 761–775.
5. Werthner P, Orlick T. (1986) Retirement experiences of successful Olympic athletes. *International Journal of Sport Psychology* **17**, 337–363.
6. Stambulova NB. (1997) Crisis of sports career. *Theory and Practice of Physical Training* **10**, 13–17.
7. Lavallee D, Nesti M, Borkoles E *et al.* (2000) Intervention strategies for athletes in transition. In: Lavallee D, Wylleman P (eds.) *Career Transitions in Sport: International Perspectives*. Morgantown: Fitness Information Technology Inc, pp. 111–130.
8. Coakley JJ. (1983) Leaving competitive sport: Retirement or rebirth? *Quest* **35**, 1–11.
9. Wylleman P, De Knop P, Menkehorst H *et al.* (1993) Career termination and social integration among elite athletes. In: Serpa S, Alves J, Ferreira V *et al.* (eds.) *Proceedings of the 8th World Congress of Sport Psychology*. Lisbon: Universidade Tecnica de Lisboa, pp. 902–906.
10. Allison MT, Meyer C. (1988) Career problems and retirement among elite athletes: The female tennis professional. *Sociology of Sport Journal* **5**, 212–222.
11. Young JA, Pearce AJ, Kane R *et al.* (2006) Leaving the professional tennis circuit: Exploratory study of experiences and reactions from elite female athletes. *British Journal of Sports Medicine* **40**(5), 477–483.
12. Kerr G, Dacyshyn A. (2000) The retirement experiences of elite female gymnasts. *Journal of Applied Sport Psychology* **12**, 115–133.
13. Taylor B, Ogilvie BC. (1994) A conceptual model of adaptation to retirement among athletes. *Journal of Applied Sport Psychology* **6**, 1–20.
14. Sinclair DA, Hackford D. (2000) The role of the sport organization in the career transition process. In: Lavallee D, Wylleman P (eds.) *Career Transitions in Sport: International Perspectives*. Morgantown: Fitness Information Technology Inc, pp. 131–142.
15. Lavellee D, Gordon S, Grove R. (1997) Retirement from sport and loss of athletic identity. *Journal of Personal and Interpersonal Loss* **2**, 129–147.
16. Shikhverdiev SN. (2007) Goals, objectives and forms of re-socialization of athletes at the final stage of professional career. *Scientific Notes of P.F. Lesgaft University* **5**(27), 97–100.
17. Coakley SC. (2006) A phenomenological exploration of the sport-career transition experiences that affect subjective well-being of former National Football League players. Unpublished doctoral dissertation, University of North Carolina, Greensboro, 219p. Available at http://libres.uncg.edu/ir/uncg/f/umi-uncg-1099.pdf. Accessed on 20 April 2012.
18. Stambulova N, Alfermann D, Statler T *et al.* (2009) ISSP position stand: Career development and transitions of athletes. *International Journal of Sport and Exercise Psychology* **7**(4), 395–412.
19. Koukouris K. (1991) Quantitative aspects if the disengagement process of advanced and elite Greek male athletes from organized competitive sport. *Journal of Sport Behavior* **14**, 227–246.

20. Bell JA, Doege TC. (1987) Athletes use and abuse of drugs. *Physician and Sports Medicine* **15**(3), 99–108.
21. Carrier C. (1993) La pratique sportive intensive en tant que conduite addictive. *Nervure* **VI**, 51–58.
22. Furst DM, Germone K. (1993) Negative addiction in male and female runners and exercisers. *Perceptual & Motor Skills* 77(1), 192–194.
23. Aidman EV, Woollard S. (2003) The influence of self-reported exercise addiction on acute emotional and physiological responses to brief exercise deprivation. *Psychology of Sport and Exercise* **4**, 225–236.
24. Seznec JC. (2002) Toxicomanie et cyclisme professionnel. *Annales Médico-psychologiques, revue psychiatrique* **60**(1), 72–76.
25. Shikhverdiev SN. (2010) Athletes' tendency to destructive behavior during final stage of sports career. *Sports Science Bulletin* **4**, 14–17.
26. Volle É, Seznec JC. (2006) L'arrêt du sport intensif: révélation d'addictions? *Annales Médico-psychologiques, revue psychiatrique* **164**(9), 775–779.
27. Meeusen R, Smolders I, Sarre S *et al.* (1997) Endurance training effects on neurotransmitter release in rat striatum: an in vivo microdialysis study. *Acta Physiologica Scandinavica* **159**(4), 335–341.
28. Di Chiara G, Tanda G, Bassareo V *et al.* (1999) Drug addiction as a disorder of associative learning. Role of nucleus accumbens shell/extended amygdala dopamine. *Annals of the New York Academy of Sciences* **877**, 461–485.
29. Koob GF. (1992) Drugs of abuse: anatomy, pharmacology and function of reward pathways. *Trends in Pharmacological Science* **13**(5), 177–184.
30. Berridge KC, Robinson TE. (1998) What is the role of dopamine in reward: Hedonic impact, reward learning, or incentive salience? *Brain Research Reviews* **28**(3), 309–369.
31. Fontes-Ribeiro CA, Marques E, Pereira FC *et al.* (2011) May exercise prevent addiction? *Current Neuropharmacology* **9**(1), 45–48.
32. Cottler LB, Abdallah AB, Cummings SM *et al.* (2011) Injury, pain and prescription opioid use among former NFL football players. *Drug and Alcohol Dependence* **116**(1–3), 188–194.
33. Rainey CJ, McKeown RE, Sargent RG *et al.* (1996) Patterns of tobacco and alcohol use among sedentary, exercising, nonathletic, and athletic youth. *Journal of School Health* **66**(1), 27–32.
34. Rodriguez D, Audrain-McGovern J. (2004) Team sport participation and smoking: Analysis with general growth mixture modeling. *Journal of Pediatric Psychology* **29**(4), 299–308.
35. Weir DR, Jackson JS, Sonnega A. (2009) "Study of Retired NFL Players" sponsored by the National Football League Player Care Foundation, September 10. Ann Arbor, MI: Institute for Social Research, University of Michigan. http://www.businessweek.com/bschools/blogs/mba_admissions/FinalReport.pdf. Accessed on 25 April 2012.
36. Lisha NE, Sussman S. (2010) Relationship of high school and college sports participation with alcohol, tobacco, and illicit drug use: A review. *Addictive Behaviors* **35**(5), 399–407.
37. Lorente FO, Souville M, Griffet O *et al.* (2004) Participation in sports and alcohol consumption among French adolescents. *Addictive Behaviors* **29**(5), 941–946.
38. Martens MP, Dams-O'Connor K, Beck NC. (2006) A systematic review of college student-athlete drinking: Prevalence rates, sport-related factors, and interventions. *Journal of Substance Abuse Treatment* **31**(3), 305–316.
39. O'Farrell AM, Allwright SP, Kenny SC *et al.* (2010) Alcohol use among amateur sportsmen in Ireland. *BMC Research Notes* **3**, 313.
40. Ishekov NS, Solovyev AG, Ishekova NI. (2003) Peculiarities of morphofunctional state in alcoholics-former sportsmen. *Siberian Gerald of Psychiatry and Addictology* **1**(27), 88–90.
41. Ishekov NS, Sidorov PI, Solovyev AG. (2000) Clinical peculiarities of chronic alcoholism in former sportsmen. *Alcoholic Disease* **12**, 1–3.

3   Doping in Sport

David A. Baron,[1,2,3] Claudia L. Reardon,[4]
and Steven H. Baron[5]

[1] International Relations and Department of Psychiatry, Keck School of Medicine at the University
of Southern California, USA
[2] Keck Medical Center at University of South California, USA
[3] Global Center for Exercise, Psychiatry, and Sports at USC, Health Sciences Campus, USA
[4] Department of Psychiatry, University of Wisconsin School of Medicine and Public Health, USA
[5] Montgomery County Community College, USA

KEY POINTS

- Virtually all doping agents are presumed to have short- and/or long-term health implications for users, but such effects have not been well studied.
- Athletes experience intense pressure to win from teammates, coaches, trainers, and family members, and this may contribute to a willingness to cheat to gain a competitive advantage.
- Sports science professionals, including sports psychiatrists, need to work with coaches, trainers, athletes, and national governing bodies to educate athletes on the effects of performance-enhancing drug use.

INTRODUCTION

Athletes compete to win. Although winning is usually defined as beating the competition, it may also be achieved by attaining personal goals, such as completing a marathon. Improving athletic performance can be achieved in a variety of ways, such as physical training, improved diet and sleep, stress reduction, and mental preparation. In addition to these "natural" performance enhancers, a number of pharmacologic interventions may also improve strength and speed. Doping, the use of banned drugs to improve athletic performance, has become an important, highly newsworthy topic in virtually every sport [1]. Doping is not restricted to highly paid professional or Olympic athletes [2–4]. It has been discovered in athletes of all ages and at every level of competition. Like it or not, doping has become one of the hottest stories in sports.

Performance-enhancing substances are not restricted to illegal drugs or prescription medications, such as anabolic steroids [5]. They include dietary supplements and a variety of compounds that are available at health food stores [6]. Despite a large number of articles and books written on the topic, the short- and long-term effects on health and athletic performance are not fully understood [1], and many of the claims that have been made are controversial [7, 8]. The goal of this chapter is to educate the reader about the history and role of doping in sport.

HISTORY OF DOPING IN SPORT

Over the past four decades, there have been few topics discussed and debated in the world-wide lay press more than doping in sports. The belief that doping is only a recent phenomenon that has arisen solely from increasing financial rewards offered to modern-day elite athletes is incorrect. In fact, doping is older than organized sports. The term "doping" is derived from the Dutch word "dop." Dop was a drink made from grape skins and was consumed by Zulu warriors to enhance their skills in battle. Ancient Greek Olympic athletes used various brandy and wine concoctions and ate hallucinogenic mush-rooms and sesame seeds to enhance performance. Various plants were used to improve speed and endurance, while others were taken to mask pain, allowing injured athletes to continue competing [9–11].

Even in ancient times, doping was considered unethical. Identified cheaters were sold into slavery and the money used to build statues honoring the Greek Gods. The statues were placed outside the Olympic Stadium as a reminder, and hopefully deterrent, to those considering cheating [1].

The modern use of doping, in the context of sports, dates back to the early 1900s with the illegal drugging of racehorses. Its use in the Olympics was first reported in 1904. Marathon runner Thomas Hicks consumed a mixture of brandy and strychnine to increase his stamina, and he nearly died as a result. Up until the 1920s, mixtures of strychnine, heroin, cocaine, and caffeine were widely used by athletes. Various coaches seemed to have their own unique, secret formula created to provide a competitive advantage [1, 7].

Although the process of doping is thousands of years old, the specific substances used to illegally enhance performance have continued to evolve. The "advances" in doping strategies have been driven, in large part, by improved drug testing detection methods. To avoid detection, various parties have developed ever more complicated doping techniques.

Historically, known adverse health consequence to users have proven to be a weak ineffective deterrent to use. The most potent driver of the use of performance-enhancing substances has been the perception of effectiveness, regardless of possible consequences. As an example, in the 1950s, the Soviet Olympic team began experimenting with testosterone supplementation to increase strength and power. This was not an individual athlete's decision, but part of a government-sponsored program of performance enhancement by national team trainers and sports medicine doctors without knowledge of short- or long-term negative consequences. Additionally, when the Berlin Wall fell, a detailed description of the East German government's program of administration of steroids and other doping agents to young elite athletes was made public. Many in the sporting world had long questioned the remarkable success of the East German athletes, particularly the women, and their rapid rise to dominance in the Olympics. As was later discovered, young female athletes responded more dramatically than males to performance-enhancing effects, but tragically suffered significant delayed adverse medical reactions, including premature death [11].

Over the past 150 years, no sport has had more high-profile doping allegations than cycling. Virtually all of the Tour de France medalists have tested positive, or been accused of doping, since 1997. The Lance Armstrong alleged doping scandal has dominated sports tabloids and talk shows for the past 15 years. Although never testing positive, Armstrong was accused of taking erythropoietin (EPO) and receiving blood transfusion. In lieu of a positive drug test (there was no available test for EPO or transfusion at the time of his seven consecutive victories), the United States Anti-Doping Agency (USADA) claimed to have multiple witnesses, including teammates, willing to testify that Mr. Armstrong had used performance-enhancing agents while competing in the Tour de France. For over a decade, he fought the allegations and offered to submit samples for analysis. In August 2012, facing arbitration with USADA that he would likely lose, he decided to stop fighting, but did not admit any wrongdoing. He maintained his claim that he had always played by the rules. Within 48 h of announcing that he would no longer contest the charges against him, USADA stripped him of his Olympic and Tour de France titles and issued a lifetime ban from competitive cycling. Regardless of guilt or not, the international reaction to this prolonged landmark case highlighted the ongoing interest in the impact of the use of banned performance-enhancing drugs.

THE CURRENT STATE OF DOPING IN SPORTS

A growing public consensus is that competing without the use of doping is the only acceptable scenario. Public skepticism has grown to the level of questioning virtually all exceptional athletic feats as possibly being the result of cheating. This current culture is unfair to the overwhelming majority of athletes who dedicate their young lives to competing by the rules, and underscores the critical need to regain public trust in the integrity of competitive sport.

The World Anti-Doping Agency (WADA) is attempting to address this concern. As doping strategies have evolved to include the use of difficult-to-test-for endogenous hormones, the need to establish individual baseline measures for athletes has emerged. WADA is now establishing a "biologic passport" for elite athletes. This passport establishes baseline hormone levels for individuals, which will be monitored before competition for significant changes. A positive test result would consist of too dramatic a change from the established individual baseline. Although final details are yet to be worked out, this is a rational approach that is intended to protect athletes from false positive tests resulting from naturally occurring high levels of endogenous substances, while catching those attempting to cheat by using naturally occurring hormones.

To date, the best specific examples of the types of doping for which it has been difficult to test and that would be detectable using the passport strategy are human growth hormone (hGH) and EPO. Both of these naturally occuring hormones are banned by WADA as performance enhancers [12], and are available over the internet (a primary source for performance-enhancing drugs). As approved medical treatments, they are also available at pharmacies. Six months prior to the 2000 Olympic Games in Sydney, a local pharmacy was robbed of 1575 multiple-dose vials of hGH. No other drugs were touched. Members of the Chinese swim team were detained on their way to Australia when vials of hGH and syringes were discovered in their luggage.

EPO is widely considered one of the most effective, and potentially deadly, doping agents for endurance athletes. It is estimated that 20 European cyclists have died from doping since 1987; all of the deaths have been attributed to EPO abuse. The difficulty in better understanding the health risks associated with doping with any agent, including EPO and hGH, lies in the fact that the doses used by athletes for performance enhancement are often 10 times or higher the doses used for therapeutic purposes. No institutional review board in the world would approve a protocol that exposed study subjects to the doses used by dopers.

Unique, supratherapeutic dosing strategies, such as "stacking" of anabolic steroids, are discovered by trial and error and reported by word of mouth through underground communication between unethical trainers and dopers. Claims of dramatic improvement in athletic performance, with little or no mention of adverse side effects, represent the engine that drives the doping train to this day.

Definitions and Terminology

Many terms are used throughout the scientific and lay press with regards to doping and are often misunderstood by both the health care community and the general public. Important terms and their definitions, along with associated information, are provided here as a resource:

Dope

Doping refers to the use of virtually any illegal or banned substance with the intent of improving athletic performance by cheating. Doping is intended to improve strength, speed, endurance, recovery time, or pain, or to mask the use of other illegal or banned drugs [13,14]. The most common examples of drugs used in doping include stimulants (e.g., amphetamines), narcotic analgesics (e.g., morphine), beta-blockers (e.g., propranolol), and the most commonly used doping agents, anabolic steroids [15]. Not all doping agents are illegal. In fact, many are prescription medications used to treat diseases. When athletes dope for performance enhancement, they usually consume far greater doses than a doctor would prescribe to treat an illness. Caffeine, found in coffee, tea, and many other beverages, is considered doping when taken in large quantities for the purpose of performance enhancement [16]. Another form of doping used by some endurance athletes (i.e., long-distance runners, cyclists, and cross-country skiers) is blood doping, which involves taking out one's own blood over time and putting back the oxygen-carrying components of the stored blood prior to competing, with the intended goal of increasing endurance. Specific sports federations, as well as WADA, maintain lists of those substances that are banned in particular sports, particularly at the elite and professional levels. Within the U.S. college system, the National Collegiate Athletic Association maintains lists of banned substances for its college athletes [1].

Doping control

These are efforts of organized sports federations or leagues to catch athletes who dope and to educate all competitors on the health risks associated with doping. The mainstay of doping control is urine drug testing. This involves the athlete providing a urine sample under strict collection procedures, with the urine then being sent to a certified laboratory that screens the urine for banned drugs. Drug testing can take place at the competition or at times other than the competition. Given the use of masking agents, testing outside of competition with no advance notice is the most effective way of catching those athletes seeking an unfair advantage. Beating drug testing (providing a drug-free urine even after doping) has become a lucrative, largely internet-based, business. Products that are sold include drug-free urine, which can be inserted into an artificial penis or vaginal pouch, and adulterants (see definition later in the chapter).

Clean urine

Clean urine is defined as a urine sample that does not contain any banned substances.

Dirty urine

Dirty urine is defined as a urine sample that tests positive for banned substances.

In-comp testing

In-comp testing is drug testing performed at the time of an athletic competition.

Out-of-comp testing

Out-of-comp testing is drug testing that takes place before or after a competition, game, or match.

Split sample

A split sample is a urine sample obtained using a drug testing procedure in which the urine sample collected is divided into two containers (A and B samples). The A sample is tested for banned substances, and the B sample is only used to confirm a positive test found in the A sample. If the A sample is clean, the B sample is not tested and is thrown out.

Chain of custody

This refers to the protocol carried out in drug testing. Once the doping control team collects a urine sample, it stays in visual contact until it is signed off to the transport service and ultimately delivered to the testing laboratory. The purpose of chain of custody is to ensure the urine sample is not tampered with before being received by the laboratory. A sign-off sheet accompanies the sample, documenting that all parties handling the sample have directly observed it. At no time can the sample not be accounted for. Lapses in the sign-off log could call into question the validity of a positive test result. In fact, any sample that has a broken chain of custody will not be tested by the lab [15].

Adulteration

Adulteration is defined as tampering with a urine sample in an attempt to invalidate a drug screen. Dopers will adulterate a urine specimen by adding contaminants to alter the pH, specific gravity, or other characteristics of the sample.

Stacking

This form of anabolic steroid doping involves a systematic increase of the dose of steroid taken over a given time frame. Doping with anabolic steroids results in dosing that far exceeds that required to treat medical illness and has serious adverse health consequences for the athlete.

Masking

Masking is the taking of a substance by an athlete with the intended goal of covering up the use of a banned drug on a urine drug screen. Masking agents, although not performance enhancing, are banned substances themselves.

CONTROVERSIES OF POSITIVE DRUG TESTS

Although most agree that knowingly taking a banned substance to gain an unfair advantage is cheating and should be punished, the issue is often less obvious. For example, if an athlete is taking a banned substance for a known medical condition or is given an illegal drug by a coach or trainer and not informed it is banned, is this cheating? The policy of all doping control agencies is that athletes are responsible for everything they put into their bodies. Although arbitration boards exist to evaluate athletes' explanations for their drug use, ignorance of the rules is rarely a successful defense.

FINANCIAL AND BUSINESS IMPLICATIONS

Drugs in sports are bad for the multibillion euro/dollar sports business. Fans admire the accomplishments of gifted athletes, but are frequently angered when a doping scandal is uncovered. In 2006, the American baseball player Barry Bonds surpassed the legend Babe Ruth in hitting home runs. A year later, he had been accused of taking steroids to gain strength and power. Despite denying the allegations, he was booed by fans outside his home city. Many have called for his records to not be acknowledged. Another example is Lance Armstrong, as mentioned above. Despite at the time being cleared of allegations of doping, he lost virtually all of his lucrative endorsements. The world loves a winner, but not one who is perceived as a cheat.

To underscore the importance and current relevance of doping in sports, Bud Selig, the current Commissioner of American Major League Baseball, ran a full-page statement in the most prestigious newspapers in the United States on 16 June 2006 [17]. In this "open letter to baseball fans," Mr. Selig addressed the use of hGH by baseball players. This action was directly related to recent reports of hGH use by a professional baseball player. In his letter, he acknowledged the revelation of a Major League player admitting to using hGH, a performance-enhancing drug. He expressed his "anger and disappointment" about someone breaking the rules. He defended the players by pointing out this is a rare event and that it is difficult to test for hGH, but "he is committed to work with testing organizations to develop a reliable test." He emphasized that Major League Baseball agreed to the "toughest drug testing and penalty program for steroids in all of professional sports." He proclaimed he was "committed to protecting our game...and the integrity of America's pastime." Of interest is the fact that performance-enhancing drug use seems to have become a priority for Major League Baseball only in recent years, after Congressional hearings were held following the Bay Area Laboratory Co-Operative (BALCO)–Barry Bonds steroid abuse allegations. It is widely acknowledged that players have used drugs for many years prior to these public proclamations.

Mr. Selig's closing statement captures the goal of doping control. He wrote, "The goal of baseball is simple. It's a game that is to be won or lost on the field as a result of the natural talents of the game's remarkable athletes. I will do everything possible to make sure that this one goal can always be met" [17]. A skeptic might question the true motivation for this action and how it is related to the business of Major League Baseball and its fan base. Regardless, it speaks volumes to the importance of doping in modern-day sports.

SHORT- AND LONG-TERM EFFECTS OF DOPING

Virtually all doping agents are presumed to present a health risk to the user, some more significant than others. Table 3.1 lists the known adverse side effects associated with use of various performance-enhancing agents. Of potentially greater concern are the *long-term* ill effects on health. By the time these effects are discovered, it may be too late for those abusing these drugs to be treated. For this reason, it is important for researchers to continue to study the short- *and* long-term side effects of all doping agents.

There are well-documented cases of athletes dying from doping, but fortunately this is relatively uncommon. Given the high doses used in doping, it is difficult to determine the short- and long-term effects on the athlete [18]. As mentioned earlier, it would not be ethical to give doses equivalent to those used "in the gym" to athletes in a research study to determine the side effects. What is known about the side effects of many of the drugs of abuse, such as anabolic steroids and growth hormone, is extrapolated from observation and reports of admitted users [18]. Additional information is derived from the existing medical literature on the effects in patients prescribed these drugs for medical reasons. There is some controversy over the reported side effect profiles of many of these compounds when used in healthy athletes. Anabolic steroids, for example, have a large number of documented adverse side effects (Table 3.1), but not every user will necessarily experience all of them. There is no way of predicting which adverse effects will develop and to what extent in a given athlete.

Much has been written about "roid rage" [18, 19]. This refers to the extreme anger reported in some steroid abusers. The clinical studies that have attempted to study this reaction have reported inconsistent findings. What most users have reported is irritability and mood lability. Aggression is not routinely reported and may be related to other factors unique to the individuals and their current life circumstances.

Given all the potential adverse side effects, why do athletes take anabolic steroids? The most obvious answer is to increase skeletal muscle mass and ultimately strength, power, and speed. These drugs do not create an athlete. They do allow the conditioned athlete to train harder by improving recovery time from strenuous workouts. The ability to "overtrain" and improve strength, power, and speed does give the user an unfair advantage over the nonusing athlete. Additionally, some investigators have reported a prominent placebo effect experienced by athletes taking anabolic steroids [18]. Regardless, there is no doubt that use of high-dose anabolic steroids combined with intense workouts will result in physical changes not achievable by training without using steroids. This is why efforts to discourage drug use through testing and education are important not only for the health of the athlete, but to promote fair competition as well.

Table 3.1 Categories of substances/methods banned by WADA, and associated common or serious side effects.

Substance/category	Side effects
Androgens (e.g., testosterone; synthetic androgens stanozolol and nandrolone; androgen precursors androstenedione and dehydroepiandrosterone; selective androgen receptor modulator andarine; exogenous hCG; antiestrogens tamoxifen, clomiphene, and raloxifene; aromatase inhibitors)	• Men: diminished spermatogenesis and fertility, decreased testicular size, gynecomastia, hastened epiphyseal closure in adolescents • Women: acne, hirsutism, temporal hair recession, clitoromegaly, voice deepening, oligomenorrhea or amenorrhea • Decreased HDL cholesterol, hepatotoxicity • Depression, mania, psychosis, aggression
Peptide hormones, growth factors (e.g., insulin and IGF-1), and related substances	• Insulin resistance, hyperglycemia, diabetes mellitus, cardiomegaly, premature epiphyseal closure, myopathy, sodium retention, hypertension, edema, carpal tunnel syndrome
Diuretics and other masking agents (e.g., diuretics hydrochlorothiazide, furosemide, acetazolamide, amiloride, spironolactone; other masking agents probenecid, epitestosterone, 5-alpha reductase inhibitors, plasma expanders, dextran, hydroxyethyl starch, mannitol)	• Dizziness, lightheadedness, muscle cramps, rash, gout, hypotension, renal insufficiency, electrolyte imbalances, gynecomastia (spironolactone)
Stimulants (e.g., amphetamine, D-methamphetamine, ephedrine, caffeine, methylphenidate, pseudoephedrine, cocaine, strychnine, modafinil)	• Headache, nausea, tremor, hypertension, tachycardia, myocardial infarction, stroke, heat stroke, rhabdomyolysis • Insomnia, anxiety, agitation, panic attacks, aggression, psychosis
Narcotics (used to increase pain threshold)	• Dependence, decreased concentration, fatigue, nausea, vomiting, constipation, loss of coordination
Cannabinoids	• Reduced alertness, impaired short-term memory, psychomotor retardation • Dysphoria, increased anxiety, paranoia
Alcohol	• Sedation, decreased concentration, loss of coordination
Glucocorticoids	• Hyperglycemia, fluid retention • Acute mood changes • Chronic use: reduced muscle mass and weakness, osteoporosis, diabetes mellitus, hypertension, weight gain, abdominal obesity, cataracts, hypomania, depression, psychosis
Beta-agonists	• Tachycardia, arrhythmias, hypokalemia, increased plasma glucose, muscle tremor
Beta-blockers	• Bradycardia, increased airway resistance, decreased endurance
Methods to increase oxygen transport (e.g., recombinant human EPO, darbepoetin alfa, transfusion)	• Myocardial infarction, stroke, thromboembolic disease, hypertension, antibody-mediated anemia, polycythemia
Gene doping	• Unknown

GENE DOPING

The capacity to manipulate the human genome is no longer science fiction. Significant advances in genetics research have made it possible to not only understand the role of genetic mutation as a core etiology of some diseases, but also to provide treatments, and possibly even cures. Gene therapy treats patients with diseases resulting from genetic mutation. The goal of gene therapy is to promote the expression of a functional gene and its protein product. The capacity to turn on, or turn off, protein synthesis has implications beyond treatment of disease. The potential to directly affect strength and endurance through gene manipulation has been demonstrated in laboratory mice. Utilizing the techniques developed for gene therapy could theoretically be used for performance enhancement in humans [20, 21].

To date, no known cases of human gene doping have been reported. However, WADA has preemptively banned gene doping as a "prohibited method of performance enhancement" in its 2013 Prohibited List. They define gene doping as "the transfer of cells or genetic elements (DNA, RNA) or the use of pharmacologic or biologic agents that alter gene expression." Gene doping offers the potential to target specific genes affecting endurance (EPO, PPAR, PEPCK), strength (IGF-1, myostatin), or tissue repair (BMP) [20, 22]. Although officially banned, testing for gene doping would be very challenging.

The likely health risks of gene doping have been demonstrated in animal models (including macaques) and humans treated with gene therapy. WADA's increasing concern for this form of doping is warranted, despite the lack of evidence that any athlete is currently using it.

CULTURAL ISSUES ASSOCIATED WITH DOPING

As the world has been united via the internet, it would be naïve to suggest that the availability of performance-enhancing drugs is not global. This is not to say that their use is equally prevalent within all nations and national sport organizations. Specific sports and specific countries have varying degrees of sport-associated "drug cultures." Consider which sports have chosen to develop and implement drug testing systems. Moreover, sports and organizations differ with regard to rigor of testing, enforcement, and punishment. Consider, for example, the Fédération Internationale de Football Association (FIFA). Recently a player tested positive and was given an immediate 1-year ban from the sport. At the same time, a player from the National Football League (NFL) tested positive and received a suspension that only lasted a few games. The clinician must be aware of the pressures to dope based on a patient-athlete's country of origin and her particular sport.

CASE STUDIES

Unfortunately, an entire text could be written of case studies of modern-day athletes and doping. It is unknown whether high-profile cases merely represent the "tip of the iceberg." Data on the prevalence of doping in sports are highly speculative and difficult to interpret. The actual number of dopers in any given sport is not known. Cheaters are unlikely to freely admit their actions, and large-scale screening on a regular basis of all athletes is currently impossible. The following real-life cases highlight a few of the issues associated with doping in sport.

Case Study 1

A 16-year-old adolescent male always dreamed of being a high school football player. Despite an aggressive workout schedule and intense weight lifting, he was only able to get his weight up to 215 pounds. The coach told him after the tryout that he liked his effort, but he would need to put on 25 additional pounds to make the team. The player asked the coach how he could possibly do it. The coach gave him the name of someone who could help him achieve his goal. Eight months later, the player returned weighing 255 pounds and looking very muscular. His strength had increased dramatically, and he was able to train at a very high level. He made the team and was very pleased. In the third game of the season, he became angry over a penalty called on him and punched the official. He was thrown off the team for his misconduct. He later confided to a teacher to whom he felt close that he had been given anabolic steroid injections by a strength and conditioning coach. The coach was subsequently fired for his actions when it was discovered he had been sending his players to a known steroid "pusher." Whether the steroids caused the violent behavior is debatable. However, the increase in weight and strength and the ability to overtrain were directly related to his steroid use. The high school did not have a drug testing program or any form of drug abuse education available to the athletes prior to this incident, but now it does.

Case Study 2

A 24-year-old world class swimmer came to a world championship meet and broke two world records. Despite being an elite swimmer, she had never challenged world records in her career. Her drop in times was remarkable, and many of her competitors questioned her dramatic improvement. In addition to her increased speed in the pool, she had a significant change in her physique. Her upper body became much more muscular, and her breasts appeared smaller. Her voice was noted to be much deeper than it had been in the past. Given her bodily changes combined with her incredible improvement in her times, many felt she had to be doping. She was drug tested following her world record swims, and no performance-enhancing drugs were detected. Despite her negative drug test, many felt she had beaten the test and, in fact, had used performance-enhancing drugs.

This case highlights a belief of many involved in doping control, namely, that the cheaters are often one step ahead of the testers. One athlete confided that current drug testing is little more than an intelligence test, since "only an idiot will get caught." Although a cynical view, it does represent a sense of failure of the doping control process by some athletes, as seen in this case.

SUMMARY

Regrettably, drugs have become an important issue in sports. Sports pages in newspapers around the globe routinely report on athletes at every level of competition using performance-enhancing substances to gain an unfair advantage over their competitors. The level of sophistication in beating drug testing, and developing "next-generation" agents, continues to grow. The relative paucity of well-designed research has been an additional factor impeding attempts to adequately address the problem. Very limited funds are currently available to conduct the necessary research. Without credible data, athletes are more vulnerable to the claims made by those benefiting from the sales of these compounds. Highly successful professional athletes are admired by many younger fans and by those dreaming of a similar future. Actions speak louder than words. Every time a successful athlete is caught using performance-enhancing drugs, every effort to diminish drug use is negatively impacted. The "win at all cost" and "second place is the first loser" mentality needs to be continually challenged by words and actions in youth sports in particular.

The war on drugs in sports must be a coordinated, well-organized international undertaking. Sports play an important role in virtually every culture. If we are to maintain the integrity of competition and protect the health of the athletes, we must dramatically increase our efforts to eliminate performance-enhancing drugs as an acceptable option for any athlete. Sports science professionals and sports psychiatrists need to work with coaches, trainers, athletes, and national governing bodies to educate athletes on the effects of performance-enhancing drug use. To achieve this important goal, everyone involved in sports needs to be knowledgeable about the negative impact this has on all aspects of organized sports. It is a difficult challenge, but one that must be addressed.

REFERENCES

1. Baron DA, Martin DM, AbolMagd S. Doping in sports and its spread to at-risk populations: an international review. *World Psychiatry* 2007; 6(2):118–123.
2. Catlin DH, Murray TH. Performance-enhancing drugs, fair competition, and Olympic sport. *The Journal of the American Medical Association* 1996; 276:231.
3. Fernandez MM, Hosey RG. Performance-enhancing drugs snare nonathletes, too. *The Journal of Family Practice* 2009; 58:16.
4. Metzl JD, Small E, Levine SR, Gershel JC. Creatine use among young athletes. *Pediatrics* 2001; 108:421.
5. Wanjek B, Rosendahl J, Strauss B, Gabriel HH. Doping, drugs and drug abuse among adolescents in the State of Thuringia (Germany): prevalence, knowledge and attitudes. *International Journal of Sports Medicine* 2007; 28:346.
6. Botrè F, Pavan A. Enhancement drugs and the athlete. *Neurologic Clinics* 2008; 26:149.
7. Sjöqvist F, Garle M, Rane A. Use of doping agents, particularly anabolic steroids, in sports and society. *Lancet* 2008; 371:1872.
8. Eichner ER. Stimulants in sports. *Current Sports Medicine Report* 2008; 7:244.
9. Yesalis CE. History of doping in sport. In: Bahrke MS, Yesalis CE (eds) *Performance Enhancing Substances in Sport and Exercise*. Champaign: Human Kinetics; 2002, pp. 1–20.
10. Landry GL, Kokotailo PK. Drug screening in athletic settings. *Current Problems in Pediatrics* 1994; 24:344–359.
11. Franke WW, Berendonk B. Hormonal doping and androgenization of athletes: a secret program of the German Democratic Republic. *Clinical Chemistry* 1997; 43:1262–1279.
12. Elliott S. Erythropoiesis-stimulating agents and other methods to enhance oxygen transport. *British Journal of Pharmacology* 2008; 154:529.
13. McDuff D, Baron D. Substance use in athletics: a sports psychiatry perspective. *Clinics in Sports Medicine* 2005; 24(4):885–897.
14. Berlin B. Steroids. Building a better you? *New Jersey Medicine* 1999; 96(3):49–51.
15. Baron D, Baron DDA, Baron SH. Laboratory testing of substances of abuse. In: Frances RJ, Miller SI, Mack AH (eds) *Clinical Textbook of Addictive Disorders*, 3rd edition. New York: Guilford Press; 2005.
16. American Academy of Pediatrics. Policy statement use of performance-enhancing substances. *Pediatrics* 2005; 115(4):1103–1106.
17. Selig AH. An open letter to baseball fans. *Los Angeles Times*, 16 June 2006.

18. Moss HB, Panzak GL, Tarter RE. Personality, mood, and psychiatric symptoms among anabolic steroid users. *American Journal on Addictions* 1992; 1(4):315–324.

19. Miller KE, Hoffman JH, Barnes GM, *et al.* Adolescent anabolic steroid use, gender, physical activity and other problem behaviors. *Substance Use & Misuse* 2005; 40(11):1637–1657.

20. McKanna TA, Toriello HV. Gene doping: the hype and the harm. *Pediatric Clinics of North America* 2010; 57:719.

21. Beiter T, Zimmermann M, Fragasso A, *et al.* Direct and long-term detection of gene doping in conventional blood samples. *Gene Therapy* 2011; 18:225.

22. Rivera VM, Gao GP, Grant RL, *et al.* Long-term pharmacologically regulated expression of erythropoietin in primates following AAV-mediated gene transfer. *Blood* 2005; 105:1424.

4   Exercise Addiction: The Dark Side of Sports and Exercise

Tamás Kurimay,[1] Mark D. Griffiths,[2] Krisztina Berczik,[3] and Zsolt Demetrovics[4]

[1] Department of Psychiatry and Psychiatric Rehabilitation, Saint John Hospital, Hungary
[2] International Gaming Research Unit, Psychology Division, Nottingham Trent University, UK
[3] Doctoral School of Psychology and Institute of Psychology, Eötvös Loránd University, Hungary
[4] Institute of Psychology, Eötvös Loránd University, Hungary

KEY POINTS

- An optimal level of regular physical activity is one of the most important factors in the maintenance of physical and mental health.
- For a minority of people, too much exercise can have adverse effects on their health and lead to exercise addiction.
- Exercise addiction can be conceptualized as a behavioral addiction.
- Exercise addiction can be characterized by salience, mood modification, tolerance, withdrawal symptoms, personal conflict, and relapse.

DEFINITIONS, SYMPTOMOLOGY, AND CLASSIFICATION

Regular exercise can be conceptualized as a set of planned, structured, and repetitive complex movement activities carried out with sufficient frequency, intensity, and duration to be effective in health promotion, while also playing a significant role in disease prevention [1, 2]. After taking into account an individual's gender, age, and fitness level, empirical research has demonstrated that regular physical exercise contributes to the maintenance of health [3–6]. The optimal level of habitual physical exercise has favorable effects on both the physical and mental well-being of the adult population [7–9], as well as on children's and teenagers' general well-being [10–12].

Glasser first introduced the concept of "positive addiction" into the psychological literature by trying to pinpoint the beneficial effects of physical exercise [13]. However, Morgan questioned Glasser's conceptualization [14], because psychiatric case studies had shown that exaggerated exercise could lead not only to physical injury, but also to the negligence of the most paramount everyday responsibilities including both work and family life. In these extreme clinical cases, the overuse of exercise has surfaced as a new form of addiction [14]. In a review of behavioral addictions, Griffiths questioned the criteria for positive addiction [15] and argued that Glasser's criteria [13] bore little resemblance to the accepted signs or components of addictions.

Clinical Sports Psychiatry: An International Perspective, First Edition. Edited by David A. Baron, Claudia L. Reardon and Steven H. Baron.
© 2013 John Wiley & Sons, Ltd. Published 2013 by John Wiley & Sons, Ltd.

Despite increased usage of the term "exercise addiction," and because it is a multidisciplinary concern, various branches of science with different research orientations still tend to use several incongruent terminologies in the discussion of the excessive exercise syndrome [16]. The most popular alternative name perhaps is *exercise dependence* [17, 18]. Nevertheless, some scholars refer to the condition as *obligatory exercising* [19] and *exercise abuse* [20], while in the media the condition is often described as *compulsive exercise* [21]. In this chapter, the term *addiction* is considered to be the most appropriate because it incorporates both dependence and compulsion. In a recent sport-related psychiatry review, exercise addiction was classified as a compulsive disorder that stressed the spectrum and process peculiarities of it [22]. Subsequently, addiction is defined as the behavioral process that can provide either pleasure or relief from internal discomfort (stress, anxiety, etc.) and is characterized by repeated failure to control the behavior (state of powerlessness) and maintenance of the behavior in spite of negative consequences [23]. This definition is then further complemented by six common symptoms of addiction as criteria for identifying the condition: salience, mood modification, tolerance, withdrawal symptoms, personal conflict, and relapse [24].

Currently, exercise addiction is not cited within any officially recognized medical or psychological diagnostic frameworks. However, it is important, on the basis of the known and shared symptoms with related morbidities, that the dysfunction receive attention in a miscellaneous category of other or unclassified disorders. Based on symptoms with diagnostic values, exercise addiction could potentially be classified within the category of behavioral addictions [25, 26].

Some disorders that are classified into different categories within certain diagnostic frameworks based on expert consensus [27] appear to resemble each other in several important ways [28]. In relation to the fifth edition of the Diagnostic and Statistical Manual of Mental Disorders (DSM-5), there is a current debate about which types of behavioral addiction have sufficient scientific evidence to appear as a distinct clinical entity in the new manual of mental disorders. At the time of this writing, it looks probable that pathological gambling will be classed as a behavioral addiction but that internet addiction will be classed as needing further scientific research to prove its status as a genuine behavioral addiction [29]. Exercise addiction – as pointed out earlier in this chapter – has not yet been classified in any diagnostic systems relating to mental and/or addictive disorders. The resemblance is evidenced not only in several common symptoms, but also in demographic characteristics, the prognosis of the disorder, comorbidity, response to treatment, prevalence in the family, and etiology [30, 31]. Hollander highlighted the obsessive, repetitive, and compulsive elements in the shared symptoms [28]. Although Hollander did not emphasize the addictive nature of the disorders with several common characteristics, it is evident that most of the cited disorders fit into the spectrum of addictions, and, more specifically, behavioral addictions. Exercise addiction could also be potentially classified into this group of disorders, because a common feature of all behavioral (and chemical) addictions is the preoccupation with the behavior when it is prevented or delayed. This is the *obsessive* facet of the dysfunction, which is accompanied by increased levels of anxiety before carrying out the behavior and decreasing anxiety, sense of relief, and satisfaction after the fulfillment of the behavior. The anxiolytic effect of the addictive behavior is often followed by feelings of guilt in the context of the behavior. The experienced relief and satisfaction are of short duration, and the urge to engage again in the behavior soon resurfaces in parallel with the progressively increasing anxiety. This is the cyclical aspect of the dysfunction, and its constituent persistent and repetitive nature is another common characteristic of addictive behaviors. A theoretical consideration of the typical symptoms and key characteristics of the syndrome reveals that exercise addiction may be closely connected to disorders encompassing obsession and impulse control [32]. This is in spite of the fact that on the continuum proposed by Hollander, it could be placed closer towards the compulsive end of the spectrum.

ASSESSMENT OF EXERCISE ADDICTION

Several instruments have been developed and adopted for the assessment of exercise addiction [16]. Two relatively early scales, namely, the *Commitment to Running Scale* [33] and the *Negative Addiction Scale* [34], are no longer used because of theoretical and methodological shortcomings that have been discussed extensively elsewhere [35]. Among the psychometrically tested instruments, the *Obligatory Exercise Questionnaire* [19], the *Exercise Dependence Scale* [36], the *Exercise Dependence Questionnaire* (EDQ) [37], and the *Exercise Addiction Inventory* [38] have proved to be both psychometrically valid and reliable instruments for gauging the symptoms and assessing the extent of exercise addiction [39].

EPIDEMIOLOGY

In the course of assessment of exercise addiction, several incongruent results have emerged. The most likely reason behind the inconsistency in findings may be connected to two issues, namely, the diversity of measurement tools and the heterogeneity of the studied populations. To date, studies of exercise addiction prevalence have been carried out on American and British samples of regular exercisers. In five studies carried out among university students, Hausenblas and Downs reported that between 3.4% and 13.4% of their samples were at high risk of exercise addiction [36]. Griffiths *et al.* [40], reported that 3.0% of a British sample of sport science and psychology students were identified as at-risk of exercise addiction. These research-based estimates are in concordance with the argument that exercise addiction is *relatively* rare [41] especially when compared to other addictions [42]. More recently, Monok *et al.* reported that 0.3–0.5% of the Hungarian general population aged 18–64 years is at risk for exercise addiction [39].

Among those who are also professionally connected to sport, the prevalence may be even higher. For example, Szabo and Griffiths found that 6.9% of British sport science students were at risk of exercise addiction [43]. However, in other studies where more involved exercisers were studied, much higher estimates have generally been found. Blaydon and Linder reported that 30.4% of triathletes could be diagnosed with primary exercise addiction, and a further 21.6% diagnosed with secondary exercise addiction [44]. In another study, 26% of 240 male and 25% of 84 female runners were classified as "obligatory exercisers" [45]. Lejoyeux *et al.* found that 42% of clients of a Parisian fitness room could be identified as exercise addicts [46]. Recently, he reported lower rates of just under 30% [47]. However, one study that surveyed 95 "ultra-marathoners" (who typically run 100-km races) reported only three people (3.2%) as at risk for exercise addiction [16].

COMORBIDITY

There is a strong link between exercise addiction and various forms of eating disorders [42]. Several studies have reported that disordered eating behavior is often (if not always) accompanied by exaggerated levels of physical exercise. The reverse relationship has also been established. Individuals affected by exercise addiction often (but not always) show an excessive concern about their body image, weight, and control over their diet [44, 48–50]. This comorbidity makes it difficult to establish which of these behaviors is the primary disorder. Related to this, it is important to clarify whether exaggerated exercise behavior is a primary problem in the affected person's life or whether it emerges as a secondary problem in consequence of another psychological dysfunction. In the former case, the dysfunction is classified as *primary exercise addiction* because it manifests as a form of behavioral addiction. In the latter case, it is termed *secondary exercise addiction* because it co-occurs with another dysfunction, typically with eating disorders such as anorexia nervosa or bulimia nervosa [51–53]. The distinguishing feature between the two is that in primary exercise addiction, the exercise is the objective, whereas in secondary exercise addiction weight loss is the objective, while exaggerated exercise is one of the primary means of achieving the objective.

In an investigation, Blaydon and Lindner examined triathletes by administering the EDQ and the Eating Attitude Test (EAT) to determine their level of exercise addiction, as well as their degree of eating disorders [44]. Based on a statistical cluster analysis, they identified four different groups. The group classified as "nondependent" showed low scores for both exercise addiction and eating disorders. The group identified as suffering from eating disorders showed high scores for eating disorders, but low scores for exercise addiction. The other two groups were described as either suffering from *primary exercise addiction* (high scores for exercise addiction accompanied by low scores for eating disorders) or from *secondary exercise addiction* (high scores for exercise addiction accompanied by high scores for eating disorders). Using cluster analysis, it was reported that 52% of the triathletes were classified as addicted to their exercise (30% suffering from primary exercise addiction and 22% suffering from secondary exercise addiction).

Since the method may not necessarily yield groups that were based on high (or at risk, or cutoff) scores, the rate of addiction established in this study – in light of the definition as harmful or destructive exercise – appears somewhat exaggerated. This speculation is also substantiated by the fact that the groups identified as primary or secondary exercise addicts did not differ significantly from each other. However, gender differences were highly apparent, as males tended to be in the majority in the primary exercise addiction group, whereas females were in the majority in the secondary exercise addiction group. The lack of symptoms of addiction and eating disorder was higher in men than in women (41% vs. 25%). This finding was consistent with Hausenblas and Downs' study [54] that also found a higher prevalence of exercise addiction in males among university students. Finally, and somewhat predictably, primary exercise addiction was more likely to be found in the professional and experienced triathletes (41%) than in the less experienced amateur triathletes (23%) [44].

In a similar study, Bamber *et al.* [51] examined the psychological profiles of women affected by primary and secondary exercise addiction and eating disorders. In addition, a nonsymptomatic control group was tested. Women classified as suffering from secondary exercise addiction did not differ significantly from the eating disorders group. However, they exhibited greater neuroticism, impulsivity, and lower self-concept as well as more preoccupation with their appearance and body weight than the participants who were classified as suffering from primary exercise addiction. Unexpectedly, the primary exercise addiction group exhibited no significant differences on those measures in comparison to the control group. In line with the results of these and other studies [55], some authors have denied the existence of primary exercise addiction as a pathological and/or a psychological dysfunction [56].

ETIOLOGY

Taking a broader view, the role of family is an important element in engaging members in regular exercise. The vast majority of the literature supports the view that family patterns contribute to a healthy lifestyle, including sports activities [57]. The main cluster of motives for engaging in regular sports activities – many of which are learned from the family – include skills that enable feelings of accomplishment (along with a sense of belonging, and social motives), fitness to improve strength, competitiveness to achieve success, and enjoyment for pleasure and fun [58, 59]. As in any potential addictive behavior, family plays an important role in exacerbating, maintaining, and helping behavioral disturbances. Theoretically, it appears obvious that since addictions and eating disorders have been studied for family influences (and/or systemic therapies), the same should be done for exercise addiction. However, there has not been any systematic study of exercise addiction within families. In clinical practice, exercise addiction, as with any behavioral addiction, can take family members by surprise, particularly because exercise is generally a positive healthy outlet. Because of the hidden pattern, excessive exercise is much easier for family members to rationalize, deny, and/or ignore [60]. Therefore, the natural consequence of this complex etiology is to incorporate family interventions into the treatment of behavioral addictions (including exercise addiction), and other sports-related disturbances [61].

As a physiological explanation for exercise addiction, perhaps the oldest, most popular, and most controversial among runners and many other exercisers – in light of the scientific evidence for it – is the *runners' high* hypothesis. It has long been reported that after intensive running, runners report an intense feeling of euphoria. The sensation has been ascribed to beta-endorphin activity in the brain. However, the changes observed in beta-endorphin levels were seen in the plasma, and because of its chemical structure, beta-endorphins cannot cross the blood–brain barrier, meaning that changes in plasma levels may not be accompanied by simultaneous changes in the brain.

From a psychological perspective, Szabo proposed a *cognitive appraisal hypothesis* as the basis for a better understanding of the etiology of exercise addiction [62]. According to this theory, once the habitual exerciser uses exercise as a means of coping with stress, the affected individual learns to depend on (and need) exercise at times of stress. The individual is convinced that exercise is a healthy means of coping with stress, as recommended in both scholastic and public media sources. Therefore, the person uses rationalization to explain the exaggerated amounts of exercise, which slowly but progressively takes its toll on other obligations and normal daily activities. If unforeseen events prevent the person from exercising or require the person to reduce the amount of daily exercise, negative psychological feelings occur. These appear in the form of irritability, guilt, anxiousness, sluggishness, etc. These collective feelings are thought to represent the withdrawal symptoms experienced due to a lack of exercise. When exercise had been used to cope with stress, apart from the negative psychological feelings, there is also a loss of the coping mechanism. Concomitantly, exercisers lose control over the stressful situation(s) with which they previously coped through exercise. The loss of the coping mechanism, followed by the loss of control over stress, generates an increased perception of vulnerability to stress, which further amplifies the negative psychological feelings associated with the lack of exercise. The mounting pressure urges the individual to resume exercise even at the expense of the other obligations in his daily life. Obviously, while exercise provides an instant reduction in the negative psychological feelings, the ignorance or superficial treatment of other social and work obligations results in conflict with people, possibly detriments at work or school, or even loss of job, which together cause further stress. The addicted exerciser is then trapped in a vicious circle needing more exercise to deal with the consistently increasing life-stress, part of which is caused by exercise itself.

The *affect regulation hypothesis* suggests that exercise has a dual effect on mood [63]. Firstly, it increases positive affect (defined as momentary psychological feeling states of longer persistence than momentary emotions) and, therefore, contributes to an improved general mood state (defined as prolonged psychological feeling states lasting for several hours or even days). Secondly, it decreases negative affect or the temporary states of guilt, irritability, sluggishness, and anxiety associated with missed exercise or training sessions. Through this relief, exercise further contributes to an improved general mood state [63]. However, the affect-regulating consequences of exercise are temporary, and the longer the interval between two exercise sessions, the more likely the experience of negative affect. In fact, after prolonged periods of abstention from exercise, these negative affective states become severe deprivation sensations and/or withdrawal symptoms that can only be relieved through further exercise. Therefore, as the cycle continues, further increasing amounts of exercise are needed to experience improvement in affect and general mood. Progressively, the interexercise rest periods decrease as a way of preventing the surfacing of withdrawal symptoms.

From a behaviorist perspective, individuals addicted to exercise may be motivated via negative reinforcement (e.g., to avoid withdrawal symptoms) as well as via positive reinforcement (e.g., to enjoy any aspect of exercise [64]). Exercise for negative reinforcement is not a characteristic of the committed exercisers who wish to improve and to enjoy their exercise [62]. Indeed, committed exercisers maintain their exercise for benefiting or gaining from their activity and, thus, their behavior is motivated via positive reinforcement. However, addicted exercisers *have to* exercise to avoid negative feelings. Their exercise may be a chore that needs to be fulfilled, or otherwise an unwanted life event would occur such as the inability to cope with stress, or gaining weight, becoming moody, etc.

Case Study

Joanna is a 25-year-old, well-educated female, from a stable family background, who realized that she had a problem surrounding exercise. She describes herself as being in excellent physical condition except for an injury sustained to her arm during a Jiu-Jitsu session. Here, we describe Joanna's behavior in terms of the main components of addiction (i.e., salience, tolerance, withdrawal, mood modification, conflict, loss of control, relapse, and negative consequences due to the behavior).

- Salience: Jiu-Jitsu is the most important activity in Joanna's life. Even when not actually engaged in the activity, she is thinking about the next training session or competition. She estimates that she spends approximately 6h a day (and sometimes much more) involved in training (e.g., weight training, jogging, general exercise, etc.). At university, she missed one of her exams to attend a Jiu-Jitsu competition in another part of the country. She fell behind in her university coursework due to exercise because she claimed she could not find the time to study.
- Tolerance: Joanna started Jiu-Jitsu at an evening class once a week during her teenage years and built up slowly over a period of about 5 years. She now exercises every single day, and the lengths of the sessions have become longer and longer

(suggesting tolerance). When not engaged in Jiu-Jitsu, she has to do some other form of exercise. This could be argued as a form of cross-tolerance.

- Withdrawal: Joanna claims she becomes highly agitated and irritable if she is unable to exercise. When her arm was bandaged up because of an arm injury, she went for 3-h jogs instead. She claims she also gets headaches and feels nauseous if she goes for more than a day without training or has to miss a scheduled session.
- Mood modification: Joanna experiences mood changes in a number of ways. She feels very high and "buzzed up" if she has done well in a Jiu-Jitsu competition (especially so if she wins). She also feels high if she has trained hard and for a long time.
- Conflict: Joanna's relationship with her long-term partner ended as a result of her exercise. She claimed she never spent much time with him and was not even bothered about their breakup. Her university work suffered because of the lack of time and concentration.
- Loss of control: Joanna claims she cannot stop herself engaging in exercise when she "gets the urge." Once she has started, she has to do a minimum of a few hours of exercise. She claims she has a total lack of concentration during lectures. She also claims she has an inability to study for exams unless she has done her exercise.
- Relapse: Joanna can only go a few days of no exercise before her day-to-day living becomes absolutely unbearable. If she misses a Jiu-Jitsu competition, she is just as bothered. The thought that she could have won a medal but was not there is particularly painful for her. She has continually tried to stop and/or cut down but claims she cannot. She becomes highly anxious if she is unable to engage in exercise and then has to go out and train to make herself feel better. She is well aware that exercise has taken over her life but feels powerless to stop it.
- Negative consequences: Joanna spends money beyond her means to maintain her exercising habit (e.g., on entrance fees for weight training, swimming, etc.). She also spends a lot of time in between two towns and therefore has several dual memberships at various health clubs. She is financially in debt not just because she is a student but also because she funds herself to attend Jiu-Jitsu competitions across the country. She has resorted to socially unacceptable means (e.g., stealing) in order to get money to fund herself. She is worried about her injured arm, which is never given enough time to heal properly before she gets the urge to take part in Jiu-Jitsu training and competitions again. Her doctor has advised her to give up the sport because he thinks she will do permanent damage to her arm. This is something she feels she is totally unable to do even if it means permanent damage.

There appears to be little doubt that Joanna is addicted to exercise and that she displays all the core symptoms of any bona fide addiction. Exercise is the most important thing in her life, and the number of hours engaged in physical activity per week has increased substantially over a 5-year period. She displays withdrawal symptoms when she does not exercise, and experiences euphoria related to various aspects of her exercising (e.g., training hard, winning competitions, etc.). She experiences conflict over exercise in many areas of her life and acknowledges she has a problem. Furthermore, she has lost friends, her relationship has broken down, her academic work has suffered, and she has considerable debt. She was advised to seek psychological help by those close to her, but she has not taken the advice.

CONCLUSION AND IMPLICATIONS

Although all addictive behaviors have idiosyncratic differences, addictions commonly share more similarities than dissimilarities [24]. However, those working in the exercise addiction field need to be careful when considering the research into excessive exercise, exercise addiction, and especially possible interventions. It should also be noted that for a diagnosis of exercise addiction to be useful, the requisite information needed includes information about etiology, process, and prognosis (i.e., within systems that assess the person's resources including a person's adaptational and functioning strengths and their limitations). Such information helps aid (i) treatment planning, (ii) technique choices, (iii) process and outcome assessments, (iv) policies to enable the development and sustaining of needed treatment alliances, and (v) staff training needs. However, while there is a need to make relevant stakeholders aware of a potential problem, there is also a need to avoid too much medicalization of the problem. Identification of excessive exercise as an addiction carries the risk of stigmatization as well due to the behavior's pejorative adjudication. In order to avoid this, all possible interventions should find a pragmatic balance between the promotion of exercise and workout, on the one hand, and prevention of excessive exercise, on the other hand. This way, similar to several other behavioral addictions (e.g., gambling, playing video games, sex, shopping), or even chemical substance use (e.g., alcohol), temperance could be the focus of communication. Possible interventions should include the message that recreational exercise is not only tolerable but a definite and desirable factor that contributes to the facilitation of health.

ACKNOWLEDGMENTS

Zsolt Demetrovics acknowledges financial support of the János Bolyai Research Fellowship awarded by the Hungarian Academy of Science. This work was supported by the Hungarian Ministry of Social Affairs and Labor (grant number: KAB-KT-09-0007) and the Hungarian Scientific Research Fund (grant number: 83884).

REFERENCES

1. Waddington I. (2000) *Sport, Health, and Drugs: A Critical Sociological Perspective*. London: Spoon Press.
2. Caspersen CJ, Powell KE, Christenson GM. (1985) Physical activity, exercise and physical fitness: Definitions and distinctions for health-related research. *Public Health Reports* 100, 126–131.
3. Blair SN, Kohl HW, Paffenbarger RS, Clark DG, Cooper KH, Gibbons LW. (1989) Physical fitness and all-cause mortality. A prospective study of healthy men and women. *The Journal of the American Medical Association* 262(17), 2395–2401.
4. Paffenbarger RS, Jr., Hyde RT, Wing AL, Hsieh CC. (1986) Physical activity, all-cause mortality, and longevity of college alumni. *The New England Journal of Medicine* 314(10), 605–613.
5. Royal College of Physicians. (1991) *Medical Aspects of Exercise. Risks and Benefits*. London: Royal College of Physicians.
6. United States Department of Health and Human Services. (1996) *Physical Activity and Health. A Report of the Surgeon General*. Atlanta: U.S. Department of Health and Human Services, Centers for Disease Control and Prevention, National Center for Chronic Disease Prevention and Health Promotion, The President's Council on Physical Fitness and Sports.

7. Folsom AR, Caspersen CJ, Taylor HL, Jacobs DR, Jr., Luepker RV, Gomez-Marin O, *et al.* (1985) Leisure time physical activity and its relationship to coronary risk factors in a population-based sample. The Minnesota Heart Survey. *American Journal of Epidemiology* 121(4), 570–579.
8. Lamb KL, Roberts K, Brodie DA. (1990) Self-perceived health among sports participants and non-sports participants. *Social Science & Medicine* 31(9), 963–969.
9. Lotan M, Merrick J, Carmeli E. (2005) A review of physical activity and well-being. *International Journal of Adolescent Medicine and Health* 17(1), 23–31.
10. Biddle SJ, Gorely T, Stensel DJ. (2004) Health-enhancing physical activity and sedentary behaviour in children and adolescents. *Journal of Sports Sciences* 22(8), 679–701.
11. Lotan M, Merrick J, Carmeli E. (2005) Physical activity in adolescence. A review with clinical suggestions. *International Journal of Adolescent Medicine and Health* 17(1), 13–21.
12. Piko BF, Keresztes N. (2006) Physical activity, psychosocial health, and life goals among youth. *Journal of Community Health* 31(2), 136–145.
13. Glasser W. (1976) *Positive Addiction*. New York: Harper & Row.
14. Morgan WP. (1979) Negative addiction in runners. *The Physician and Sportsmedicine* 7, 57–70.
15. Griffiths MD. (1996) Behavioural addictions: An issue for everybody? *Journal of Workplace Learning* 8(3), 19–25.
16. Allegre B, Therme P, Griffiths MD. (2007) Individual factors and the context of physical activity in exercise dependence: A prospective study of 'ultra-marathoners'. *International Journal of Mental Health and Addiction* 5, 233–243.
17. Cockerill IM, Riddington ME. (1996) Exercise dependence and associated disorders: A review. *Counselling Psychology Quarterly* 9(2), 119–129.
18. Hausenblas HA, Downs DS. (2002) Exercise dependence: A systematic review. *Psychology of Sport and Exercise* 3(2), 89–123.
19. Pasman LN, Thompson JK. (1987) Body image and eating disturbance in obligatory runners, obligatory weightlifters, and sedentary individuals. *International Journal of Eating Disorders* 7(6), 759–769.
20. Davis C. (2000) Exercise abuse. *International Journal of Sport Psychology* 31, 278–289.
21. Dalle Grave R, Calugi S, Marchesini G. (2008) Compulsive exercise to control shape or weight in eating disorders: Prevalence, associated features, and treatment outcome. *Comprehensive Psychiatry* 49(4), 346–352.
22. Reardon CL, Factor RM. (2010) Sport psychiatry: A systematic review of diagnosis and medical treatment of mental illness in athletes. *Sports Medicine* 40(11), 961–980.
23. Goodman A. (1990) Addiction: Definition and implications. *British Journal of Addiction* 85(11), 1403–1408.
24. Griffiths MD. (2005) A 'components' model of addiction within a biopsychosocial framework. *Journal of Substance Use* 10, 191–197.
25. Demetrovics Z, Griffiths MD. (2012) Behavioral addictions: Past, present and future. *Journal of Behavioral Addictions* 1(1), 1–2.
26. Grant JE, Potenza MN, Weinstein A, Gorelick DA. (2010) Introduction to behavioral addictions. *The American Journal of Drug and Alcohol Abuse* 36(5), 233–241.
27. American Psychiatric Association. (2000) *Diagnostic and Statistical Manual for Mental Disorders*, 4th edition. Washington, DC: American Psychiatric Publishing.
28. Hollander E. (1993) Obsessive-compulsive spectrum disorders: An overview. *Psychiatric Annals* 23, 355–358.
29. American Psychiatric Association. (2012) Gambling Disorder, May 28. http://www.dsm5.org/ProposedRevisions/Pages/proposedrevision.aspx?rid=210. Accessed on December 7, 2012.
30. Bartz JA, Hollander E. (2006) Is obsessive-compulsive disorder an anxiety disorder? *Progress in Neuro-Psychopharmacology & Biological Psychiatry* 30(3), 338–352.
31. Castle DJ, Phillips KA. (2006) Obsessive-compulsive spectrum of disorders: A defensible construct? *The Australian and New Zealand Journal of Psychiatry* 40(2), 114–120.
32. Shaffer HJ, LaPlante DA, LaBrie RA, Kidman RC, Donato AN, Stanton MV. (2004) Towards a syndrome model of addiction: Multiple expressions, common etiology. *Harvard Review of Psychiatry* 12, 1–8.
33. Carmack MA, Martens R. (1979) Measuring commitment to running: A survey of runners' attitudes and mental states. *Journal of Sport Psychology* 1, 25–42.
34. Hailey BJ, Bailey LA. (1982) Negative addiction in runners: A quantitative approach. *Journal of Sport Behavior* 5(3), 150–154.

35. Szabo A, Frenkl R, Caputo A. (1997) Relationships between addiction to running, commitment to running, and deprivation from running. *European Yearbook of Sport Psychology* 1, 130–147.
36. Hausenblas HA, Downs DS. (2002) How much is too much? The development and validation of the exercise dependence scale. *Psychology and Health* 17(4), 387–404.
37. Ogden J, Veale DM, Summers Z. (1997) The development and validation of the Exercise Dependence Questionnaire. *Addiction Research* 5(4), 343–355.
38. Terry A, Szabo A, Griffiths MD. (2004) The exercise addiction inventory: A new brief screening tool. *Addiction Research and Theory* 12(5), 489–499.
39. Monok K, Berczik K, Urbán R, Szabo A, Griffiths MD, Farkas J, Magi A, Eisinger A, Kurimay T, Kokonyei G, Kun B, Paksi B, Demetrovics Z. (2012) Psychometric properties and concurrent validity of two exercise addiction measures: A population wide study in Hungary. *Psychology of Sport and Exercise* 13, 739–746.
40. Griffiths MD, Szabo A, Terry A. (2005) The exercise addiction inventory: a quick and easy screening tool for health practitioners. *British Journal of Sports Medicine* 39(6), 30–31.
41. Szabo A. (2000) Physical activity as a source of psychological dysfunction. In: Biddle SJ, Fox KR, Boutcher SH (eds) *Physical Activity and Psychological Well-Being.* London: Routledge, 130–153.
42. Sussman S, Lisha N, Griffiths MD. (2011) Prevalence of the addictions: A problem of the majority or the minority? *Evaluation and the Health Professions* 34, 3–56.
43. Szabo A, Griffiths MD. (2007) Exercise addiction in British sport science students. *International Journal of Mental Health and Addiction* 5(1), 25–28.
44. Blaydon MJ, Lindner KJ. (2002) Eating disorders and exercise dependence in triathletes. *Eating Disorders* 10(1), 49–60.
45. Slay HA, Hayaki J, Napolitano MA, Brownell KD. (1998) Motivations for running and eating attitudes in obligatory versus nonobligatory runners. *International Journal of Eating Disorders* 23(3), 267–275.
46. Lejoyeux M, Avril M, Richoux C, Embouazza H, Nivoli F. (2008) Prevalence of exercise dependence and other behavioral addictions among clients of a Parisian fitness room. *Comprehensive Psychiatry* 49(4), 353–359.
47. Lejoyeux M, Guillot C, Chalvin F, Petit A, Lequen V. (2012) Exercise dependence among customers from a Parisian sport shop. *Journal of Behavioral Addictions* 1(1), 28–34.
48. Klein DA, Bennett AS, Schebendach J, Foltin RW, Devlin MJ, Walsh BT. (2004) Exercise "addiction" in anorexia nervosa: Model development and pilot data. *CNS Spectrums* 9(7), 531–537.
49. Lyons HA, Cromey R. (1989) Compulsive jogging: Exercise dependence and associated disorder of eating. *Ulster Medical Journal* 58(1), 100–102.
50. Sundgot-Borgen J. (1994) Eating disorders in female athletes. *Sports Medicine* 17(3), 176–188.
51. Bamber DJ, Cockerill IM, Carroll D. (2000) The pathological status of exercise dependence. *British Journal of Sports Medicine* 34(2), 125–132.
52. Blaydon MJ, Lindner KJ, Kerr JH. (2002) Metamotivational characteristics of eating-disordered and exercise-dependent triathletes: An application of reversal theory. *Psychology of Sport and Exercise* 3(3), 223–236.
53. de Coverley Veale DM. (1987) Exercise dependence. *British Journal of Addiction* 82(7), 735–740.
54. Hausenblas HA, Downs DS. (2002) Relationship among sex, imagery, and exercise dependence symptoms. *Psychology of Addictive Behaviors* 16(2), 169–172.
55. Basson CJ. (2001) Personality and behaviour associated with excessive dependence on exercise: Some reflections from research. *South African Journal of Psychology* 31(2), 53–59.
56. Yates A, Shisslak CM, Allender J, Crago M, Leehey K. (1992) Comparing obligatory to nonobligatory runners. *Psychosomatics* 33(2, Spring), 180–189.
57. Trost SG, Loprinzi PG. (2011) Parenting influences on physical activity behavior in children and adolescents: A brief review. *American Journal of Lifestyle Medicine* 5(2), 171–181.
58. Buonamano A, Cei A, Mussino A. (1995) Participation motivation in Italian youth sport. *The Sport Psychologist* 9, 265–281.
59. Lowry R, Kremer J, Trew K. (2007) Young people: Physical health, exercise and recreation. In: Coleman J, Hendry L, Kloep M (eds) *Adolescence and Health Understanding Adolescence.* Chichester: John Wiley & Sons, Ltd, pp. 19–40.
60. Simmons LL. (2008) *The Everything Health Guide to Addiction and Recovery: Control Your Behavior and Build a Better Life.* Avon: Adams Media Corporation.

61. Hellstedt J. (2005) Invisible players: A family systems model. *Clinics in Sports Medicine* 24, 899–928.
62. Szabo A. (1995) The impact of exercise deprivation on well-being of habitual exercisers. *The Australian Journal of Science and Medicine in Sport* 27, 68–75.
63. Hamer M, Karageorghis CI. (2007) Psychobiological mechanisms of exercise dependence. *Sports Medicine* 37(6), 477–484.
64. Pierce EF, Eastman NW, Tripathi HL, Olson KG, Dewey WL. (1993) Beta-endorphin response to endurance exercise: Relationship to exercise dependence. *Perceptual & Motor Skills* 77(3, Pt 1), 767–770.

5 Eating Disorders in Athletes

Antonia L. Baum

Department of Psychiatry and Behavioral Sciences, George Washington University School of Medicine and Health Sciences, USA

KEY POINTS

- Eating disorders occur more often in sports that emphasize aesthetics, in which low body weight enhances performance, that are subdivided into weight classes, or in which there is a need to make weight for competition.
- Eating disorders are seen in both female and male athletes.
- Female athletes with disordered eating are susceptible to the female athlete triad.
- Education and prevention are the first steps in treatment; other important elements of treatment include consideration of the importance of return to play for the athlete, and balancing that with safety.
- Further epidemiologic research will be helpful in understanding the scope of the problem of disordered eating among athletes.

INTRODUCTION

There are unique aspects to eating disorders in the athlete. Etiology is optimally understood through a biopsychosocial formulation. While there are emerging data from family, twin, and molecular genetic studies to support a significant genetic influence in the genesis of anorexia nervosa (AN), bulimia nervosa (BN), and traits of these disorders [1], it is also important to consider the possible predisposing factors of the eating disordered individual that may propel him or her towards athletics in general, and towards specific sports, and the role specific sports may play in the genesis or exacerbation of an eating disorder. It is also important to consider the health risks to an eating disordered athlete, general treatment approaches, some of which must be tailored to the athlete, and, finally, the prevention of disordered eating in the athlete. Areas of future research are always fruitful to contemplate; there are still many frontiers in the relatively nascent field of sports psychiatry.

The assessment of an eating disorder in the athlete is complicated by the necessary focus on intake and nutrition in those for whom the body is the instrument. This very focus, which may be interpreted to be pathological in the nonathlete, may be adaptive in the athlete, and even necessary in the elite athlete. Determining when discipline gives way to pathology is an inexact

Clinical Sports Psychiatry: An International Perspective, First Edition. Edited by David A. Baron, Claudia L. Reardon and Steven H. Baron.
© 2013 John Wiley & Sons, Ltd. Published 2013 by John Wiley & Sons, Ltd.

science. In those athletes already predisposed to eating disorders through genetics, family environment, or past personal history of an eating disorder predating their athletic history, this very focus in the pursuit of sport may tip the scales and lead to disordered eating behavior.

The question often asked is whether eating disorders manifest more often in the athlete than in the general population. Though there are some data, the more relevant questions may be: Are there predisposing factors that may lead an already vulnerable individual into sports? Are there aspects of eating disorders in the athlete that are unique and that differentiate them from eating disorders in nonathletes? Are there sports-specific factors that may play a role in the development or perpetuation of an eating disorder?

As with eating disorders in general, athletes may cover the spectrum of disordered eating, from restrictive patterns, to bingeing, to abnormal compensatory behaviors. The obsessional focus and drive required to attain elite status as a competitive athlete are traits frequently seen in eating disorders, particularly the restricting and overexercise that are common to AN. Overexercise can also be a means to purge in BN. It may be that these premorbid traits, or the presence of an eating disorder, cause an individual to seek athletics, a socially sanctioned environment for some of their inherent pathology. It is, however, far more common to see unhealthy eating attitudes and the practice of unhealthful weight control techniques among athletes than it is to see athletes who meet criteria for an eating disorder [2]. Often, athletes with disordered eating will suffer recurrent injury, inconsistent performance, and abbreviated athletic careers [3]. Early recognition of disordered eating can be accomplished by addressing eating disorder signs and symptoms during an athlete's preparticipation sports physical.

Some sports engender disordered eating behavior by their very nature. These include sports where athletes need to make weight for competition, sports in which low body fat is advantageous for performance, and aesthetic sports where there is an emphasis on the appearance of the body.

EPIDEMIOLOGY

It can be theorized that involvement in athletics may be a protective factor, preventing the occurrence of eating disorders [4]. This protection may be afforded through improvement in body image in the athlete, an overall enhancement of psychological well-being, and possibly, less of a tendency to diet [5]. Nonetheless, eating disorders do occur in the athlete, sometimes clearly fostered by involvement in sport. Attempts to quantify these problems, particularly in the athletic arena, are complicated by the possibility of athletes' masking, denying, normalizing, or minimizing symptoms. Some studies suggest the possibility that disordered eating actually occurs more in athletes than in nonathletes. A large Norwegian study of elite athletes ($N = 1620$) revealed that 13.5% had clinical or subclinical eating disorders (AN, BN, or eating disorder not otherwise specified (ED NOS)), compared with 4.6% of the control group ($N = 1696$). The prevalence in male athletes was 8% and in female athletes 20%. This study, published in 2004, was the most ambitious to date, not only in its scope, and the inclusion of male athletes, but also in that the questionnaires used were validated through clinical interviews [6].

ED NOS is the most prevalent eating disorder, both in the general population and almost certainly in the athletic population as well. It is associated with significant psychological and physiological morbidity, and should not be discounted as a less important clinical condition [7].

A 2011 study of over 2000 male and female French athletes revealed that 4.9% had an active eating disorder, most meeting criteria for ED NOS [8].

THE ROLE OF SPORTS IN THE GENESIS OF EATING DISORDERS AND SPORTS-SPECIFIC EATING DISORDERS

Sports in which there is a need to make weight

Sports in which there is a need to make weight create an emphasis on acquisition and expenditure of calories. These sports include wrestling, rowing – particularly lightweight rowing, boxing, some of the martial arts, including Taekwondo and judo, and jockey-style horse racing. The pathologic means by which athletes drop weight prior to weigh-ins and competition cover the gamut, including: fasting; overexercise; self-induced vomiting; working out in saunas, rubber suits, and heavy clothing in hot and humid conditions; and laxative, diuretic, and stimulant abuse. In these particular sports, the weight fluctuations can be dramatic and occur in a cyclical fashion within a single season. The resulting dehydration and electrolyte disturbances, including hypokalemia, can obviously endanger the health of the athlete, leading to syncopal episodes, seizures, and cardiac events, with the risk of sudden death, particularly in those who are nutritionally compromised. These metabolic imbalances are particularly problematic in those who are still growing and developing. Sometimes a multisport athlete will have to make a significant transition in his weight and body makeup as he goes from one season to the next, for example, a fall football player who must morph into a winter wrestler.

The subculture in some sports is that there is team-wide bingeing and purging, with often tacit condonation or outright rejection of education or treatment, by coaches for whom the goal is victory. One wrestler described finding himself in line at a drugstore with teammates purchasing laxatives when their coach happened upon them. He looked the other way. A wrestler might hover at the margins of being malnourished in an effort to compete at a lower weight class, rather than seeking the weight class that might be optimal for his natural strength and size. After the weigh-in, the athlete has a short window in which to quickly consume calories to regain some strength for the match. This is all done in the interest of gaining an advantage over a lighter opponent. In this male-dominated sport, muscularity is equated with masculinity, and this may be a possible reinforcer for losing body fat [9]. In 1997, three college wrestlers died secondary to these types of rapid weight loss strategies [10].

Case Study

The father of a 5-year-old wrestler himself was a former wrestler. He pressured his son to fast for 2 days prior to his weigh-in, and to sit in a sauna the evening before in order to lower his body weight by 2.27 kg (10% of this young boy's body weight) so that he could wrestle at a lower weight class [11].

Male horse jockeys experience eating disorders far more often than their female counterparts, who are naturally smaller and lighter. Low weight is clearly advantageous when on the back of an animal trying to get to the finish line first. Jockeys must weigh in with their substantial saddles. One jockey described the misery of chronic starvation and bouts with donning a rubber suit and sitting in his car with the heat turned up. He would habitually gain significant weight in the off-season, only to have to drop it when racing season began.

Those who row crew and need to weigh in – a more problematic phenomenon when rowing light weight, where again, there is an effort to maximize strength-to-size ratio – are all too familiar with putting on several pairs of sweats and running in hot conditions, in addition to the usual methods of dropping weight.

Sports in which low body fat is advantageous

A second category of sport, which may either attract those with already unhealthy eating patterns or those with premorbid risk factors, consists of sports in which low body fat is advantageous for superior performance. Long-distance running has been described as an analog of AN. The body types of some ethnic groups, lean and with an orthogonal stride, render them more successful at long-distance running events, such as the marathon. If an athlete is not naturally ideally shaped for such distances he might try to alter his fat to lean muscle mass ratio. The calorie burn from distance workouts designed to establish a base can lead to a cycle of further weight loss. It is interesting to contemplate the convergence of the endorphin-induced runner's high with the endorphin-mediated euphoria that has been associated with the starved state; patients will describe this, and it has been demonstrated in rats, who can, indeed, get "hooked" on starving themselves to death. Triathletes, with their often extreme brick workouts, seem susceptible to the cycle of restriction and overexercise. One could speculate that ultramarathoners and other ultradistance athletes might be another population prone to disordered eating behavior.

Competitive swimming can also engender pathological eating behaviors. One study (age range 9–18 years) revealed that 15.4% used pathogenic weight control techniques [12]. In a group of elite female swimmers from 14 to 30 years of age, nearly 70% of their coaches had instructed them to lose weight [13]. It is not uncommon for team weigh-ins to occur in a public and potentially humiliating forum. Interestingly, most coaches make these recommendations not through a specific knowledge base, or by objective measures, but rather by the athlete's physical appearance. Coaches were also noted to recommend weight loss more often for female athletes than for male athletes [14, 15].

Sports in which athletes are judged on aesthetics

The third category of sport that is a lightning rod for eating disorders, again, either engendered through the sport or sought out due to premorbid pathology or risk factors, includes those sports in which judging is based on aesthetics, for example, gymnastics, diving, figure skating, and synchronized swimming. Though not numerically judged, classical ballet also fits into this category, as do numerous other genres of dance. Members of the Royal Ballet of Canada were reported to have ingested toilet paper to create a sense of satiety, which they would later purge (Personal communication (1993) St. Paul's Hospital, University of British Columbia, Vancouver). Even sports not typically thought of as aesthetic, such as tennis and swimming, can engender eating disorders. One tennis player described her discomfort in being in front of crowds in her revealing tennis dress.

Wendy Williams, an Olympic gold medalist in diving, has described her BN, as she struggled to maintain weight during her diving career. The required clean lines and flawless entries into the water necessitate a near-obsessional focus on the body's contours. The body-revealing suits worn by the divers add another dimension to the concerns a diver might experience before spectators and judges.

Aspiring Olympic gymnast Christy Henrich, whose weight eventually dropped below 50 lbs, died of complications of AN. She said: "In gymnastics they're always telling you, 'Don't eat that, don't eat that.' Pretty soon you become so paranoid that everyone is watching what you eat, and you feel everything is bad. You felt like you were really, really doing something wrong if you ate" [16]. She was a tragic statistic among many who are never brought to anyone's attention. It is adaptive for a gymnast to stave off puberty and the associated change in shape and increase in weight and height, in an effort to perform at her peak, from a physics perspective. A smaller, more compact body with a lower center of gravity can leap, spin, and maintain balance better than the pubescent or postpubescent athlete. Ludmilla Tourischeva, in spite of her grace and maturity, fell from the top of the podium as she grew. Gymnasts can lose points if their hair is not expertly coiffed and sprayed into place, or if their leotard does not fit perfectly, so any excess body fat does not go unnoticed. In female college gymnasts, there is a high prevalence of at least one pathologic weight-control behavior, ranging in various studies from 62% to 74% [17, 18]. Out of the members of a national rhythmic gymnastics team, 16.7% were diagnosed with AN [19]. The prevalence of AN and BN among ballet dancers was found to be as high as 25.7% [20] and 19% [21], respectively.

Competitive figure skating is renowned for the unusual attention to aesthetics, including elaborate costumes and makeup. Athletes have been known to resort to plastic surgery, including rhinoplasty in one competitive figure skater in an effort to improve her appearance on the ice "…when a judge said her nose was distracting" [16]. (It is worthwhile to consider a diagnosis of body dysmorphic disorder, where relevant.) It is not difficult to imagine how scrutiny can lead to an overemphasis on body shape and weight. Those figure skaters who excel at jumping require strong gluteal muscles and quadriceps to propel them off the ice, but this look is not considered ideal aesthetically, thus favoring those longer, naturally leaner skaters, causing some with a more "solid" build to struggle with eating disorders. Figure skater Chantal Bailey decried her natural build for years, developing BN, diagnosed at age 14, before realizing she could not make her body fit the archetype, and eventually finding success as a speed skater. In the latter sport, her build was advantageous, and she made the 1994 Olympic team.

How does one distinguish the "epidemic" of sport subculture-induced pathologic eating behavior from an intrinsic eating disorder? One distinction may be that those who have other risk factors and are therefore more susceptible are unable to shed these pathologic eating behaviors at season's end, and may find themselves in an unhealthy cycle that can last for years, or even for life.

EATING DISORDERS IN THE MALE ATHLETE

Eating disorders do occur in the male athlete. However, there is more danger that an eating disorder in a male athlete will go unrecognized, as eating disorders are more common in females and in female athletes. There are some sports in which males are particularly vulnerable. It is important to be mindful of this when evaluating a male athlete. Because eating disorders among males are less common, there can be more of a sense of shame, and even more effort to conceal the pathological behaviors.

In males, partial syndrome eating disorders are more common than full syndrome eating disorders [22]. While not exclusive to males, the phenomenon of muscle dysmorphia, a form of body dysmorphic disorder, has been described more extensively in males. It is characterized by an unhealthy preoccupation with muscularity. Those afflicted spend inordinate amounts of time lifting weights, dieting, and mirror checking. There is a predisposition to the abuse of anabolic steroids among athletes with muscle dysmorphia. Those sports in which muscle dsymorphia appears to be more common are bodybuilding and weight lifting [23].

THE FEMALE ATHLETE TRIAD

The female athlete triad – low energy availability, menstrual dysfunction, and low bone mineral density (BMD) [24] – is a serious consequence of restrictive eating and/or chronic malnourishment. Here it is important to note that the disordered eating that results in low energy availability does not imply psychopathology, and can include the *inadvertent* failure to take in as many calories as are being expended through physical training [25]. The body responds differently to the energy deficit that results from exercise and to the energy deficit that results from dietary restriction [26]. As Truswell has explained, "...there is no strong biological imperative to match energy intake to activity-induced energy expenditure" [27].

High volume training and low energy intake can lead to disruption of the hypothalamic–pituitary axis. This can result in amenorrhea with a subsequent drop in estrogen levels, which can in turn lead to low BMD, specifically osteopenia or osteoporosis, with the former being much more common in female athletes than the latter. The attendant risks associated with the female athlete triad include infertility and stress fractures [28].

Radiographs of young female gymnasts can mimic those of women in their ninth decade of life. Unfortunately, even with refeeding, baseline bone density cannot be restored. BMD can be improved in athletes with menstrual disturbance through weight-bearing exercise [28]. A large study of elite athletes demonstrated higher BMD compared to their nonathletic controls, and that higher-impact sports are associated with higher BMD than middle- and low-impact sports. Further, the nonathlete premenopausal women in this study were two to three times more likely to have *low* BMD than the elite athletes [29]. Interestingly, a more recent study of high-school athletes versus sedentary students revealed that one or more components of the triad were present in 78% of the athletes and 65% of the sedentary students [24].

TREATMENT

The first step in the treatment of the eating disordered athlete is prevention. Psychoeducation is the cornerstone of prevention. There is still a lot of work to be done in this area. Psychoeducational talks designed for coaches, athletic trainers, athletes, and parents are a good place to start. A 2004 survey of National Collegiate Athletic Association (NCAA) Division I Head Athletic Trainers demonstrated that though nearly all had encountered female athletes with eating disorders, just one quarter felt able to identify the psychopathology themselves, and only one third felt comfortable asking the athlete if she had an eating disorder [30].

A physiologic screening test for eating disorders geared to competitive female college athletes was developed and can be included in a preparticipation sports physical. This screening test combines self-report interview items (including the number of hours spent exercising outside of practice, a weight history addressing perception of weight, and a history of menstrual irregularity) with actual physiologic measurements (including percent body fat, waist-to-hip ratio, standing diastolic blood pressure, and presence or absence of parotid gland enlargement) [31].

For effective treatment of eating disorders in the athletic arena, there must be easy access to a sports psychiatrist. The ideal is the consultation liaison model, wherein a sports psychiatrist is embedded in a sports organization, perhaps literally in the training room, available for formal – and curbside – consultations, working alongside the orthopedists [32]. Normalizing the presence and utility of a psychiatrist goes a long way in minimizing the stigma often associated with this specialty – a stigma that tends to be pronounced in the athletic arena. Athletes are taught to reject any sense of mental frailty, a trait associated with psychiatric illness.

Part of the educational process is encouraging athletes, particularly at elite levels of competition, to select sports for which their body type is well-suited, rather than attempting to alter their physique to enhance sports performance. This process is often one of natural selection. However counterintuitive it might seem, the most important – and difficult – role a sports psychiatrist might play in an eating disordered athlete's life is to recommend that they quit their sport, a suggestion often met by resistance from coaches, parents, and the athletes themselves. Often a more constructive approach, and one more easily embraced, is to encourage alternative sports for which the patient's body type is more ideally suited.

Early diagnosis is an important factor in conquering eating disorders. The longer a behavior pattern is entrenched, the more difficult it becomes to eradicate.

Treatment can be challenging. Not only is one facing the ego-syntonic aspects of an eating disorder, the adaptive role that disordered eating behavior and overexercise might play for an athlete, and denial, but there may be collusion in this denial. Coaches, parents, and agents have a disincentive to address the problem; they may fear that arresting these behaviors could detract from an athlete's chance of victory. By acknowledging the presence of eating disorders, major sports organizations could jeopardize their image, and the promotion of their particular sport [15].

Among psychiatric disorders, eating disorders – specifically AN – are associated with the highest mortality rate. Treatment can be a matter of urgency. The initial determination must be whether an inpatient medical hospitalization is required to stabilize the athlete from a cardiac standpoint, to rehydrate, renourish, and reverse any electrolyte imbalances. Then the question of inpatient or outpatient psychiatric (including day hospital) treatment must be addressed. Factors to be considered include the duration and severity of the symptoms and the degree of support from family, coaches, trainers, teammates, and friends.

As noted earlier, while participation in athletics may contribute to the development of an eating disorder, the converse is also true. Exercise can be a valuable therapeutic tool in the treatment of an eating disorder. In the relatively newly described binge eating disorder, it is easy to see the role exercise can play in treatment [4]. Whether an athlete can continue in their athletic training during treatment is an important consideration. While a respite from training may be necessary, the athlete may experience this as punitive; a return to working out and competition can clearly be used as a strong incentive to overcome his symptoms. 'Food as fuel' can be a useful motif in restoring nutrition and healthy attitudes towards eating. The drive and determination that can be a part of the genesis of an eating disorder in the athlete can be the very traits the treatment team can enlist in the patient/athlete to attain victory over his psychopathology.

Treatment of comorbid psychiatric disorders is a necessary aspect of treatment. Common comorbidities include affective disorders and anxiety spectrum disorders. In AN, a malnourished state can present as depression, and refeeding may be necessary before effectively evaluating a patient for a mood disorder.

There is no clearly effective psychopharmacologic intervention in the treatment of AN. There is a body of literature to support the use of serotonin-specific reuptake inhibitors in BN, with evidence for impact on the impulse to binge and purge. Nonpharmacologic treatments cover the gamut, and must be tailored to the individual patient and their situation, from group, to family, to individual therapy. The latter might include supportive, cognitive behavioral, and insight-oriented approaches.

The National Athletic Trainers' Association position statement created guidelines to assist in the prevention, diagnosis, and treatment of eating disorders in athletes [33].

FUTURE RESEARCH

Additional epidemiologic studies focusing on specific sports are needed, so that we may get a sense of the scope of the problem. More data to quantify the etiologic factors unique to eating disorders in athletes will be useful in prevention. Illuminating the prevalence of eating disorders among male athletes will help to bring attention to this problem. Ideally, these data will serve to reduce the stigma, and ultimately help those athletes struggling with disordered eating to get the treatment they require.

REFERENCES

1. Bulik CM (2005) Exploring the gene-environment nexus in eating disorders. *Journal of Psychiatry & Neuroscience* 30(5), 335–339.
2. Plaisted V (1994) Gender and sport. In: Morris T, Summers J (eds.) *Sport Psychology: Theory, Applications and Issues*. John Wiley & Sons, Inc., New York.
3. Currie A, Phil M, Morse ED (2005) Eating disorders in athletes: managing the risks. In: Tofler IR, Morse ED (eds.) *Clinics in Sports Medicine: The Interface Between Sports Psychiatry and Sports Medicine*. Saunders, Philadelphia. *Clinics in Sports Medicine* 24(4), 871–884.
4. Baum AL (2006) Eating disorders in the male athlete. *Sports Medicine* 36(1), 1–6.
5. Cooper M (2003) *The Psychology of Bulimia Nervosa: A Cognitive Perspective*. Oxford University Press, Oxford, pp. 122–123.
6. Sundgot-Borgen J, Torstveit MK (2004) Prevalence of eating disorders in elite athletes is higher than in the general population. *Clinical Journal of Sport Medicine* 14(1), 25–32.
7. Thomas JJ, Vartanian LR, Brownell KD (2009) The relationship between eating disorder not otherwise specified (EDNOS) and officially recognized eating disorders: meta-analysis and implications for DSM. *Psychological Bulletin* 135(3), 407–433.
8. Schaal K, Tafflet M, Nassif H *et al.* (2011) Psychological balance in high level athletes: gender-based differences and sport-specific patterns. *PLoS One* 6(5), e19007.
9. Hargreaves J (1984) Women and the Olympic phenomenon. In: Tomlinson A, Whannel G (eds.) *Five-Ring Circus: Money, Power and Politics in the Olympic Games*. Pluto Press, London, p. 68.
10. Guilherme GA, Franchini E, Nicastro H *et al.* (2010) The need of a weight management control program in judo: a proposal based on the successful case of wrestling. *Journal of International Society of Sports Nutrition* 7, 15.
11. Sansone RA, Sawyer R (2005) Weight loss pressure on a 5 year old wrestler. *British Journal of Sports Medicine* 39, e2.
12. Dummer GM, Rosen LW, Heusner WW *et al.* (1987) Pathogenic weight-control behaviors of young competitive swimmers. *The Physician and Sports Medicine* 15, 75–84.
13. Benson R (1991) Weight control among elite women swimmers. In: Black DR (ed.) *Eating Disorders among Athletes*. American Alliance of Health, Physical Education, Recreation and Dance, Reston.
14. Griffin J, Harris MB (1996) Coaches' attitudes, knowledge, experiences and recommendations regarding weight control. *Sports Psychology* 10, 180–194.
15. Baum AL (1988) Young females in the athletic arena. *Child and Adolescent Clinics of North America* 7(4), 745–755.

16. Ryan J (ed.) (2000) They stole her soul and they still have it: eating disorders. In: *Little Girls in Pretty Boxes*. Warner Books, New York, pp. 4, 93.

17. Rosen LW, Hough DO (1988) Pathogenic weight control behaviors of female college gymnasts. *Physician Sportsmedicine* 16, 140–144.

18. Rosen LW, McKeag DB, Hough DO *et al.* (1986) Pathogenic weight control behavior in female athletes. *Physician Sportsmedicine* 14, 79–86.

19. Sundgot-Borgen J (1996) Eating disorders, energy intake, training volume, and menstrual function in high-level modern rhythmic gymnasts. *International Journal of Sport Nutrition* 6, 100–109.

20. Garner DM, Garfinkel PE, Rockert W *et al.* (1987) A prospective study of eating disturbances in the ballet. *Psychotherapy and Psychosomatics* 48, 170–175.

21. Hamilton LH, Brooks-Gunn J, Warren MP (1985) Sociocultural influences on eating disorders in professional female ballet dancers. *International Journal of Eating Disorders* 4, 465–477.

22. Woodside DB, Garfinkel PE, Line E *et al.* (2001) Comparisons of men with full or partial eating disorders, men without eating disorders, and women with eating disorders in the community. *American Journal of Psychiatry* 158, 570–574.

23. Pope HG Jr., Gruber AJ, Choi P *et al.* (1997) Muscle dysmorphia: an underrecognized form of body dysmorphic disorder. *Psychosomatics* 38, 548–557.

24. Hoch AX, Pajewski NM, Moraski L *et al.* (2009) Prevalence of the female athlete triad in high school athletes and sedentary students. *Clinical Journal of Sport Medicine* 19(5), 421–428.

25. Loucks AB (2007) Refutation of "the myth of the female athlete triad." *British Journal of Sports Medicine* 41(1), 55–57.

26. Hubert P, King NA, Blundell JE (1998) Uncoupling of the effects of energy expenditure and energy intake: appetite response to short-term energy deficit induced by meal omission and physical activity. *Appetite* 19, 309–319.

27. Truswell AS (2001) Energy balance, food and exercise. *World Review of Nutrition & Dietetics* 25, 9013–9025.

28. Birch K (2005) Female athlete triad. *British Medical Journal* 330(7485), 244–246.

29. Torstveit M, Sundgot-Borgen J, Wark J (2005) Low bone mineral density is two to three times more prevalent in non-athletic premenopausal women than in elite athletes: a comprehensive controlled study. *British Journal of Sports Medicine* 39(5), 282–287.

30. Vaughan JL, King KA, Cottrell RR (2004) Collegiate athletic trainers' confidence in helping female athletes with eating disorders. *Journal of Athletic Training* 39(1), 71–76.

31. Black DR, Larkin LJS, Coster DC *et al.* (2003) Physiologic screening test for eating disorders/disordered eating among female collegiate athletes. *Journal of Athletic Training* 16(4), 286–297.

32. Baum AL (1998) Sports psychiatry: an outpatient consultation-liaison model. *Psychosomatics* 39(4), 395–396.

33. Bonci CM, Bonci LJ, Granger LR *et al.* (2008) National Athletic Trainers' Association position statement: preventing, detecting, and managing disordered eating in athletes. *Journal of Athletic Training* 43(1), 80–108.

6 Personality and Personality Disorders in Athletes

Heba M. Fakher M. Hendawy[1] and
Ezzat Abdelazeem A. Awad[2]

[1] Department of Neuropsychiatry, Faculty of Medicine, Institute of Psychiatry, Ain Shams University, Egypt
[2] NTNU Norway, Hail, Kingdom of Saudi Arabia

KEY POINTS

- The most common personality traits in athletes are extraversion, perfectionism, and narcissism.
- Personality traits have been found to have an association with athletes' performance.
- Athletic identity is the degree to which an individual views himself within the athlete role and looks to others for confirmation of that role.
- Personality disorders in athletes follow the usual classification in the Diagnostic and Statistical Manual of Mental Disorders (DSM), with the presence of personality disorders potentially affecting athletic performance.

INTRODUCTION

Personality is one of the most attractive fields of study in psychology, with many definitions and theories developed in an attempt to explain its different aspects. For instance, Allport defined personality as "the dynamic organization of the individual's psychophysical systems that determine unique adjustments to his environment" [1]. Personality can be comprehensively defined as the unique total characteristics of an individual that colors his or her behavior [2, 3], thoughts, and emotions most of the time and in most situations. Personality is characterized by being stable, consistent, and coherent in a way that influences our thinking, emotions, and behaviors. These characteristics are integrated in a unique fashion that differentiates individuals and shapes the identity of the person [2]. For example, extroverts are characterized by having positive emotions such as happiness, liveliness, optimism, and high levels of energy and activity [3], whereas neuroticism predicts negative emotions like fear, worry, hastiness, anger, and guilt feeling [3, 4].

Clinical Sports Psychiatry: An International Perspective, First Edition. Edited by David A. Baron, Claudia L. Reardon and Steven H. Baron.
© 2013 John Wiley & Sons, Ltd. Published 2013 by John Wiley & Sons, Ltd.

PERSONALITY TRAITS IN ATHLETES

In the field of sports psychology, research has been conducted to determine the difference between personality traits among athletes and nonathletes, and even between different types of sports. In other words, psychologists have tried to answer the question: is there any connection between sports and personality? [5]. However, these efforts have not yielded conclusive results on personality profiles that distinguish athletes from nonathletes. Thus, what distinguishes athletes from nonathletes is not a single profile [1].

Some authors have concluded that research has not proven that athletes possess unique personality characteristics [1, 6], while other studies have yielded results that support the presence of characteristics of competitive athletes that discriminate them from nonathletes [1]. It is worth mentioning that even the studies refuting the athletic personality showed discrepancy between athletes and nonathletes and even among athletes themselves in categorizing athletes by different sports types [6]. It was found that athletes show more positive personality characteristics than nonathletes [5, 7], with better effect on their mental health [7]. With regards to the five-factor personality model characteristics (neuroticism, extraversion, openness to experience, agreeableness, and conscientiousness), athletes show higher scores for extraversion and conscientiousness and less neuroticism, yet they do not show differences in openness to experience and agreeableness [5]. The five-factor model was used to study the interpersonal relations between athletes and their coaches. In an actor–partner interdependence model, Jackson and others [8] found that divergence between partners regarding extraversion and openness was negatively associated with commitment and relatedness for coaches and athletes. Favorable interpersonal relationships were detected when partners had high conscientious and/or agreeable factors. High-risk sport athletes were examined regarding the big five trait model and were found to have higher scores on conscientiousness, energy (extraversion), and emotional stability (less neuroticism) than the nonathletes and to a lesser degree than the nonrisk sport athletes. The nonrisk sport athletes scored highest for openness [9].

McKelvie and his group [10] compared athletes and nonathletes using the Eysenck model and found that athletes have less neuroticism. On the other hand, extraversion did not vary significantly between athletes and nonathletes in general or between contact and noncontact athletes, but extraversion was higher for athletes compared to American college norms. As extraversion and neuroticism were enduring and persistent during the 4-year study, they concluded that people higher in extraversion and lower in neuroticism are attracted to university sports. Contact sport athletes show higher scores on sensation seeking than noncontact sport athletes [11].

Research shows that professional athletes have higher self-esteem, sensation seeking, and mental health than do amateur athletes, who rank higher in those realms than do nonathletes. These characteristics were shown to be negatively correlated with anxiety and depression levels, social anxiety disorder, and presence of physical symptoms [7]. According to Zuckerman, "sensation seeking is defined as the need for complicated, new, and different feelings and the tendency for accepting physical and social perils for these experiences" [12]. Rosenberg *et al.* [13] defined self-esteem as "the individual's positive or negative attitude towards the self as a totality." Another study has shown that athletes score higher on sensation seeking than nonathletes, with males having higher scores than females [11].

When comparing populations of athletes and nonathletes based on self-satisfaction, social orientation, labor effort, inhibition, irritability, aggressiveness, fatigability, physical complaints, health concerns, frankness, extroversion, and emotionality, research has shown that athletes demonstrated significantly higher levels of inhibition, irritability, aggressiveness, fatigability, physical complaints, frankness, and emotionality and lower only in health concerns than non-athletes. The same differences were found in male and female subgroups of athletes and nonathletes. Also, team sports and individual sports participants were compared, showing again significant differences in the same variables together with self-satisfaction and social orientation. Specifically, the individual sport athletes had higher levels of inhibition, irritability, aggressiveness, fatigability, physical complaints, frankness, and emotionality and lower levels of self-satisfaction, social orientation, and health concerns [1].

When comparing athletes' personality characteristics in individual and team sports, Nia and Besharat [3] also concluded that athletes' personality characteristics are different for individual and team sports. Their results showed that individual sport athletes scored significantly higher on conscientiousness and autonomy (combination of beliefs, behavioral tendencies, and attitudes that lead people to focus on their own uniqueness, physical functioning, and control over their environment) than did team sport athletes. In contrast, the team sport athletes scored significantly higher on agreeableness and sociotropy (combination of beliefs, behavioral tendencies, and attitudes that lead a person to attend to and depend on others for personal satisfaction) than did the individual sport athletes. No significant differences were found between the two groups with regards to neuroticism, extraversion, and openness.

Athletic satisfaction represents "a positive affective state resulting from a complex evaluation of the structures, processes, and outcomes associated with the athletic experience" [14]. It is related to higher levels of commitment, lower intentions of quitting, increased job performance, and more organizational citizenship behaviors. Athletic satisfaction also appears to play a role with regard to player motivation, social-loafing, and athlete-related turnover. Satisfied athletes experience fewer emotional problems and increased well-being [14].

Another characteristic that has recently attracted research is "mental toughness." Mental toughness is one of the most widely used and least understood terms within the literature on athlete personalities. It has been defined as the ability of a person to cope with the demands of training and competition with increased determination, focus, confidence, and maintenance of control under pressure [15]. Clough *et al.* [16] developed a model and measurement scale for mental toughness that consisted of four main domains: (i) control (emotional and life), a tendency to feel and act as if one is influential, (ii) commitment, a tendency to involve oneself in rather than experience alienation from an activity, (iii) challenge, belief that life is changeable and to view this as an opportunity rather than a threat, and (iv) confidence (interpersonal and in abilities), a high sense of self-belief and unshakable faith concerning one's ability to achieve success. Mental toughness is correlated with better coping and more optimism. Higher levels of mental toughness are associated with more "approach"-coping strategies (mental imagery, effort expenditure, thought control, and logical analysis) and less use of avoidance coping strategies (distancing, mental distraction, and resignation) [17]. Coaches working with mentally tough athletes are advised to consider emphasizing training and instructive leadership behaviors that are targeted to improve performance rather than emphasizing social support, democratic behaviors, autocratic behaviors, or positive feedback leadership styles [18].

Another related characteristic is "hardiness." Hardiness is the ability of people to cope with stressors. It is believed to buffer major life stressors and is assumed to decrease the likelihood of stress-related physical illnesses, mental illnesses, and decrements in performance, conduct, and morale [19]. It associates positively with sport achievement and psychological well-being [20].

PERFECTIONISM

Perfectionism has been one of the most frequently studied traits in athletes in the past decades, yet it is still one of the most controversial topics, especially when it comes to its relation to sports [21, 22]. Some consider it a trait that helps to excel and improve performance [23], while others see it as an obstacle that consumes athletes' efforts, overloads them, and hinders their progress, as it can lead to anxiety and burnout [22, 24].

Perfectionism can be defined as an achievement-related personality trait that includes setting and compulsive pursuit of excessively high standards of performance in conjunction with a tendency to make harsh, overly critical self-evaluations [24, 25]. Perfectionism is hypothesized to be either (i) normal, healthy perfectionism that can be adaptive, or (ii) unhealthy neurotic perfectionism, which is maladaptive [26, 27]. Positive (normal) perfectionism can be defined as the motivation to achieve a certain goal in order to obtain a favorable outcome. Negative (neurotic) perfectionism can be defined as the motivation to achieve a certain goal in order to avoid adverse consequences [26]. Positive perfectionism is negatively associated with cognitive and somatic anxiety and positively associated with self-confidence [21], but it also can predict disturbed eating attitudes in male athletes [28]. Negative reaction to imperfection (negative perfectionism) is positively associated with cognitive and somatic anxiety [21, 29] and social physique anxiety together with disturbed eating attitudes in female athletes [28], and negatively associated with self-confidence [21, 29]. Self-esteem as well can influence the pattern of perfectionism in athletes; athletes with high self-esteem that is "internally based" more often exhibit positive patterns of perfectionism, whereas those whose self-esteem derives from external factors show more negative perfectionism [29]. Some researchers differentiate between striving for perfection and negative reaction to imperfection as traits [30]. In their study, Stoeber and his colleagues [30] found that negative reactions to imperfection were associated with anxiety while striving for perfection was related to higher self-confidence and less anxiety during competitions. Apparently both positive and negative aspects of perfectionism contributed to the development of eating disorders in athletes. The converse held true as well: eating disorders themselves could modify the direction and amplitude of perfectionist thinking. Furthermore, the challenging environment that focuses on physique and weight in athletic life adds complexity to the pathway of interaction between perfectionism and eating disorders [31].

Several dimensional approaches have been introduced by researchers to help in studying perfectionism. Flett and Hewitt defined three dimensions: self-oriented perfectionism (directed to oneself), other-oriented perfectionism (demanding perfection from others), and socially prescribed perfectionism (others require perfection from the individual) [22]. Both self-oriented and socially prescribed forms of perfectionism have the potential to render young athletes vulnerable to the development of the "burnout syndrome." Both dimensions of perfectionism have been negatively related to unconditional self-acceptance, which is associated with a reduced sense of accomplishment and the emotional and physical exhaustion dimensions of burnout [24]. Another study showed that socially prescribed perfectionism demonstrated a significant positive association, while self-oriented perfectionism a significant negative association, with burnout dimensions [32].

Parents and coaches can play a significant role, either directly or indirectly, in the development of athlete perfectionism. Perfectionism can be acquired by social learning and social expectation [23, 24, 26, 33]. Athletes' perfectionism has been predicted by parents' perfectionism. Athletes' perceptions of their parents' perfectionism, but not parents' self-reported perfectionism, emerged as a significant predictor of athletes' own perfectionism [33].

The source of perfectionism could determine the affective reaction in the athlete. Externally originating perfectionism, that is, that which is encouraged or reinforced by a parent, coach, teammate, or significant other, is associated with a variety of negative mood states including total mood disturbance, sadness, depression, fatigue, tension, anxiety, anger, and hostility. When perfectionism is driven internally, however, no association with negative mood states is seen [34].

ANGER AND AGGRESSION

Anger has been described as a negative feeling associated with specific cognitive and perceptual distortions and deficiencies [35]. Trait anger is defined as the tendency for some individuals to feel anger more intensely, more often, and for a longer period of time than others [36]. Anger could be constructive (assertive) or destructive (aggressive) [37]. A three-factor model of trait anger consisting of angry emotions, aggressive behaviors, and cynical cognition has been used to research the relation between anger and other personality traits. It was found that angry emotions were most strongly related to neuroticism, while aggressive behaviors were associated with low agreeableness, and cynical cognition associated with both neurotic and disagreeable characteristics [38]. It is worth mentioning that anger is usually goal directed to correct a provoking situation [37]. Aggression is behavior intended to inflect harm deliberately to another individual who is motivated to avoid being harmed [37]. In one meta-analytic study [37], trait aggressiveness and trait irritability were found to influence both provoked and unprovoked aggressive behavior, while other personality variables, for example, trait anger, influenced aggressive behavior only under provoking conditions. Moreover, they also found that neuroticism may be more likely to be positively associated with aggressive behavior only in response to provocation.

ATHLETIC IDENTITY

Identity was proposed by Erikson [39] as the organizational process that determines how individuals act and behave in the social world surrounding them. In different situations, individuals use the suitable identity for given circumstances [40]. Athletic identity can be defined as the degree to which an individual views himself within the athlete role and looks to others for confirmation of that role [41]. Although athletic identity can be conceptualized differently by individuals, it generally relates to one's view of self in relation to physical activity and involvement in sport [42].

Athletic identity includes three main factors: social identity, exclusivity, and negative affectivity [41, 43]. Social identity focuses on the extent to which the athlete views herself as occupying the athlete role in others' eyes. Exclusivity is the degree to which an athlete evaluates herself exclusively according to her implementation of the athlete role. Negative affectivity is the extent to which individuals worry about poor performance or not being able to fulfill their athletic role and how they generalize that negative affect to overall self-evaluation [40, 42]. Athletic social identity and negative affectivity were positively related to athlete satisfaction while the exclusivity facet of athletic identity was negatively related to athlete satisfaction [40].

Some athletes have strong athletic identities that dominate their behavior and conceal other important facets of their lives [41]. Hughes and Coakley [44] identified "sport ethic" and viewed it as the code accentuating values of dedication to the game, uniqueness, taking risks, and challenging limits. They described abuse of sport ethic as the situation that occurs when this ethic becomes the only guide for behavior for a given athlete. The importance of abuse of sport ethic was argued against by Horton and Mack [45], who found no evidence that athletes with high athletic identity were neglecting other aspects of life in order to fulfill the role of an athlete. Strength of athletic identity has been correlated with higher physical activity as measured by two variables: stage of exercise behavior and exercise frequency per week [46]. Additionally, relative to low athletic identity, high athletic identity was associated with better athletic performance, more commitment to sport, expanded social network, and relatively more frequent experience of both positive and negative effects of training [45].

In contrast, several studies have found that strong athletic identity does include some drawbacks. Overinvolvement in one's athletic role can lead to two types of hazards: (i) deviance in the athletic role itself resulting in several psychiatric hazards to the athletes [45]; this includes overtraining, anxiety on absence of training, and use of performance-enhancing drugs [44, 47]; and (ii) restriction in the development of a multidimensional self-concept [45]. Strong exclusive athletic identity has been linked to vulnerability to depression. It has been suggested that self-concept complexity can protect against depression, perceived stress, and physical symptoms when facing life stressors or major changes that affect one of the identity dimensions, as in retirement or severe injury [48]. A strong athletic identity may lead to poor lifelong development of various identity alternatives, role flexibility, and proper socialization. Such a strong athletic identity may lead to lack of effective adjustment and emotional vulnerability upon athletic career termination [42, 49]. Moreover, identity limitations and strong athletic identity have been inversely related to career maturity, suggesting that failure to explore alternative roles and identifying strongly and exclusively with the athlete role are associated with delayed career development in athletes [50]. This has also been associated with poor physical and emotional health, social isolation [41], and less interest in academic achievement [42]. It is worthwhile to clarify that although there are recognized potential negative aspects of athletic identity, it is not necessarily related to dysfunctional commitment [45].

PERSONALITY DISORDERS IN ATHLETES

Although there are plenty of psychological studies on personality traits in athletes, the psychiatric literature on personality disorders in athletes based on the DSM-IV is very scarce. However, personality disorders in athletes follow the same regular classification in DSM-IV (Table 6.1).

Table 6.1 Classification of personality disorders according to DSM-IV.

Cluster A personality disorders	Cluster B personality disorders	Cluster C personality disorders
The odd and eccentric cluster:	Dramatic, emotional, erratic:	Anxious cluster:
Paranoid	Histrionic	Avoidant
Schizoid	Narcissistic	Dependent
Schizotypal	Antisocial	Obsessive compulsive
	Borderline	

Table 6.2 Frequencies and percentages of personality disorders "threshold" and subthreshold traits detected in a sample of actively competing Egyptian athletes via use of the SCID II interview instrument [51].

Personality disorder/measure		Number of athletes	Percentage of athletes surveyed
SCID II	No personality disorder	46	45.5
	Single personality disorder	42	41.6
	>One personality disorder	13	12.9
Avoidant	No	96	95.0
	Threshold	5	5.0
Dependent	No	98	97.0
	Subthreshold	2	2.0
	Threshold	1	1.0
Obsessive	No	61	60.4
	Subthreshold	24	23.8
	Threshold	16	15.8
Passive aggressive	No	96	95.0
	Subthreshold	1	1.0
	Threshold	4	4.0
Depressive	No	88	87.1
	Subthreshold	10	9.9
	Threshold	3	3.0
Paranoid	No	81	80.2
	Subthreshold	14	13.9
	Threshold	6	5.9
Schizotypal	No	100	99.0
	Subthreshold	1	1.0
Schizoid	No	97	96.0
	Subthreshold	2	2.0
	Threshold	2	2.0
Histrionic	No	100	99.0
	Subthreshold	1	1.0
Narcissistic	No	77	76.2
	Subthreshold	17	16.8
	Threshold	7	6.9
Borderline	No	76	75.2
	Subthreshold	9	8.9
	Threshold	16	15.8
Antisocial	No	95	94.1
	Subthreshold	5	5.0
	Threshold	1	1.0
Mixed personality disorder	No	94	93.1
	Threshold	7	6.9

A recent study on Egyptian athletes was done by Heba Hendawy, with the rates of different personality disorders in actively competing Egyptian athletes as given in Table 6.2 [52]. This study was conducted on 101 athletes recruited from several sports including team and individual sports (basketball, volleyball, handball, badminton, tennis, judo, karate, running, and throwing). The participants were interviewed using Structured Clinical Interview for DSM-IV Axis II (SCID II) to diagnose personality disorders. The results showed that many Egyptian athletes have at least one personality disorder. The most common personality disorders detected were obsessive compulsive, borderline, narcissistic, and mixed. Sport might attract such people for a variety of reasons, including that it can satisfy a desire for being at the center of attention, increase self-esteem, or provide a venue for obsessive compulsive behavior.

CASE STUDIES

Case reports of athletes with personality disorders or problematic or pathological traits can be found, but larger trials have not been conducted. The following cases are presented as examples of mixed personality disorders in professional athletes, and of how their personality affected their performances and hindered their careers.

Case Study 1

Mr. I is a 31-year-old professional soccer player who was advised to consult a psychiatrist after a marked career drift. He started his professional career at the age of 18 as a member of an Egyptian championship team. He had a sparkling start with his team, became one of the most popular stars in a couple of years, and was called for the national team. The player changed his appearance for each match, with frequent changes in his hair cut and color. He was uncooperative with his team partners and sometimes got into quarrels with his coaches. He tried to attract the attention of media and the fans with his behavior on the soccer field, for example, by harassing the other team, engaging in arguments with the referees, and provoking the crowds during the matches. Later, the verbal aggression turned to physical aggression against other teams' players. This was associated with decreased concentration and performance in games. Off the field, he was known for his deviant manners, as he drank alcohol against his coaches' instructions and was easily provoked with uncontrollable bursts of anger. Mr. I has also beaten his wife and cheated on her frequently. He was suspended several times for his behavior. Despite his repeated apologies and frequent requests for forgiveness, he continued to make the same mistakes. Ultimately his team had to terminate his contract. He would go on to join five other first-class teams with no improvement in his behavior. He became known as a troublemaker and had to play for less-ranked clubs for the duration of his career.

Comment: In this case, we can detect the enduring nature of the athlete's personality characteristics as the cause of his occupational and social dysfunction. The condition was diagnosed as mixed personality disorder with symptoms of cluster B disorders, namely, borderline, histrionic, and antisocial. Mr. I never sought psychiatric help during his career, and his personality traits were attributed to the effect of rapid fame and wealth from a young age. This case illustrates the apparent resistance to involving psychiatrists in sports (since no psychiatrists were involved in his care), and how that resistance can end the professional athletic life of the most talented athletes.

Case Study 2

Mr. K is a 28-year-old professional wrestler and an Olympic gold medal winner. He was advised to consult a psychiatrist after a striking decline in his career. His trainer told the psychiatrist that he exhibited inflated self-confidence and exaggerated self-importance. He had always seemed quite self-assured, but that tendency appears to have increased lately. He reported that Mr. K had been missing a lot of his recent training, and, when there, had not been training well. Additionally, Mr. K had been losing several matches against modest or nonprofessional players. At the psychiatrist's clinic, Mr. K reported feeling that other players were jealous of him. He also admitted that he felt irritable and angry in reaction to criticism, and he even had attacked a journalist who described him as a showy player with a big reputation but bad results. He admitted that he was not training much lately as he thought he had the ability to win any game without training, since he was the world champion. He disclosed that he felt the media should focus on him as he was the world champion and Olympic Games gold medalist. Recently, Mr. K was suspended from play after he engaged in a violent attack against a waiter in a restaurant who treated him as an ordinary guest in the restaurant.

Comment: In this case we can find the characteristics of narcissistic personality disorder in the form of a grandiose sense of self-importance, preoccupation with fantasies of power and success, the feeling of being an excessively special person, requirement for excessive admiration, and aggression, especially against criticism. However, the history should differentiate if this case is a genuine narcissistic personality disorder, personality changes after exposure to media or an acute manic episode.

Case Study 3

Miss S is a 19-year-old professional basketball player who was admitted to the psychiatric hospital after acute agitation and violence against one of her teammates, whom she attacked with a knife. The trainer said that Miss S is a known troublemaker but is also quite talented. Her trainer mentioned that he has been her coach since she was 14 years old and attested that Miss S has always tended to start fights. She never obeys orders and is frequently impulsive. He also explained that she has similar difficulties in school. The police officer told the psychiatrist that Miss S was convicted 3 years ago of stealing sport clothes, shoes, and money from her classmates and teammates. He also mentioned that her father is an alcoholic and often hits her or otherwise punishes her with or without a reason. Her brother is 9 years old and was recently diagnosed with conduct disorder.

Comment: In this case study, we can identify the enduring nature of the athlete's personality characteristics as the cause of her occupational and social dysfunction. The condition was diagnosed as antisocial disorder with symptoms of other cluster B personality disorders. Miss S never sought psychiatric help during her career (other than the hospitalization described earlier), despite many recommendations from her trainer to visit a psychiatrist to address her abnormal and violent behavior. In this case, we can find the characteristic criteria for antisocial personality in the form of manifestation before the age of 15 years, irritability, aggression, and failure to respect norms in society. Moreover, Miss S has a family history of familial punishment and a brother with conduct disorder, which are common associations with antisocial personality disorder. We can see how her career was affected by the personality disorder, as she was suspended and even admitted to a psychiatric hospital because of her abnormal actions.

SUMMARY

Personality can be comprehensively defined as the unique total characteristics of an individual that colors her behavior. Extraversion, perfectionism, and narcissistic personality traits have been found to be the most common personality traits in athletes. Moreover, personality traits have been found to correlate with athletes' performance. Researchers have shown that professional athletes have higher self-esteem, sensation seeking, and mental health than do amateur athletes. Athletic identity is the degree to which an individual views himself within the athlete role and looks to others for confirmation of that role. Athletic identity includes three main factors: social identity, exclusivity, and negative affectivity. Personality disorders in athletes follow the usual classification in DSM-IV and may impact many athletes' careers in sport.

REFERENCES

1. Filho MGB, Ribeiro LCS, García FG. Comparison of personality characteristics between high-level Brazilian athletes and non-athletes. *Revista Brasileira de Medicina do Esporte* (2005);11(2):114–118.
2. Smith ER. Advances in cognitive-social personality theory: applications to sport psychology. *Revista de Psicología Del Deporte* (2008);17(2):253–276.
3. Nia ME, Besharat MA. Comparison of athletes' personality characteristics in individual and team sports. *Procedia – Social and Behavioral Sciences* (2010);5:808–812.
4. Robinson MD, Ode S, Moeller SK, Goetz PW. Neuroticism and affective priming: evidence for a neuroticism linked negative schema. *Personality and Individual Differences* (2007);42(7):1221–1231.
5. Shariati M, Bakhtiari S. Comparison of personality characteristics athlete and non-athlete student, Islamic Azad University of Ahvaz. *Procedia – Social and Behavioral Sciences* (2011);30:2312–2315.
6. Weinberg RS, Gould D. Personality and sport. In: Weinberg RS, Gould D (eds.), *Foundation of Sport and Exercise Psychology*, 5th edn. Champaign: Human Kinetics (2011), pp. 27–50. http://www. amazon.co.uk/Foundations-Exercise-Psychology-Robert-Weinberg/dp/0736064672. Accessed on 18 January 2013.
7. Samadzadeh M, Abbasi M, Shahbazzadegan B. Comparison of sensation seeking and self-esteem with mental health in professional and amateur athletes, and non-athletes. *Procedia – Social and Behavioral Sciences* (2011);15:1942–1950.
8. Jackson B, Dimmock J, Gucciardi D, Grove JR. Personality traits and relationship perceptions in coach athlete dyads: do opposites really attract? *Psychology of Sport and Exercise* (2011);12:222–230.
9. Kajtna T, Tusak M, Baric R, Burnik S. Personality in high risk sports athletes. *Kinesiology* (2004);36(1):24–34.
10. McKelvie SJ, Lemieux P, Stout D. Extraversion and neuroticism in contact athletes, no contact athletes and non-athletes: a research note. *Athletic Insight – The Online Journal of Sport Psychology* (2003);5(3):19–27.
11. Schroth ML. A comparison of sensation seeking among different groups of athletes and nonathletes. *Personality and Individual Differences* (1995);18(2):219–222.
12. Zuckerman M. Sensation seeking: a comparative approach to a human trait. *Behavioral and Brain Sciences* (1984);7(3):413–434.
13. Rosenberg M, Schooler C, Schoenbach C, Rosenberg F. Global self-esteem and specific self-esteem: different concepts, different outcomes. *American Sociological Review* (1995);60(1):141–156.
14. Chelladurai P, Riemer HA. A classification of the facets of athlete satisfaction. *Journal of Sport Management* (1997);11:133–159.
15. Jones G, Hanton S, Connaughton D. What is this thing called mental toughness? An investigation of elite performers. *Journal of Applied Sport Psychology* (2002);14:205–218.
16. Clough P, Earle K, Sewell D. Mental toughness: the concept and its measurement. In: Cockerill I (ed.). *Solutions in Sport Psychology*. London: Thomson (2002), pp. 32–45.
17. Nicholls AR, Polman RCJ, Levy AR, Backhouse SH. Mental toughness, optimism, pessimism, and coping among athletes. *Personality and Individual Differences* (2008);44:1182–1192.

18. Crust L, Azadi K. Leadership preferences of mentally tough athletes. *Personality and Individual Differences* (2009);47:326–330.
19. Golby J, Sheard M. Mental toughness and hardiness at deferent levels of rugby league. *Personality and Individual Differences* (2004);37:933–942.
20. Nezhad MAS, Besharat MA. Relations of resilience and hardiness with sport achievement and mental health in a sample of athletes. *Procedia – Social and Behavioral Sciences* (2010);5:757–763.
21. Hamidia S, Besharat MA. Perfectionism and competitive anxiety in athletes. *Procedia – Social and Behavioral Sciences* (2010);5:813–817.
22. Flett GL, Hewitt PL. The perils of perfectionism in sports and exercise. *Current Directions in Psychological Science* (2005);14(1):14–18.
23. Gould D, Dieffenbach K, Moffett A. Psychological characteristics and their development in Olympic champions. *Journal of Applied Sport Psychology* (2002);14(3):172–204.
24. Hill AP, Hall HK, Appleton PR, Kozub SA. Perfectionism and burnout in junior elite soccer players: the mediating influence of unconditional self-acceptance. *Psychology of Sport and Exercise* (2008);9: 630–644.
25. Frost RO, Marten P, Laharat C, Rosenblate R. The dimensions of perfectionism. *Cognitive Therapy and Research* (1990);14(5):449–468.
26. Soenens B, Elliot J, Goossens L, Vansteenkiste M, Luyten P, Duriez B. The intergenerational transmission of perfectionism: parents' psychological control as an intervening variable. *Journal of Family Psychology* (2005);19(3):358–366.
27. Terry-Short LA, Owens RG, Slade PD, Dewey ME. Positive and negative perfectionism. *Personality and Individual Differences* (1995);18(5):663–668.
28. Haase AM, Prapavessis H, Owens RG. Perfectionism, social physique anxiety and disordered eating: a comparison of male and female elite athletes. *Psychology of Sport and Exercise* (2002);3:209–222.
29. Koivula N, Hassmén P, Fallby J. Self-esteem and perfectionism in elite athletes: effects on competitive anxiety and self-confidence. *Personality and Individual Differences* (2002);32:865–875.
30. Stoeber J, Otto K, Pescheck E, Becker C, Stoll O. Perfectionism and competitive anxiety in athletes: differentiating striving for perfection and negative reactions to imperfection. *Personality and Individual Differences* (2007);42:959–969.
31. Forsberg S, Lock J. The relationship between perfectionism, eating disorders and athletes: a review. *Minerva Pediatrica* (2006);58:525–536.
32. Appleton PR, Hall HK, Hill AP. Relations between multidimensional perfectionism and burnout in junior-elite male athletes. *Psychology of Sport and Exercise* (2009);10:457–465.
33. Appleton PR, Hall HK, Hill AP. Family patterns of perfectionism: an examination of elite junior athletes and their parents. *Psychology of Sport and Exercise* (2010);11:363–371.
34. Stirling AE, Kerr GA. Perfectionism and mood states among recreational and elite athletes. *Athletic Insight – The Online Journal of Sport Psychology* (2006);8(4):13–27.
35. Maxwell JP, Visek AJ. Unsanctioned aggression in Rugby union: relationships among aggressiveness, anger, athletic identity, and professionalization. *Aggressive Behavior* (2009);35:237–243.
36. Deffenbacher JL, Oetting ER, Thwaites GA, Lynch RS, Baker DA, Stark RS, Thacker S, Eiswerth-Cox L. State-trait anger theory and the utility of the Trait Anger Scale. *Journal of Counseling Psychology* (1996);43(2):131–148.
37. Bettencourt BA, Talley A, Benjamin AJ, Valentine J. Personality and aggressive behavior under provoking and neutral conditions: a meta-analytic review. *Psychological Bulletin* (2006);132(5):751–777.
38. Martin R, Watson D, Wan CK. A three-factor model of Trait anger: dimensions of affect, behavior, and cognition. *Journal of Personality and Social Psychology* (2000);68(5):869–897.
39. Erikson EH. *Identity, Youth and Crisis.* New York: W. W. Norton Company (1968).
40. Burns GN, Jasinski D, Dunn SC, Fletcher D. Athlete identity and athlete satisfaction: the nonconformity of exclusivity. *Personality and Individual Differences* (2012);52(3):280–284.
41. Brewer BW, Van Raalte JL, Linder DE. Athletic identity – Hercules muscles or Achilles heel. *International Journal of Sport Psychology* (1993);24(2): 237–254.
42. Groff DG, Zabriskie RB. An exploratory study of athletic identity among elite alpine skiers with physical disabilities: issues of measurement and design. *Journal of Sport Behavior* (2006);29(2):126–141.
43. Hale BD, James B, Stambulova N. Determining the dimensionality of athletic identity: a "Herculean" cross-cultural undertaking. *International Journal of Sport Psychology* (1999);30(1):83–100.
44. Hughes R, Coakley J. Positive deviance among athletes: the implications of over-conformity to the sport ethic. *Sociology of Sport Journal* (1991);8(4):307–325.

45. Horton RS, Mack DE. Athletic identity in Marathon runners: functional focus or dysfunctional commitment? *Journal of Sport Behavior* (2000);23(2):101–110.
46. Anderson CB. Athletic identity and its relation to exercise behavior: scale development and validation. *Journal of Sport and Exercise Psychology* (2004);26(1):39–56.
47. Coen SP, Ogles BM. Psychological characteristics of the obligatory runner: a critical examination of the anorexia analogue hypothesis. *Journal of Sport and Exercise Psychology* (1993);15(3):338–354.
48. Linville PW. Self-complexity as a cognitive buffer against stress-related illness and depression. *Journal of Personality and Social Psychology* (1987);52(4):663–676.
49. Blinde EM, Greendorfer SL. A reconceptualization of the process of leaving the role of competitive athlete. *International Review for the Sociology of Sport* (1985);20(1):287–294.
50. Murphy GM, Petitpas AJ, Brewer BW. Identity foreclosure, athletic identity, and career maturity in intercollegiate athletes. *The Sport Psychologist* (1996);10(3):239–246.
51. Bronisch T. The typology of personality disorders – diagnostic problems and their relevance for suicidal behavior. *The Journal of Crisis Intervention and Suicide Prevention* (1996);17(2):55–58.
52. Hendawy HMF, Baron DA, Sei-Eldawla AE, Fekry M, Hwidi DH. Prevalence of psychiatric disorders and coping processes in a sample of Egyptian competitive athletes. Faculty of Medicine, Ain Shams University (2012); pp. 60–62.

7 Assessing and Treating Depression in Athletes

David A. Baron,[1,2,3] Steven H. Baron,[4]
Joshua Tompkins,[5] and Aslihan Polat[6]

[1] International Relations and Department of Psychiatry, Keck School of Medicine at the University of Southern California, USA
[2] Keck Medical Center at University of Southern California, USA
[3] Global Center for Exercise, Psychiatry, and Sports at USC, Health Sciences Campus, USA
[4] Montgomery County Community College, USA
[5] Keck School of Medicine at the University of Southern California, USA
[6] Department of Psychiatry and Women's Mental Health Unit, Kocaeli University School of Medicine, Turkey

KEY POINTS

- Depression in athletes is a relatively new field of study that is becoming increasingly relevant as professional and scholastic sports become more competitive.
- Athletes with depression may present with signs and symptoms such as increased irritability, poor performance in practice and in competition, lack of enjoyment in competing, overtraining, or drug and alcohol use.
- Few studies have investigated the effects of antidepressants on athletic performance, with varied results.

INTRODUCTION

A significant amount of time and money is spent on the treatment of physical injury and illness in athletes [1]. Sports sections of newspapers all over the world report extensively on the physical health of athletes. Video footage of injuries sustained on the playing field is replayed ad nauseam during the coverage of a game or match. Sideline reporters cover the status of an athlete's injury in minute detail, and every serious fan knows the devastating consequences of a torn rotator cuff or a ruptured anterior cruciate ligament (ACL).

Conversely, it is rare for the emotional state of an athlete to be mentioned. The status of an athlete's depression would appear to be a taboo topic to cover. Glick and Horsfall [1] and Begel [2] offer a number of compelling explanations for this absence, the most prominent being the significant social stigma associated with psychiatric/psychological illness . The ongoing stigma associated with mental illness globally in the general population is even greater in the world of sport. Thus, the diagnosis and treatment of depression in athletes offer a unique challenge for the sports mental health professional.

Clinical Sports Psychiatry: An International Perspective, First Edition. Edited by David A. Baron, Claudia L. Reardon and Steven H. Baron.
© 2013 John Wiley & Sons, Ltd. Published 2013 by John Wiley & Sons, Ltd.

DEFINING DEPRESSION

Depression is a widely used term that describes a person's mood as being reduced from what is perceived as being normal. The word *depression* is used to describe a below-average mood state (i.e., sadness) as well as a psychiatric syndrome. Descriptions of depression can be found in documents dating back to antiquity. In fact, Hippocrates used the term *melancholia*, a word we now use to describe a severe depressed state, and the Roman physician Celsus described melancholia in his work *De re medicina* as depression caused by black bile.

Some 2000 years later, the first edition of the Diagnostic and Statistical Manual of Mental Disorders was created in 1952 and allowed communication between psychiatrists (especially in different countries) to be uniform. After five revisions, the current version is the Diagnostic and Statistical Manual of Mental Disorders (DSM-IV-TR), published in 2000. It describes a major depressive episode as having five or more of the following symptoms present during a 2-week period (and representing a change from previous functioning): (i) depressed mood most of the day, nearly every day; (ii) markedly diminished interest in or pleasure from all, or almost all, activities most of the day, nearly every day; (iii) significant weight loss (when not dieting), weight gain (e.g., a change of more than 5% of total body weight in a month), or decrease or increase in appetite nearly every day; (iv) insomnia or hypersomnia nearly every day; (v) psychomotor agitation or retardation nearly every day; (vi) fatigue or loss of energy nearly every day; (vii) feelings of worthlessness or excessive or inappropriate guilt nearly every day; (viii) diminished ability to think or concentrate nearly every day; and (ix) recurrent thoughts of death, recurrent suicidal ideation without a specific plan, or a suicide attempt or a specific plan for committing suicide.

Under the DSM-IV-TR description of a major depressive episode, the lowered mood varies little from day to day, is unresponsive to circumstances, and may be accompanied by so-called somatic symptoms, such as waking in the morning several hours before the usual time, depression worse in the morning, marked psychomotor retardation, agitation, loss of appetite, weight loss, and loss of libido.

Depending upon the number and severity of the symptoms, a depressive episode may be specified as mild, moderate, or severe. In a mild depressive episode, few, if any, symptoms in excess of those required to make the diagnosis are present, and the patient is distressed by these but will probably be able to continue with most regular activities. Moderate depression is defined by the number and severity of symptoms somewhere between mild and severe. A severe depressive episode occurs when most of the symptoms mentioned earlier are present and several of them are marked and distressing. Suicidal thought and acts are common and a number of somatic symptoms are usually present in a severe depressive episode.

SYMPTOMS AND PRESENTATION

From the few epidemiological studies done to date, it is believed that athletes suffer from psychiatric illness, including depression and other mood disorders, at the same rate as the rest of the population [3]. Common situational triggers of depression in athletes may include overtraining (OT), injury, pain, competitive failure, aging, retirement from sport, and the same psychosocial factors that can cause depression in nonathletes [4].

As useful as the *DSM-IV-TR* is for mental health clinicians, the typical symptoms of depression do not necessarily hold true for special subgroups of individuals such as athletes.

Namely, athletes suffering from depression may not present with the classic symptoms, such as sad mood. Their symptoms may manifest in the form of increased irritability, poor performance in practice and in competition, lack of enjoyment in competing, overtraining, or drug and alcohol use. Weight loss is not uncommon, making depression in athletes easy to confuse with anorexia nervosa. Injured athletes with depression may catastrophize about the premature end of their careers while recently retired athletes may feel a loss of control and a self-perceived inability to function in the working world.

Athletic trainers are instructed to watch for possible signs of a depressed athlete, which include a slumped posture, lack of enthusiasm, being tardy or missing practice, and failing to exhibit a satisfactory level of participation in the practice sessions. Another indication that the athlete is having trouble may be excessive self-criticism or the setting of unrealistically high standards for herself. These are possible indicators of athlete depression of which mental health professionals must be aware.

OT merits special consideration as it can be either a cause of or a symptom of depression [5]. Indeed, it can be difficult to distinguish OT from major depressive disorders. OT and depression have many symptoms in common (fatigue, insomnia, appetite change, weight loss, amotivation, and diminished concentration), but there are important physiological differences: in OT, patients also exhibit rapid heart rate and elevated blood pressure, muscle soreness, and changes in serum hormone levels [6–9]. An even more important distinction lies in the course of the illness upon cessation of training: in OT, mood subsequently tends to improve, whereas in depression the idle athlete's symptoms grow worse.

Risk factors for a depressive episode include being female, over the age of 65, a family history of mood disorders, having a previous diagnosis of depression, and having any chronic or serious medical illness. An especially important risk factor for depression in the athlete is injury. In particular, an injury that precludes the athlete from participating in practice or competition for an extended period of time can be a risk factor. Finally, a person potentially susceptible to a depressive episode would be a marginal athlete who is not living up to his or her own expectations; such situations have been correlated with chronic fatigue and depression in athletes.

Depression impairs the ability of athletes to train and compete. The disorder is often underappreciated by athletes, coaches, and the community. Given the pivotal role of coaches in athletes' lives, it is important for coaches and trainers to be aware of the signs and symptoms of depression in their athletes and encourage them to seek appropriate treatment. The ongoing stigma against mental health disorders is more acute in the world of sports. Around the world, denial by athletes that emotional problems may be present delays diagnosis and treatment of the problem.

DIAGNOSTIC ISSUES

Considering the often atypical presentation of depression in athletes, diagnosis can be difficult. The psychiatrist must be mindful of risk factors such as high-level defeats, injury, performance slumps, and recent or impending retirement. Because the vegetative signs of depression in athletes may present only within the context of their athletic pursuits (i.e., apathy toward practice), depressed athletes are sometimes sent to sports psychologists for performance enhancement while the root cause goes unrecognized.

A key challenge lies in distinguishing (i) adjustment disorder with depressed mood, (ii) major depressive disorder, and (iii) an organic affective disorder stemming from multiple concussions. Thus, consideration of the patient's situation is essential. For example, an organic affective disorder would be likely in an older athlete who is a veteran of contact sports but not in a young athlete or a tennis star. Neuroimaging modalities such as MRI can aid the diagnosis. A player who until recently was performing at his or her optimum level before losing a championship match is likely suffering from adjustment disorder with depressed mood, whereas an athlete exhibiting anhedonia, hopelessness, or helplessness toward his or her sport in the context of a long-standing slump should be suspected of having major depressive disorder.

DIAGNOSTIC TOOLS

No studies have examined the sensitivity or specificity of any psychometric screening instrument for diagnosing depression in athletes. The Beck Depression Inventory is a 21-item self-report questionnaire that covers symptoms such as hopelessness and irritability, guilt or feelings of being punished, fatigue, weight loss, and lack of interest in sex. Other depression screening tools include the Zung Self-Rating Depression Scale, the Wechsler Depression Rating Scale, the Raskin Depression Rating Scale, the Inventory of Depressive Symptomatology, the Patient Health Questionnaire (PHQ-9), and the Quick Inventory of Depressive Symptomatology.

The Baron Depression Screener for Athletes (BDSA) (Box 7.1) is the only depression screening tool designed specifically for use with athletes. It is a 10-question self-report questionnaire that addresses mood, sports-related anhedonia, weight loss, fatigue, self-image, substance abuse, suicidality, and other parameters. Of note, this is a screening and not a diagnostic tool. Thus, there are no cutoff scores that automatically suggest a diagnosis of major depressive disorder. However, an athlete with a score of greater than 5 should be evaluated by a mental health professional.

Box 7.1 Baron depression screener for athletes

Please respond to the following questions utilizing the following scale.

    0 – Never
    1 – Some of the time (over a 2-week period)
    2 – Most of the time (over a 2-week period)

_____ 1. I feel sad even after a good practice session or successful competition
_____ 2. I rarely get pleasure from competing anymore and have lost interest in my sport
_____ 3. I get little or no pleasure from my athletic successes
_____ 4. I am having problems with my appetite and weight
_____ 5. I do not feel rested and refreshed when I wake up
_____ 6. I am having problems maintaining my focus and concentration during training and competition
_____ 7. I feel like a failure as an athlete and person
_____ 8. I cannot stop thinking about being a failure and quitting sports
_____ 9. I am drinking alcohol or taking supplements to improve my mood
_____10. I have thoughts of ending my life

TREATMENT

Athletes with mental health problems tend to avoid seeking professional help because of two factors: (i) social stigma surrounding mental illness and (ii) fear of appearing weak in the eyes of their coaches and teammates [10, 11]. Affected athletes may also fear that their mental problems, if diagnosed by a physician, would necessitate the use of psychotropic medications and that such medications could adversely impact their athletic performance.

Elite athletes – by definition, athletes with Olympic potential – are a small and challenging subset of the athlete-patient population, and their circumstances and mindsets can make them even less willing to accept psychiatric help. They are accustomed to being the center of attention, with fawning entourages of agents, family members, and coaches orbiting around them. Many are wealthy yet often receive goods and services for free, making a psychiatrist's fee a possible barrier to care. An expectation of VIP treatment can be anticipated. Yet, conversely, they have likely been taught by coaches that physical pain is a natural consequence that should be ignored or "worked through," and due to a lack of other coping skills they may express stoicism in the face of emotional distress as well. For these reasons, the treating psychiatrist must engage not only the patient but the entourage members who form the athlete's social support network [12].

The use of psychopharmacologic agents to treat depression in athletes requires careful forethought for two reasons. First, many sports impose strict bans on the use of many substances, both legal and illicit. The World Anti-Doping Agency (WADA) maintains a list of prohibited substances, but the list is not exhaustive – many categories also forbid the use of any substance chemically or effectively similar to those on the list [13]. Moreover, many sports maintain their own lists of banned substances. For example, the International Archery Federation forbids the use of anxiolytics, antidepressants, antipsychotics, and commonly prescribed mood stabilizers. It is the responsibility of the psychiatrist to be intimately familiar with all relevant prohibitions imposed on competitors of the sport in question when considering pharmacotherapy [4].

Second, as mentioned earlier, an athlete's apprehension over any potential adverse impact of antidepressant therapy on performance is a legitimate concern. No large, systematic studies have been performed on the use of any psychotropic medications in athletes [4], but several small-scale studies have examined the effects of some antidepressants on athletic performance. See Chapter 15 for details of those studies.

Thus, given the lack of robust data on the impact of antidepressants on athletic performance and the risk of inadvertently prescribing a banned substance, it is our belief that pharmacotherapy should not be a first-line treatment for athletes with depression. Conventional psychotherapy or cognitive behavior therapy (CBT) should be attempted initially. CBT may be especially effective given the particular mindset generally ascribed to high-performance athletes. Popular culture has long acknowledged the routinized preparation methods and superstitious, almost obsessive belief systems of elite athletes regarding jersey numbers, good-luck charms, and other irrational factors. Many athletes will catastrophize after a major defeat, potentially triggering a self-fulfilling prophecy in the form of additional losses. Such a series of misfortunes can have devastating ramifications for a star player in the professional sports world, where the public's memory of triumphs is fleeting and its patience for failure is equally brief.

Although no studies have examined the use of CBT in athletes with depression, CBT is an effective and well-validated modality for treating depression which has already been used successfully in depressed athletes by several sports psychiatrists and psychologists. Developed by physician Aaron T. Beck in 1952, CBT seeks out a patient's unrealistic negative thoughts about recent personal events, the world in general, and the anticipated future. The therapist's objective is to challenge these exaggerated beliefs with alternative explanations and to show the patient how changing thoughts and behaviors can impact emotions [19].

This approach is well-suited to the athletic realm for several reasons. First, athletes are accustomed to receiving and relying on advice and support from coaches, and the role of the CBT therapist is to listen, teach, and encourage. Second, just as athletes are instructed to train on their own between supervised workouts, CBT patients are often given "homework" by therapists to reinforce the strategies imparted during sessions. Third, CBT typically involves a relatively short course of treatment when compared to other forms of psychotherapy, making it well-suited for depressed athletes seeking rapid results [19]. See Chapter 11 for more information.

Regardless of the therapy used, treating elite athletes requires careful management of all aspects of the psychiatrist–patient relationship due to the expectations and behaviors that are identified in this population. In a recent paper on the psychiatric diagnosis and treatment of athletes, Glick *et al.* [12] embraced a principle of "flexibility with appropriate boundaries" when determining treatment. In a list of recommended "dos" and "don'ts," the authors advise being flexible within reason about the timing of sessions in recognition of an elite athlete's other obligations. Other tips include involving family members in the therapy when appropriate (and insisting on the participation of significant others of athletes with severe mental illness), using discretion when prescribing psychiatric medications, and counseling athletes on the inappropriate nature of sexual relations between athletes and their coaches and hazards of dietary demands made by coaches that may contribute to eating disorders. The authors caution against allowing consistent canceling of sessions by the patient, compromising on the delivery of appropriate treatment out of deference to the athlete's celebrity status, agreeing to see a surrogate instead of the actual patient, giving experimental treatments and banned substances, and continuing psychotherapy with an athlete with evidence of a substance abuse problem without insisting that the patient undergo substance abuse treatment before resuming therapy [12].

Case Study

Ms. A is 23 years old. Because of her top performance in figure skating nationwide, she was offered a scholarship 5 years ago at a well-known School of Physical Education and Sport. Unfortunately, for the last 2 years, she seems overtrained each competition season. She complains of fatigue, even at rest, with a loss of purpose, energy, and competitive drive. Last year, her performance was mediocre by her own standards, and her coach was disappointed in her. She was thought to be suffering from overtraining syndrome and was even out of practice for several weeks prior to an important tournament. This year, she consulted with a mental health professional for performance enhancement. Ms. A explained that she came from a highly educated family, middle-to-upper socioeconomic status, and was supported in pursuing figure skating since childhood. Her mother, she said, was a very lively woman who has always been very supportive of her. However, during winter, she becomes cheerless and inactive. This has never been considered a problem by the family, but, rather, simply a character trait of the mother. Ms. A. then explained that for the last 2 years, she too had felt very tired just before the winter tournaments. She wanted to sleep all the time and experienced lack of energy and motivation. She did not feel physically prepared to compete but had not informed her coach. After a month or so, her energy returned. She suspected that these symptoms had started with an injury 2 years ago, which was actually not very severe but kept her out of practice for several weeks prior to an important tournament. Following her meeting with the psychiatrist, she was diagnosed with seasonal affective disorder, presumably as her mother had. Although she disputed a psychiatric diagnosis initially, with her coach's encouragement, she finally accepted treatment with an antidepressant.

SPECIAL CONSIDERATIONS

Depression in injured athletes

It does not take an injured athlete to understand an injured athlete; it is easy to imagine how a serious injury to an active player could lead to negative emotional states such as depression, anxiety, and anger. Being sidelined by injury may trigger a complex array of responses, including frustration at not contributing to team victories (or failing to prevent team defeats), regret over missed opportunities for individual achievements such as awards and record setting, and anxiety concerning the long-term consequences of the injury (e.g., impaired performance, loss of athletic job prospects, and the possible premature end of one's career). Whereas the psychological response to athletic injury was once viewed as a series of stages similar to those found in the prevalent theories regarding grief and loss, more recent work has focused on the athlete's cognitive appraisal of the injury, which can be affected by personal factors (e.g., age and self-esteem) as well as situational factors (injury severity, injury duration, pain, and social support) [20].

The evidence for increased depression in injured athletes continues to accumulate. A recent study of high school and college athletes with a diagnosed concussion found a substantially higher level of depression from baseline at 2 days, 7 days, and 14 days post concussion. The depressed athletes also displayed impaired neurocognitive function as evidenced by impaired reaction time and visual memory, suggesting a possible usefulness of assessing for depression soon after concussion as a method of screening for neurocognitive dysfunction [21]. Other studies have found evidence of depression in retired professional boxers [22] and football players [23] with a history of concussion.

The type of injury suffered by the athlete can have a marked impact on any subsequent mental health problems. In a study of college athletes from a wide variety of competitive sports, those who had suffered injury to the ACL in one of their knees were found to have a sevenfold increase in depression symptoms over their baseline emotional status, whereas athletes who had experienced a concussion were only three times more likely to be depressed than before their injury. The emotional dysregulation also lasted longer in the ACL injury group than in the concussion group, with the ACL group displaying increased depression 11 days post injury while the concussion group's depression had generally resolved after

1 week. Suspecting that the status of being "benched" by their injuries, with all the associated frustrations, might underlie the depression in the concussion group, the authors investigated and made a surprising discovery: the depression symptoms typically resolved long before the athlete had been cleared to resume play, effectively eliminating the psychological impact of being sidelined as a causative factor of their depression [24].

In cases of depression associated with concussion, what is the neurological mechanism of the emotional dysregulation? Because previous functional imaging studies have identified the prefrontal area of the brain as a possible locus of both major depression and concussive injury, subsequent research has sought to uncover a shared pathophysiology. In a recent study of 56 male college hockey and football players, functional MRI scanning of athletes with concussion as well as depression symptoms revealed reduced activation in the dorsolateral prefrontal cortex and striatum and attenuated deactivation in medial frontal and temporal regions. Athletes with symptoms of depression also showed less reduction in activity in the parahippocampal gyrus and several other areas relative to a control group during the performance of a working memory task. The authors concluded that depressed mood after a concussion could stem from a neural mechanism consistent with a limbic-frontal model of depression [25].

Depression in young athletes

The mentally and physically protective effects of youth sports have been well documented by various studies dating back to the early 1980s [26]. Researchers have concluded that exercise and sports may promote psychological coping mechanisms such as autonomy, self-efficacy, and optimism [27, 28] and can actually buffer stress-related psychopathological problems [29]. Other authors have credited leisure and recreation – among which sports and exercise are the most popular choice by young people – for helping adolescents develop a sense of achievement and mastery [18, 30].

A central question is whether these protective effects are found in youth who participate in competitive sports at an elite level. Concerns about the potentially deleterious effects of intensely competitive youth sports were first raised in the 1970s, with special attention given to issues such as too many competitions and unwarranted emphasis on winning [31]. It is generally understood that competing at an elite level requires a large investment of time and energy, and researchers have noted the mental strain this could place on young athletes, who may face pressure to excel from parents, coaches, and others. In such situations, the athlete may be implicitly or explicitly informed that quitting or reducing participation are not permitted. Earlier studies have demonstrated that some adolescents are unable to cope with these demands successfully [32].

Unfortunately, only one study to date has scrutinized the relationship between high-performance youth sports and depression. A 2011 study [Gerber] of teen Swiss athletes (both Olympic trainees and less elite players) produced several discoveries, among them that stress was indeed associated with depression, but that participation in elite sports was not a source of additional stress. In fact, the Olympic-level competitors reported less stress, better sleep, and decreased depressive and anxious symptoms than their less elite counterparts [33].

Other research on youth athlete depression has focused on the impact of excessive training. OT, as mentioned earlier, is a concept that lacks a consensus definition but has been described as a long-term performance decrease with multifactorial causes that may include excessive physical overload and incomplete recovery. Full-blown OT syndrome is believed to be preceded in many cases by the equally ill-defined nonfunctional overreaching (NFO), which has been associated with a prolonged period (i.e., more than 1 month) of reduced performance, psychological distress, and hormonal disturbances. In one recent study of soccer players and distance runners, most of whom were teenagers, this prolonged reduction of performance coincided with elevated depression and anger scores, as well as a blunted cortisol response. Because the depression was associated with both tension and fatigue, the authors suggested using field performance tests to screen for early signs of OT in young athletes to possibly avert the emotional sequelae [34].

Case Study

Ms. B is a 19-year-old handball player. She moved to a big city from a rural part of her country after winning a scholarship in sports 2 years ago. The team coach was a very rigid man who even forbade players from using mobile phones in order to control their private lives. Ms. B was feeling very lonely and homesick. Having grown up in a small town, she was having adaptation problems with the new culture. She described feeling like an outsider and began to isolate herself from the outer world. As a lonely "big girl" from the countryside, a "negative stigma" was attached to her, she said. Her teammates were questioning her sexual orientation. Feeling helpless, she also started drinking alcohol to overcome sleep problems. She had been an honor student in high school, but in college her academic performance was very poor. She was dragging herself to practice because she had to, but was unable to do much else. Not only was she behaving aggressively toward others, but she was also struggling with suicidal ideas. While competing as a professional athlete, she decided to quit playing. A careful female coach recognized that something was wrong with her. Even for such a careful and thoughtful coach, it was hard to imagine that such a "tough" girl could become severely depressed for no apparent reason. A psychiatrist was consulted. After a diagnosis of severe depression, antidepressant treatment along with psychotherapy aiming to improve her coping skills was started. It was explained to her coach that her physical skills did not make her any less human, and that no human being is immune to depression.

Depression in female athletes

While the benefits of participating in sports outweigh the risks for most women, it is reported that increasing numbers of female athletes are struggling with depression [35]. Depression may affect many parts of an athlete's life, including sport performance. Beyond the biological factors, possible male–female differences in preference for certain types of relationships, a differential investment in reproduction and offspring, as well as social options (or the lack thereof) all contribute to the fact that women are more vulnerable to mood disorders than are men. In addition, there is a great pressure that accompanies elite-level athletics. Female athletes experience even more stressors because of the multiple roles they balance. The morbidity associated with depression in women is also greater. Not only is the lifetime prevalence of depression nearly twice as high among women as it is among men, but a higher rate of depression-associated comorbid conditions is seen. From the age of menarche, many women also suffer from specific mood disorders, including premenstrual dysphoria and depression associated with pregnancy and the postpartum period as well as mood disorders associated with infertility and pregnancy loss [36].

Not every athlete who experiences a difficult event will develop depression, of course, but in susceptible persons, especially when there is a family history of depression, the clinician should be careful. Even though they experience more stress, female athletes often believe that they should be strong enough to cope as independently as their male counterparts and may not want to acknowledge any psychological concerns. Sometimes the family and social network supporting the women interpret depression as an expected response to recent stress.

As a result it is assumed that the depression does not require formal treatment. Individuals without serious stress before the onset of depressive symptoms may have difficulty recognizing the presence of the disorder or may believe it will abate shortly without the need for professional help. In addition, for many female athletes the idea of taking medications is quite undesirable because of possible side effects, potential performance impairment, or concerns about drug testing. Sometimes maladaptive coping behaviors (e.g., self-medication with alcohol) may be found in female athletes who develop subthreshold levels of depression [37, 38].

The failure to recognize depression in female athletes is not only due to the fact that they present less frequently to health-care providers but also that their presentation might be atypical (e.g., with more somatic complaints). Women tend to report reversed vegetative, or atypical, symptoms (e.g., appetite and weight increase) as well as anxiety and somatic symptoms more often than men. Symptom presentation also shows difference by gender, with women endorsing feelings of increased hostility and loss of libido more frequently than men. Seasonal affective disorder is more prevalent in women than in men and is characterized by depressive symptoms, hypersomnia, hyperphagia, and weight gain localized to a particular season, usually the winter months [39, 40].

When approaching a female athlete for psychiatric assessment, gender-specific aspects of the situation should be taken into account. It is important to conduct a careful assessment of the relationship of the patient's symptoms to her menstrual cycle, to inquire about the possibility that she may be pregnant, and to ask about her use of contraception. Contraceptive pills may themselves cause depression. Because they may influence the choice of treatment, the patient's plans regarding pregnancy should also be asked. Previous pregnancy losses or infertility treatments are also important issues. Seasonality of mood symptoms should be explored, because, as mentioned earlier, seasonal affective disorder is more common in women than in men. Women who are preoccupied with their weight should be asked about ritualistic or restrictive eating patterns and bingeing and purging behaviors, including use of laxatives, diuretics, and appetite suppressants. Sexual preference, relationship styles, and level of satisfaction with current relationships should also be inquired. Tendency to take on certain roles in relationships (e.g., caregiver, nurturer, or dependent or helpless roles) should be documented. Because reproduction-related mood symptoms often run in families, a family history regarding premenstrual dysphoric disorder and depression should be obtained [41, 42].

The psychiatrist should also be aware that social roles and pressures may influence a woman's resilience, coping capacity, and vulnerability to psychopathology. Feeling guilty or disloyal about expressing her own needs when they conflict with those of family members, a woman may need some encouragement to discuss strains in her life, such as family or marital conflict, domestic violence, or exhausting caretaking responsibilities. It is important to ask for suicidal ideation and intent. Like men, women are generally uncomfortable with talking about death or suicide [42].

People with mental disorders have been discriminated against and stigmatized worldwide throughout history. Being a woman with mental illness puts somebody under a double burden of discrimination. Stigma surrounding the use of psychiatric services plays a discouraging role in the patient's recovery processes [43]. It is sometimes difficult to convince some coaches that the mental health of their athletes is as critical as their physical well-being. In fact, we must be as quick to confront emotional issues as we would confront a physical athletic injury. Considering the costs and morbidity associated with depression, programs specially designed to screen for depression in female players should be implemented wherever needed. Educational programs incorporating resilient coping strategies observed in many women athletes could be designed to garner more support for those in need of help.

Depression in retired athletes

The sense of loss and helplessness that an elite athlete might feel after the end of his or her career is easy to envision. The premature end of a career due to injury or lack of employment could leave a professional athlete especially vulnerable to feelings of worthlessness due to losses both real (e.g., further playing opportunities, awards, income, physical fitness, and media attention) and perceived (e.g., life purpose, public adoration, and vitality). For these reasons, the subject of depression in retired athletes warrants special attention.

Statistically, it is not known whether retired athletes experience depression at a lower, equivalent, or higher rate than the general public. In a 2007 survey of more than 3000 retired U.S. National Football League (NFL) players, 84.5% of respondents were judged to have no depression or mild depression (using a standard PHQ-9 questionnaire), and 14.7% gave responses consistent with moderate to severe depression. Seven percent of respondents indicated that their depressive symptoms made their work or home life extremely difficult. The relatively young retirement age of NFL players makes comparison to the general population of U.S. retirees problematic, but most studies have indicated that older American retirees experience depression at rates roughly similar to those found in the former NFL players. Former players having moderate to severe depression were much more likely to report trouble sleeping, loss of fitness, and financial difficulties. They were also more likely to cite barriers to seeking help for their depression such as embarrassment, anticipated loss of self-respect, and failure to recognize the severity of the problem [44].

Chronic pain was also reported by many of the NFL retirees, cited as "very common" by 25.2%, "quite common" by 22.7%, and "not common" or "somewhat common" by 52.1%. Previous studies have established the common comorbidity of pain and depression in the general population, and in the NFL survey former players reporting both severe depression and moderate pain had elevated odds ratios for prescription medication use, alcohol intake, and financial difficulties [44]. In a different study, researchers examined the quality of life of former professional football players in the United Kingdom and discovered a strong correlation between anxiety/depression and joint pain caused by osteoarthritis, for which former football players are at increased risk [45]. For patients with both depression and chronic pain, other researchers have looked at combined treatment strategies using both medication and psychotherapy, and the authors of the NFL survey suggested developing educational and clinical outreach programs for new retirees to help them adjust to life after football and the symptoms that so often accompany it [44]. The biological and psychological mechanisms of the connection between pain and depression have been examined in detail by other researchers, and it is believed that chronic pain usually precedes depression, not vice versa.

Other studies of depression in former athletes have turned up dichotomous results. One report showed that former male distance runners were less likely to be depressed than control subjects [46]. Likewise, in a survey of former Finnish Olympians, the athletes reported less depression than control subjects. The authors of the Finnish study then delved into the possible contributing – and protective – factors for depression in former athletes, starting with current activity level. Respondents citing moderate or low physical activity were more likely to be depressed than those engaging in high physical activity. A search for confounding traits and behaviors discovered several curious correlations. For example, retired athletes tended to be more extraverted than controls, and a high level of extraversion was associated with less likelihood of depression. Retired athletes were also more likely than controls to have executive jobs and less likely to work as skilled laborers – a job category associated with a twofold increase in depression prevalence [47]. From these results, it should be clear that no clear-cut association can be drawn between the end of an athletic career and the late onset of depression. Given the numerous confounding variables, future studies should strive to isolate the specific causative factors in an effort to improve the mental health of former athletes.

Case Study

A recently retired professional football (American Soccer) player is referred for evaluation and treatment of increasing dysphoria, decreased appetite, low energy, restless sleep, poor concentration, and increasing irritability. The symptoms began 6 months after retiring. The unplanned retirement resulted from a career-ending knee injury sustained in practice. The patient reports a recurring nightmare in which he drives to a championship match and is unable to get out of his car when he arrives at the stadium. He reports one prior depressive episode 15 years ago after he failed to qualify for the national U-18 team. He has never been treated for depression, but admitted to excessive alcohol use during his initial depression. He reports three prior sports-related concussions and a possible family history of depression and alcohol dependence in an uncle.

The psychiatrist determined that the symptoms of depression in this patient are likely the result of a number of factors. The adjustment to life after sports, the effect of multiple sports-related concussions, and genetic loading are all relevant factors to consider. The patient was closely monitored for suicidal ideation, given the self-reported dysphoria and impulsivity. Treatment interventions included CBT and consideration of pharmacotherapy if symptoms would not have resolved. Evaluation of headache and altered cognition was included in every therapy session along with assessment of hopelessness and worthlessness.

CONCLUSION

Diagnosing and treating depression in athletes is a relatively new psychiatric endeavor that serves a vital function in both the scholastic and professional sports realms. Depression can have a devastating effect on a player, impacting both athletic performance and personal life, as recent media stories on the mental health of athletes have demonstrated. Longitudinal studies on the potential impact of selective serotonin reuptake inhibitors (SSRIs) and other psychiatric drugs are needed in order to address the concerns of athletes, and future discoveries in the field of genomic medicine will help to identify athletes predisposed to depression and to guide the selection of the most efficacious therapies [14]. As the nascent field of sports psychiatry evolves into a boarded psychiatric subspecialty with fellowships at the world's leading academic medical centers, we predict that depression in athletes will be a major focus of both research and clinical work.

REFERENCES

1. Glick ID, Horsfall JL (2001) Psychiatric conditions in sports: diagnosis, treatment, and quality of life. *The Physician and Sportsmedicine* 29, 44–55.
2. Begel D (1992) An overview of sport psychiatry. *American Journal of Psychiatry* 149(5), 606–614.
3. Burton RW (2000) Mental illness in athletes. In: Begel D, Burton RW (eds.), *Sport Psychiatry: Theory and Practice*. New York: W. W. Norton & Company.
4. Reardon CL, Factor RM (2010) Sport psychiatry: a systematic review of diagnosis and medical treatment of mental illness in athletes. *Sports Medicine* 40(11), 961–980.
5. Armstrong LE, VanHeest JL (2002) The unknown mechanism of the overtraining syndrome: clues from depression and psychoneuroimmunology. *Sports Medicine* 32, 185–209.
6. McCann S (1995) Overtraining and burnout. In: Murphy SM (ed.), *Sport Psychology Interventions*. Champaign: Human Kinetics, 347–365.
7. Callister R, Callister RK, Fleck SJ, *et al.* (1989) Physiological and performance responses to overtraining in elite judo athletes. *Medicine & Science in Sports & Exercise* 22, 816–824.
8. Costill DL, Flynn MG, Kirwin JP, *et al.* (1998) Effects of repeated days of intensified training on muscle glycogen and swimming performance. *Medicine & Science in Sports & Exercise* 20, 249–254.
9. Hackney AC, Pearman SN, Nowacki JM (1990) Physiological profiles of overtrained and stale athletes: a review. *Journal of Applied Sport Psychology* 2, 21–33.
10. Glick ID, Horsfall JL (2005) Diagnosis and psychiatric treatment of athletes. *Clinics in Sports Medicine* 24(4), 771–781.
11. Linder DE, Brewer BW, Van Raalte JL, *et al.* (1991) A negative halo for athletes who consult sport psychologists: replication and extension. *Journal of Sport & Exercise Psychology* 13, 133–148.
12. Glick ID, Stillman MA, Reardon CL, *et al.* (2012) Managing psychiatric issues in elite athletes. *Journal of Clinical Psychiatry* 73(5), 640–644.
13. World Anti-Doping Agency. http://www.wada-ama.org/en/. Accessed on 29 July 2012.
14. Parise G, Bosman MJ, Boecker DR (2001) Selective serotonin reuptake inhibitors: their effect on high-intensity exercise performance. *Archives of Physical Medicine and Rehabilitation* 82, 867–871.
15. Meeusen R, Piacentini MF, van Den Eynde S, *et al.* (2001) Exercise performance is not influenced by a 5-HT reuptake inhibitor. *International Journal of Sports Medicine* 22, 329–336.
16. Wilson WM, Maughan RJ (1992) Evidence for a possible role of 5-hydroxytryptamine in the genesis of fatigue in man: administration of paroxetine, a 5-HT re-uptake inhibitor, reduces the capacity to perform prolonged exercise. *Experimental Physiology* 77, 921–924.
17. Strachan AT, Leiper JB, Maughan RJ (2004) Paroxetine admin administration fails to influence human exercise capacity, perceived effort or hormone responses during prolonged exercise in a warm environment. *Experimental Physiology* 89(6), 657–664.
18. Waslick BD, Walsh BT, Greenhill LL, *et al.* (1999) Cardiovascular effects of desipramine in children and adults during exercise testing. *Journal of the American Academy of Child and Adolescent Psychiatry* 38(2), 179–186.
19. Baron DA, Baron SH, Foley T (2009) Cognitive and behavioral therapy in depressed athletes. In: Christodoulou GN, Jorge M, Mezzich JE (eds.), *Advances in Psychiatry*, Volume 3. Athens: Beta Medical Publishers.
20. Brewer BW, Linder DE, Phelps CM (1995) Situational correlates of emotional adjustment to athletic injury. *Clinical Journal of Sport Medicine* 5, 241–245.
21. Kontos AP, Covassin T, Elbin RJ, *et al.* (2012) Depression and neurocognitive performance after concussion among male and female high school and collegiate athletes. *Archives of Physical Medicine and Rehabilitation* 93, 1751–1756.
22. Erlanger DM, Kutner KC, Barth JT, *et al.* (1999) Neuropsychology of sports-related head injury: dementia pugilistica to postconcussion syndrome. *Clinical Neuropsychology* 13, 193–209.

23. Guskiewicz, Marshall SW, Bailes J, *et al.* (2007) Recurrent concussion and risk of depression in retired professional football players. *Medicine & Science in Sports & Exercise* 39(6), 903–909.

24. Mainwaring LM, Hutchison M, Bisschop SM, *et al.* (2010) Emotional response to sport concussion compared to ACL injury. *Brain Injury* 24(4), 589–597.

25. Chen JK, Johnston KM, Petrides M, *et al.* (2008) Neural substrates of symptoms of depression following concussion in male athletes with persisting postconcussion symptoms. *Archives of General Psychiatry* 65(1), 81–89.

26. Kobasa SC, Maddi SR, Puccetti MC (1982) Personality and exercise as buffers in the stress-illness relationship. *Journal of Behavioral Medicine* 5, 391–404.

27. Weiss MR, Smith AL (2002) Friendship quality in youth sport: relationship to age, gender, and motivation variables. *Journal of Sport & Exercise Psychology* 24, 420–437.

28. Ekeland E, Heian F, Hagen KB (2005) Can exercise improve self-esteem in children and young people? A systematic review of randomised controlled trials. *British Journal of Sports Medicine* 39, 792–798.

29. Roth DL, Holmes DS (1985) Influence of physical fitness in determining the impact of stressful life events on physical and psychological health. *Psychosomatic Medicine* 47, 164–173.

30. Frydenberg E, Lewis R (1993) *Adolescent Coping Scale: Administrator's Manual.* Hawthorn: The Australian Council for Educational Research.

31. Patriksson G (1988) Theoretical and empirical analyses of dropouts from youth sports in Sweden. *Scandinavian Journal of Sports Science* 10, 29–37.

32. Szabo A (2000) Physical activity as a source of psychological dysfunction. In: Biddle SJ, Fox KR, Boutcher SH (eds.), *Physical Activity and Psychological Well-Being.* London: Routledge, 130–153.

33. Gerber M, Hosboer-Trachsler E, Puhse U, *et al.* (2011) Elite sport is not an additional source of distress for adolescents with high stress levels. *Perceptual and Motor Skills* 112, 581–599.

34. Schmikli SL, Brink MS, de Vries WR, *et al.* (2010) Can we detect non-function overreaching in young elite soccer players and middle-long distance runners using field performance tests? *British Journal of Sports Medicine* 45, 631–636.

35. Appaneal RN, Levine BR, Perna FM, *et al.* (2009) Measuring postinjury depression among male and female competitive athletes. *Journal of Sport & Exercise Psychology* 31, 60–76.

36. O'Keane V (2000) Unipolar depression in women. In: Steiner M, Yonkers K, Eriksson E (eds.), *Mood Disorders in Women.* London: Martin Dunitz, 119–135.

37. Cogan KD (2000) The sadness in sports: working with a depressed and suicidal athlete. In: Anderson MB (ed.), *Doing Sport Psychology.* Champaign: Human Kinetics, 107–119.

38. Alyson S (2010) Phenomenological Examination of Depression in Female Collegiate Athletes. Master's thesis, California.

39. Berryman JC (2000) Older mothers and later motherhood. In: Sherr L, St. Lawrence J (eds.), *Women, Health and the Mind.* Chichester: John Wiley & Sons, Ltd.

40. Burt VK (2002) Women and depression: special considerations in assessment and management. In: Lewis-Hall F, Williams TS, Panetta JA, *et al.* (eds.), *Psychiatric Illness in Women: Emerging Treatments and Research.* Washington, DC: American Psychiatric Publishing.

41. Polat A, Yücel B (2001) Psychiatric assessment of female patients (Kadın hastaların psikiyatrik değerlendirmesi). *Journal of Psychiatry, Psychology and Psychopharmacology* (in Turkish) 9, 609–610.

42. Burt VK, Hendrick VC (2005) *Clinical Manual of Women's Mental Health.* Washington, DC: American Psychiatric Publishing.

43. Kuey L (2010) Stigma, women and mental health. In: Kohen D (ed.), *Oxford Textbook of Women and Mental Health.* Oxford, UK: Oxford University Press.

44. Schwenk TL, Gorenflo DW, Dopp RR, *et al.* (2007) Depression and pain in retired football players. *Medicine & Science in Sports & Exercise* 39(4), 599–605.

45. Turner AP, Barlow JH, Heathcote-Elliott C (2000) Long term health impact of playing professional football in the United Kingdom. *British Journal of Sports Medicine* 34, 332–337.

46. Morgan WP, O'Connor P, Ellickson K, *et al.* (1988) Personality structure, mood states and performance in elite male distance runners. *International Journal of Sport Psychology* 19, 247–263.

47. Bäckmand H, Kaprio J, Kujala U, *et al.* (2003) Influence of physical activity on depression and anxiety of former elite athletes. *International Journal of Sports Medicine* 24, 609–619.

8 Suicide in Athletes

Antonia L. Baum

Department of Psychiatry and Behavioral Sciences, George Washington University School of Medicine and Health Sciences, USA

KEY POINTS

- Athletes do commit suicide. Several of the possible etiologies are unique to the athletic arena.
- Steps to prevent athlete suicide include an awareness of risk factors and warning signs.
- Involvement in sports and exercise may be useful as treatment to prevent suicide.

INTRODUCTION

That athletes commit suicide has been well established, however unlikely such a self-destructive act might seem in someone who is focused on bettering her physical being through involvement in athletics. The effort to increase attention to the existence of psychopathology in this population has been upstream, such that to make the case for the most devastating and tragic outcome, that of suicide, has been ever more against the current. Once it is on the radar screen, it is remarkable to see that suicide is not an uncommon experience in the athletic arena.

Extreme sports can also be conceptualized as existing on a continuum toward suicidal behavior. Parachuting deaths have occurred due to failure to pull the ripcord. BASE (an acronym for building/antenna/span [bridge]/earth [cliffs]) jumping, a sport wherein the athlete propels himself off a structure and parachutes to the ground, has one of the highest fatality rates in the athletic arena. Other sports involving significant risk taking include extreme skiing, mountaineering, gliding, bungee jumping, race car driving, and scuba and cave diving [1].

Suicide accounts for almost 13% – it is the third leading cause – of deaths in the United States in the 15–24-year-old age group. The relationships between depression, anxiety, involvement in sports and exercise, and suicidality are complex. There is a suggestion that participation in organized sports may confer some protection against hopelessness, depression, and suicidal ideation and attempts, and that exercise is usually associated with less depression and less frequent suicidal ideation in males. However, other evidence suggests that frequent exercise might actually be associated with increased risk in females (hypothesized to be secondary to low self-esteem tied to negative body image) [2]. Overall, results have been inconclusive [1].

Clinical Sports Psychiatry: An International Perspective, First Edition. Edited by David A. Baron,
Claudia L. Reardon and Steven H. Baron.
© 2013 John Wiley & Sons, Ltd. Published 2013 by John Wiley & Sons, Ltd.

In a 2005 study, Baum [2] reviewed the medical literature over a 35-year period, and the periodical literature over a 20-year period. These searches revealed 71 athletes who had either contemplated, attempted, or completed suicide, the latter occurring in 66 of the 71 reported cases. The average age was 22.3 years, with 61 males and 10 females. Football was the most heavily represented sport, with basketball, swimming, track and field, and baseball following, and an occasional case in a variety of other sports. It must be considered that there was underreporting of such cases, given the stigma of suicide in general, and the stigma associated with psychiatric illness in the sports world enduring. By inference, some etiologic possibilities were presented.

ETIOLOGY

Injury

MSK injuries

Optimal fitness and function are vital to the success of the competitive athlete. The repetition and overuse that occur through training, and the adrenalinized mishaps during races or collisions on the field, lead to injury, which can result in significant depression. Physical injury may be the single most devastating event in the career of an athlete. In a small study of five injured athletes who attempted suicide, the commonalities identified included the achievement of significant success prior to the injury, an injury severe enough to require surgery followed by a prolonged and challenging rehabilitation necessitating restriction from their sport, the inability to return to their preinjury level in their sport, and having their positions usurped by teammates. Each of these five athletes were in that 15–24-year-old age group associated with a relatively high risk of suicide. The authors of that study noted that the Emotional Responses of Athletes to Injury Questionnaire (ERAIQ) may be used to assess the risk for suicidal thoughts or behavior in an injured athlete [3].

The potential significance of injury to a professional athlete and to his livelihood might be accompanied by still greater depression and susceptibility to suicidal ideation and behavior.

Case Study

In 2010, two professional athletes committed suicide within a 4-month period following injuries. A 25-year-old LGPA Tour Golfer, Erica Blasberg, who had left college after 2 years to turn professional, sustained a back injury in 2009 and lost her tour card. She killed herself the following year by asphyxiation, and was found to have toxic levels of anxiolytics and prescription headache, cough, and pain medications. Her father stated that she had been depressed [4].

Denver Broncos receiver Kenny McKinley suffered a knee injury in 2010, which led to his second knee surgery of the year, and prematurely ended his season. In the immediate postoperative period, as he felt he had no alternative to playing football, he said: that he "should just kill [himself]." Just 4 weeks later he shot himself in the head [4].

Central nervous system injuries

There is a unique relationship between head injury and suicide. A number of studies have identified an association between traumatic brain injury (TBI) of any severity and major depression. Postconcussive symptoms can include depression, anxiety, agitation, irritability, and aggression. Although most patients with mild TBI have fairly rapid and complete resolution of symptoms, some will go on to have a more chronic course with significant disability, including neurodegenerative diseases. This outcome can be minimized by acting quickly through patient education and referral for treatment [5].

What is now known as chronic traumatic encephalopathy (CTE), previously known as dementia pugilistica and associated with boxing, is a form of neurofibrillary degeneration, a distinct and slowly progressive tauopathy [6] secondary to repeated head trauma. It can also be associated with sports such as football, hockey, soccer, and professional wrestling. Behavioral manifestations include apathy, depression, irritability, impulsiveness, and suicidality [7]. See Chapter 9 for more information.

Case Study

In April 2012, Ray Easterling, former Atlanta Falcons safety, committed suicide following a 20-year progression of depression, insomnia, and dementia. His wife described that "He had been feeling more and more pain. He felt like his brain was falling off. He was losing control." He was in the process of suing the NFL over his head injuries, and was the second NFL player in a short period of time to commit suicide with symptoms suggestive of CTE; Dave Duerson of the New York Giants and the Chicago Bears had committed suicide 14 months earlier, and in a suicide note he described memory loss and headaches, and requested that his brain be given to Boston University's Center for the Study of Traumatic Encephalopathy [8].

RETIREMENT

The career of an elite or professional athlete is generally brief, as the body's peak performance tends to occur early in life. Women's gymnastics is at one end of the spectrum, where optimum performance might occur prepubertally. While the career of a rookie position player in major league baseball is 5.6 years on average, one out of five position players will play for just 1 year [9]. The sacrifices involved – financial, emotional, moving away from family, investment of time, missing out on socializing, and singular focus – are significant, and often leave an athlete ill-equipped for any future beyond retirement. Depression and even suicidal ideation can occur in the wake of retirement.

Mike Wise, an ex-NFL lineman for the Los Angeles Raiders and the Cleveland Browns, committed suicide 3 weeks after his waiver by Cleveland. Several days prior to his death, he had told his fiancee that he equated having his name on the waiver wire with having it in an obituary [10].

PSYCHOLOGICAL TRAITS

Perfectionism is a character trait not infrequently observed in a successful athlete. Repetition and attention to detail may distinguish the victor from the second spot on the podium. Extreme perfectionism, "…where anything less than perfect is unacceptable, can leave individuals vulnerable to depression" [11], which can, in turn, lead to suicidal behavior. Psychological characteristics including anger, confusion, fatigue, tension, and depression have been associated with injury [12], which leaves an athlete vulnerable to suicidal behavior.

Freud understood the self-loathing of depression to stem from anger toward a love object turned inward. Suicide could then be viewed as a past drive to kill someone else [13]. Aggression on the field can be a necessary ingredient for success in an athlete. When turned toward the self, such powerful aggression can translate into suicidal behavior.

SUBSTANCE ABUSE/ANABOLIC STEROID ABUSE

Substance abuse or dependence, including performance-enhancing drugs, is a part of the subculture of certain sports and particular teams. Interestingly, aggression has been associated with a developing cultural norm described as the "jock" [14], or even "toxic jock," as distinguished from the so-called student-athlete. The former group, though it has a sport-related identity, is also associated with masculinity and risk taking. Consumption of energy drinks such as Red Bull and other stimulant beverages has been associated with this subgroup [15]. Both in the military and the civilian world, there has been increasing concern that these energy drinks are associated with the use of other stimulants, sometimes prescribed for attention deficit hyperactivity disorder (ADHD), as well as with the use of other drugs of abuse, and that their use has been noted in cases of suicide. The hypothesis is that the sleep deprivation secondary to a combination of a prescribed stimulant in conjunction with significant doses of caffeine could result in impulsivity [16]. There are some personality characteristics shared by members of the military and athletes. This is an important reminder to include a caffeine intake history routinely.

The abuse of or dependence upon alcohol and recreational drugs increases the risk of suicidal behavior, and athletes are not an exception. Not only is recreational drug use encouraged among some groups of athletes, but the chronic pain due to injury in athletes predisposes them to the abuse of narcotics, and often alcohol. Stimulants might then be abused to counteract the effects of the narcotics.

Psychostimulants, with their attendant risks, can also be used as performance-enhancing drugs among athletes, as are anabolic–androgenic steroids (AAS). The abuse of the latter is not infrequently seen in muscle dysmorphia, a form of body image disturbance characterized by an unhealthy preoccupation with muscularity. AAS do meet criteria for a drug of dependence. This dependency has been hypothesized to develop through (i) an "addiction" to the anabolic effects, (ii) an effort to reverse the dysphoria or major depression resulting from hypogonadism during anabolic steroid withdrawal, and (iii) their hedonic effects, not unlike other "classical" addictive drugs, especially opioids [17]. The crash into depression following cessation of AAS and the so-called roid rage associated with their use have both been implicated in cases of athlete suicide. "Roid rage" might be best understood through alterations in brain testosterone (increased) and allopregnanolone synthesis (decreased), so that the abuse of AAS may result in irritability, impulsive aggression, and signs of major depression [18]. A survey of 163 weight lifters showed that of those using AAS, 7% reported suicidal ideation within a month of stopping the drug [19].

It has been increasingly recognized that AAS abuse and dependence are not limited to elite or professional athletes. Not only are they used in nonathletes, and in association with other drugs [20], but they are perhaps used more often by those aspiring to be athletic but disenfranchised from organized sports. In a large survey of Icelandic high school students, the biggest risk group for AAS use were those students involved in fitness and informal athletic training, apart from organized athletic programs [21].

AXIS I PSYCHOPATHOLOGY

Eating disorders

There appears to be some overlap between the abuse of AAS and bodily preoccupation, such as that observed in muscle dysmorphia [22], or in the eating-disordered athlete [23].

Athletes have lost their lives through what might be considered the self-destructive or suicidal behavior of starvation. Anorexia nervosa, which has been linked to a number of sports, is the psychiatric disturbance with the highest rate of mortality, 9–12%. One third of these deaths are a direct result of suicide.

Case Study

A Georgetown track scholarship athlete developed an eating disorder following a hamstring injury. The inactivity while injured led to a fear of weight gain. She became focused on what she felt was necessary for a serious runner; thinness was synonymous with speed. The thoughts that eventually propelled her toward a suicide attempt centered on food. She jumped from a railroad bridge, and, tragically, lost the use of her legs [24].

Affective disorders/anxiety disorders

Affective disorders, both unipolar and bipolar, as well as anxiety spectrum disorders, not infrequently co-occurring with substance abuse or dependence, and all of which are associated with an increased risk of suicide, can occur in athletes. Greater than 90% of those who commit suicide suffered from depression. When taking a history, a family history of suicide should be elicited.

Case Study

Jeret Peterson was a 29-year-old seven-time World Cup Champion and the U.S. 2010 Olympic silver medalist in freestyle aerial skiing, known for his signature "Hurricane," a risky and technically difficult jump attempted by few in the sport. In the 2006 Olympic Games, he risked the Hurricane in lieu of a more conservative jump, and committed an error on his landing, likely sacrificing the gold medal. That night, he punched his best friend during a bar fight, causing the U.S. Ski Team to ask him to leave the games. Other stressors that presumably contributed to his ongoing difficulties with depression and abuse of alcohol included his report that he had been molested as a child, the 1987 death of his half-sister by a drunken driver, and the 2005 suicide by a gunshot to the head of a friend in front of him. He killed himself in 2011 by a gunshot wound to the head just days after appearing in court to plead not guilty to drunken driving charges [25].

Attention deficit hyperactivity disorder

ADHD may predispose an individual to seek involvement in sports, an area where they may enjoy success over academics or over other more sedentary pursuits. The athletic arena may then become a refuge for a patient struggling with an attentional deficit or with hyperactivity. If an athlete loses that area of competence or comfort, he might begin to feel adrift.

Case Study

Kenny Wright had a history that was consistent with a diagnosis of ADHD. He opted out of college: "…as much as the boy adored football, he knew that he couldn't take four more years of studying … but to be in sports, to be active – that was always what motivated him, diverted him from the less active pleasures in life … He could not sit and read or even remain long before the TV … Sports put a lot of structure into Kenny's existence … his grades were invariably better during the football season … his temper was contained during football … And it's true that the only time Kenny really floundered in his life was after he finished school and there was no more football to point to in the fall" [26]. He shot himself when he was 24 years old.

Another important issue to consider is that the stimulant medications commonly used in the treatment of ADHD – for which therapeutic use exemptions can be attained when stimulants are banned as potential performance-enhancing drugs – may be dangerous or even lethal when taken in overdose.

PRESSURE TO WIN

The pressure to win in the athletic arena is a more distilled and tangible measure of success than in many other aspects of life. For the elite athlete, one-hundredth of a second can separate the victor from the number two position, the latter often viewed as the "loser" [27]. A gold versus a silver medal in the Olympic Games can mean the difference between career-making endorsements and being rapidly forgotten. Winning and losing in the professional sports world can dictate multimillion dollar contracts won or lost.

Case Study

Nadia Comaneci, the Romanian gymnast who distinguished herself in 1976 at age 14, not only as the Olympic champion, but also as the one who set the bar higher than anyone else with her unprecedented perfect tens, attempted suicide when she was 15 years old by drinking bleach. This afforded her the opportunity to rest in the hospital for 2 days. She reported feeling tired and that she was "glad. Glad because I didn't have to go to the gym for 2 days, so I am happy" [28]. Since that incident, she has denied that it represented a suicide attempt.

SEXUAL ABUSE

The unique emphasis on the physical in the athletic arena, in settings where athletes are often scantily clad and in physical contact with their coach or trainer – with the inherent power imbalances – creates sexual situations where there may be the opportunity for abuse to occur. Frequently there are institutional and competitive pressures to hide this abuse, in addition to denial. Suicides have occurred in both victims and in the accused. On-field aggression has at times expressed itself in sexual aggression or rape off the field [1]. In 2010, the U.S. Olympic Committee convened a working group to educate and to address and attempt to prevent such abuses in sport following allegations that one of USA Swimming's coaches had sexually abused some of his athletes. See Chapter 16 for more information.

HOMOSEXUALITY

Homosexuals in the high risk demographic for suicide of ages 15–24 are at a two to three times higher risk of attempting suicide compared to age-matched heterosexuals. Homophobia is rampant in professional sports, particularly the more violent sports [1]. "The most brutal sports, including football, have the tightest locks on the closet door … The vulnerability implied in men loving men is not part of the game plan" [29].

Case Study

The Olympic champion diver Greg Louganis was teased as a child because of his pre-dilection for dance, acrobatics, and theater. He attempted suicide three times before he was 18 years old [30]. Eight years after his 1976 Olympic debut at age 16, he was still not secure in making his sexual orientation public knowledge; during the 1988 Seoul Olympics, while attempting the difficult reverse two-and-a-half pike in the prelimi-nary round, he hit his head on the board, sustaining a concussion and a scalp laceration requiring sutures. It would be six more years before he announced to the world that he was gay, and that he was HIV positive, and had been at the time of his injury, creating a controversy over the fact that the nondisclosure of his HIV status could theoretically have put others at risk [31].

FIREARMS

The access to firearms, particularly in the context of substance abuse, elevates the risk for suicide. Because of their high profile, it has become increasingly common for professional athletes to carry guns for protection. In 1994, in an effort to educate their athletes, the NBA Player's Association created a security division [32].

CULTURAL INFLUENCES

"Cultural attitudes toward suicide may influence behavior in the athletic arena. In Japan, the marathon is a more visible and respected athletic event than it is in many western cultures; 'the perfect marathon' is seen as 'draining one's body,' a form of 'ritual suicide'" [33]. "Maybe it's the pain in a society that admires the bearing of pain … The Japanese tend to be very moved by those who try to accomplish something that involves a lot of pain and suffering" [1, 34].

Case Study

"Kokichi Tsubaraya was on medal pace in the 1964 Tokyo Olympic marathon when he was overtaken, thus losing the bronze medal. He felt he had let his country down, and committed suicide 4 years later" [1, 35].

"Marathon coach Kiyoshi Nakamura, who died by drowning, was thought to have committed suicide in response to his protégé's defeat (he placed fourteenth) in the Los Angeles Olympics" [1, 36].

PREVENTION

An awareness of the factors that may put athletes at risk for suicide, including competitive pressures, injury, retirement, risk-taking personality profiles, Axis I psychopathology, sexual abuse and orientation, and the increasing availability of firearms, can help prevent tragedies from occurring. Education is an important step in raising this awareness. Athletes, coaches, trainers, and athletes' families need to learn that athletes are not immune to suicide, and what the warning signs might be.

SPORTS AS THERAPY

Involvement in sports can be therapeutic for those suffering from Axis I disorders and coping with stress and retirement. Athletics can therefore play a significant role in the prevention of suicidal ideation and behavior. Sports participation can help to develop self-esteem through mastery, esprit de corps, and enhanced body image. Athletic involvement in adolescent females is associated with an older age for first sexual experience, less overall sexual activity, and a lower rate of pregnancy [37]. Teen pregnancy is associated with an increase in the rate of suicide and attempted suicide [38], so arguably, sports participation may play a specific protective role in this population.

FUTURE RESEARCH

Because of the stigma associated with psychiatric illness, strongly held in the world of sports, with suicidal ideation and behavior perhaps most antithetical to the athletic ideal, unconscious denial and deliberate obfuscation have made it difficult to compile accurate statistics on the rate of suicide among athletes. Increasing awareness will pave the way to gather these data. We will also get a clearer picture of the magnitude of recreational and performance-enhancing drugs in the sports world, and their contributions to suicidal ideation and behavior. Understanding the scope of the problem will be an important building block in prevention.

REFERENCES

1. Baum AL (2005) Suicide in athletes: a review and commentary. In: Tofler IR, Morse ED (eds.) *Clinics in Sports Medicine: The Interface Between Sports Psychiatry and Sports Medicine* Saunders, Philadelphia. *Clinics in Sports Medicine* 24(4), 853–869.
2. Miller KE, Hoffman JH (2009) Mental well-being and sport-related identities in college students. *Sociology of Sport Journal* 26(2), 335–356.
3. Smith AM, Milliner EK (1994) Injured athletes and the risk of suicide. *Journal of Athletic Training* 29(4), 337–341.
4. Image CPR (2010) Two pro athletes commit suicide following serious injuries. www.imagecpr. com/?p=2611. Accessed on 12 December 2012.
5. Blyth BJ, Bazarian JJ (2010) Traumatic alterations in consciousness: traumatic brain injury. *Emergency Medicine Clinics of North America* 28(3), 571–594.
6. McKee AC, Cantu RC, Nowinski CJ *et al.* (2009) Chronic traumatic encephalopathy in athletes: progressive tauopathy following repetitive head injury. *Journal of Neuropathology & Experimental Neurology* 68(7), 709–735.
7. Gavett BE, Stern RA, McKee AC (2011) Chronic traumatic encephalopathy: a potential late effect of sport-related concussive and subconcussive head trauma. *Clinical Journal of Sport Medicine* 30(1), 179–188.
8. Associated Press (2012) Ray Easterling, former Atlanta Falcons safety who was suing NFL over head injuries, committed suicide. http://query.nytimes.com/search/sitesearch/#/Ray+Easterling%2C+former +Atlanta+Falcons+safety+who+was+suing+NFL+over+head+injuries%2C+committed+suicide. Accessed on 13 December 2012.
9. Witnauer WD, Rogers RG, Saint Onge JM (2007) Major league baseball career length in the twentieth century. *Population Research and Policy Review* 26(4), 371–386.
10. Salguero A (1997) NFL retirees cope with many difficulties after playing days are over. *Knight-Ridder Tribune News Service*, April 5, 405K4688.
11. Melrose S (2011) Perfectionism and depression: vulnerabilities nurses need to understand. *Nursing Research and Practice*, 2011, 1–7.
12. Galambos S, Terry P, Moyle G *et al.* (2005) Psychological predictors of injury among elite athletes. *British Journal of Sports Medicine* 39(6), 351–354.
13. Freud S (1995) *Mourning and Melancholia.The Freud Reader.* W. W. Norton, New York.
14. Pokhrel P, Sussman S, Black D *et al.* (2010) Peer group self-identification as a predictor of relational and physical aggression among high school students. *Journal of School Health* 80(5), 249–258.
15. Miller KE (2008) Wired: energy drinks, jock identity, masculine norms, and risk taking. *Journal of American College Health* 56(5), 481–489.
16. Tyson AS, Jaffe G (2009) Generals find suicide a frustrating enemy. *Washingtonpost.com*, May 23.
17. Kanayama G, Brower KJ, Wood RI *et al.* (2010) Treatment of anabolic-androgenic steroid dependence: emerging evidence and its implications. *Drug and Alcohol Dependence* 109(1–3), 6–13.
18. Pinna G, Costa E, Guidotti A (2005) Changes in brain testosterone and allopregnanolone biosynthesis elicit aggressive behavior. *Proceedings of the National Academy of Science USA* 102(6), 2135–2140.
19. Bower B (1991) Pumped up and strung out: steroid addiction may haunt the quest for bigger muscles. *Science News* 140, 30–31.
20. Skarberg K, Nyberg F, Engstrom I (2008) The development of multiple drug use among anabolic-androgenic steroid users: six subjective case reports. *Substance Abuse Treatment, Prevention, and Policy* 3, 24.
21. Thorlindsson T, Halldorsson V (2010) Sport, and use of anabolic-androgenic steroids among Icelandic high school students: a critical test of three perspectives. *Substance Abuse Treatment, Prevention, and Policy* 5, 32.
22. Pope HG Jr., Gruber AJ, Choi P *et al.* (1997) Muscle dysmorphia: an underrecognized form of body dysmorphic disorder. *Psychosomatics* 38, 548–557.
23. Hildebrandt T, Lai JK, Langenbucher JW *et al.* (2011) The diagnostic dilemma of pathological appearance and performance enhancing drug use. *Drug and Alcohol Dependence* 114(1), 1–11.
24. Levin E (1983) A lethal quest for the winning edge; a runner's grim battle with anorexia nervosa underscores the peril of athletes on starvation diets. *People* 20, 18–22.
25. Slotnik DE (2011) Jeret Peterson, skier known for a daring move, dies at 29. http://www.nytimes. com/2011/07/28/sports/jeret-peterson-skier-known-for-a-daring-move-dies-at-29.html?_r=0. Accessed on 13 December 2012.

26. Deford F (1981) Kenny dying young. *Sports Illustrated* 30, 2.
27. Lapchik R (1994) Losing out on their time to shine. *The Sporting News* 217, 8.
28. Harrison BG (1990) The fall from grace of an angel named Nadia. *Life* 13, 24–32.
29. Foster RD (2000) Still short of the goal. *Advocate* 60.
30. Dolen C (1999) In his own words…Greg Louganis. *Knight-Ridder/Tribune News Service*, November 1, KO485.
31. Cichocki M (2008) In to the pool and out of the closet: a word about HIV positive Olympic diving champion Greg Louganis. *About.com*, October 25.
32. Shappell L (1994) As world becomes more dangerous, increasing numbers of athletes say carrying a handgun has become a necessity. *Arizona Republic Knight-Ridder/Tribune News Service* April 2, 0402K1935.
33. Burfoot A (1991) Home run. *Runner's World* 26(12), 90.
34. Struck D (2000) They're in it for the long run; Japanese see marathon as a symbol for life. *Washington Post*, August 20.
35. Beech H (1998) Medalists with mettle. *Time International* 150, 48.
36. Neff C (1987) Money talked, nobody walked. *Sports Illustrated* 66, 34–35.
37. Baum AL (1998) Young females in the athletic arena. *Child & Adolescent Psychiatric Clinics of North America* 7(4), 745–755.
38. Jorgensen SR, Potts V, Camp B (1993) Project taking charge: six-month follow-up of a pregnancy prevention program for early adolescents. *Family Relations* 42, 373–380.

9 Concussion in Sports

David A. Baron,[1,2,3] Claudia L. Reardon,[4]
Jeremy DeFranco,[5] and Steven H. Baron[6]

[1] International Relations and Department of Psychiatry, Keck School of Medicine at the University of Southern California, USA
[2] Keck Medical Center at the University of Southern California, USA
[3] Global Center for Exercise, Psychiatry, and Sports at USC, Health Sciences Campus, USA
[4] Department of Psychiatry, University of Wisconsin School of Medicine and Public Health, USA
[5] Department of Psychiatry, Keck School of Medicine at the University of Southern California, USA
[6] Montgomery County Community College, USA

KEY POINTS

- Concussion results from a sudden impact to the brain induced by (direct or indirect) traumatic biomechanical forces.
- Concussion does not require loss of consciousness.
- Repeated concussions can result in significant cognitive, behavioral, and emotional symptoms, both acutely and years after the initial injury.
- Returning to play too soon after brain injury may result in irreversible neuropsychiatric symptoms and (rarely) severe neurologic consequences.

INTRODUCTION

On June 20, 2012, nine newspapers across the United States printed stories on head injury prevention in sports [1]. Likewise, it has become difficult to keep up with the volume of scientific articles being written addressing this problem globally. A Google search of "sports concussion" on that same 2012 date resulted in over 3 760 000 hits [2].

The term "concussion" is derived from the Latin *concutere*. The English translation is "to shake violently" [3]. This is an accurate description of what happens to the brain of concussed individuals. Although an accepted consequence of participation in contact sports such as boxing, soccer, and American football, the clinical significance of head and neck trauma in many other sports is only recently being fully appreciated [4]. In addition, the long-term consequences of repeated "subclinical" concussions are emerging as a highly significant clinical concern, especially in youth athletes [5, 6]. Prior clinical reports have focused on the immediate and short-term neurologic symptoms, with little (if any) discussion of mood lability, depression, sleep problems, and attention deficit hyperactivity disorder (ADHD)-like symptoms [7]. The importance of delayed neuropsychiatric symptoms, often presenting a decade or more after the initial brain injury, has become a major focus of current and proposed future clinical investigation [8].

WHAT IS CONCUSSION AND TRAUMATIC BRAIN INJURY?

Concussion literature prior to 2008 commonly employed the terms concussion and mild traumatic brain injury (mTBI) interchangeably. There was not a universally agreed-upon definition of concussion up to that point. Research findings were often not transferable from study to study, and the field of concussion research had encountered a stymie. At the 2008 Third International Conference on Concussion in Sport in Zurich [3], researchers from around the world convened to address this issue, and several others, within the field of concussion research. A panel discussion regarding the definition of concussion and its separation from mTBI was held. It was acknowledged that the terms concussion and mTBI represent separate injury constructs and should not be used interchangeably. Furthermore, unanimous agreement about the definition of concussion was made. The most recent sports psychiatry literature utilizes the term mTBI to describe head trauma in athletes, despite the work of the International Conference on Concussion in Sport [9].

Concussion has been defined as a pathophysiological process affecting the brain that is induced by traumatic biomechanical forces. Several common features that incorporate clinical, pathologic, and biomechanical injury constructs that may be utilized in defining the nature of a concussive head injury include:

1. Concussion may result directly from a hit to the head, face, or neck, or it may indirectly result from a hit to another part of the body and subsequent "impulsive" force that is transmitted to the head.
2. Concussions tend to be rapid in onset, and resolutions of short-term functional neurological impairments tend to be spontaneous.
3. Concussion may result in neuropathological changes, but acute clinical symptoms represent a *functional* disturbance rather than a *structural* injury.
4. Concussion results in a graded set of clinical symptoms, which may or may not involve a loss of consciousness. Resolution of clinical and cognitive symptoms typically follows a sequential course, although a small percentage of cases (10–20%) have a prolonged course of post-concussive symptoms.
5. No abnormality is present on standard structural neuroimaging studies in concussion.

The definition of concussion has not been the only area of concussion research in need of consensus. There have been three international conferences on concussion and sport to date. Topics brought up for consensus include definition, classification, evaluation, management, modifying factors (i.e., factors that alter evaluation and management and factors that predict prolonged or persistent symptoms), special populations (e.g., children and adolescents, elite vs. non-elite athletes), protective equipment, rule changes, and athlete and coach education. The group of individuals participating in the three international conferences on concussion and sport is known as the Concussion in Sports Group (CISG). If nothing else, these conferences brought together the global leaders in the field and helped to create the existing momentum of clinical and research interest. Credit should be given to this group for initiating a change in the current culture, which does not take sport concussion seriously. Despite the lack of full consensus on many key issues, such as how to diagnose, determine return-to-play criteria, and effective treatment strategies, these conferences helped initiate the process of better understanding the need to address these fundamental clinical questions.

Researchers have made attempts to classify concussion into severity-based systems. In fact, there are at least 25 different grading systems currently in use that have been identified within the literature. Ideally, these classification schemes would hold prognostic value and guide return-to-play decisions. These systems have been based on little more than personal experience and opinion, and have limited scientific evidence to validate any of them.

The three most commonly utilized and best studied concussion grading scales are the Cantu Concussion Grading Scale, the Colorado State Medical Society (CMS) grading scale, and the American Association of Neurology (AAN) grading scale. None of these systems are intended for use specifically in sports concussion and are more appropriate for more severe head trauma.

The CISG does not endorse any single concussion severity grading system. In reality, concussion severity can only be determined in retrospect, after all concussion symptoms clear, neurological exam returns to normal, and cognitive function returns to baseline. Concussion severity is highly individualized and ultimately determined by combined measures of recovery. Most initial concussion symptoms (80–90%) are thought to resolve in a short period of 7–10 days. However, the effects of multiple, mild concussions may persist for months to years. The later onset mental status changes, often not recognized by sports medicine physicians or reported by athletes, can result in significant long-term functional disability [6, 10].

PATHOPHYSIOLOGY OF CONCUSSION

The pathophysiology of concussion has not been completely elucidated, although several pathophysiological processes are known to occur. Concussion is known to involve impaired neurotransmission, dysregulation of ions, the creation of a hypermetabolic state, and the reduction of cerebral blood flow. Impaired neurotransmission includes the excessive release of the excitatory neurotransmitter glutamate, which leads to neurotoxicity and the opening of ion channels. The opening of ion channels then leads to dysregulation of ions in the brain. Dysregulation of ions in turn places strain on ion pumps, which leads to increased energy demand. This then leads to a hypermetabolic state in the brain, wherein larger than normal amounts of glucose are consumed. This hypermetabolic state is combined with a reduction of cerebral blood flow, which results in an "energy crisis." Ongoing research with animal models of concussion are helping to elucidate additional etiologic factors [3, 11].

DIAGNOSIS OF CONCUSSION

The diagnosis of concussion has been another major topic addressed by the CISG. The CISG proposed the following four-part protocol: clinical history, evaluation, neuropsychological testing, and brain imaging. Within this protocol, an initial abbreviated sideline assessment is followed by a more comprehensive assessment.

Clinical history should include a detailed concussion history, and ideally the performance of a preparticipation examination. This baseline exam should include assessment of neurocognitive and core mental status functioning. Results from baseline tests can be compared to postinjury assessment to better determine functional recovery. The ImPact test is an excellent example of this strategy, and is the most widely used standardized preassessment tool [12]. Many youth sports programs around the globe now require a preseason ImPact test to be administered to all participants. This has been a major advance and has raised brain trauma awareness in athletes, coaches, trainers, and parents. Unfortunately, athletes have reported "sand bagging" (consciously underperforming on the baseline test) in an attempt to "beat" the test and avoid being denied permission to return to play post head injury. It is estimated that 50% of all athletes fail to report concussive symptoms. Many players either want to keep playing for fear of losing their position on the team to a backup player, do not want to be perceived as "weak," or both. Furthermore, an estimated 33% of athletes do not even know the symptoms of concussion. Returning to play too soon after a concussion places the athlete at risk of second impact syndrome should a subsequent hit involving any "impulsive" force transmitted to the brain occur [13]. This is discussed further later in this chapter.

A preparticipation examination in total ideally should include a baseline cognitive assessment, a baseline neuropsychiatric assessment, a physical examination, and a concussion history. One should bear in mind that many players are unable, or unwilling, to identify a concussion when undergoing a concussion history. A thorough concussion history should therefore include assessment of previous signs and symptoms. Likewise, one should also inquire about protective gear worn during previous concussions.

Evaluation of concussion should begin with an on-site medical examination using standard emergency management principles. Attention should be given to excluding a cervical spine injury. A neurological examination should be administered, along with a mental status exam. When assessing mental status, it has been found that orientation questions involving person, place, and time are unreliable, while memory assessment has been found to be more reliable. A brief neuropsychological battery should also be performed during initial concussion evaluation. Reliable brief neuropsychological batteries include Maddock's questions and the Standardized Assessment of Concussion (SAC).

A determination of the need for emergent neuroimaging must also be made. Indications for imaging include suspicion for structural abnormality, worsening post-concussion symptoms, presence of focal neurological deficits, loss of consciousness lasting more than 1 min, presence of seizures, and a history of multiple concussions. The appropriate disposition of the player must be determined by the treating healthcare provider in a timely manner [9]. If no healthcare provider is available, the player should be safely removed from practice or play, and an arrangement for urgent referral to a physician should be made. This is an unlikely scenario during competition, but could happen during a practice session or outside training, when sports medicine personnel are unavailable.

It takes just one symptom to diagnose a concussion. Likewise, the appearance of concussion symptoms may be delayed several hours following a concussive episode. The clinician should always err on the side of safety and remember the phrase, "When in doubt sit 'em out." The player should not be left alone following injury, and serial monitoring for deterioration of clinical status is essential over the initial few hours following head injury.

Once initial evaluation and any necessary urgent management and/or urgent neuroimaging have been completed, a comprehensive neuropsychiatric examination and balance testing should be performed. These postinjury tests will be referenced, along with future tests, to guide clinical management decisions. A commonly employed balance test is the balance error scoring system (BESS), which provides a thorough evaluation of motor function. A further supplemental evaluation called the sports concussion assessment tool (SCAT-2) may also be performed at this point in time. This test was developed at the Third International Conference on Concussion in Sport [3]. Follow-up clinical evaluation should be set up for the following day, if possible. Headache, sleep disturbance, problems with concentration and memory, and sensitivity to light and noise are common initial symptoms, and should be monitored [9, 14].

EPIDEMIOLOGY AND ETIOLOGY OF CONCUSSION

Sports-related concussions tend to differ from nonsports concussion, such as those sustained in motor vehicle accidents, as the former often result from multiple lower-velocity impacts and result in transient disorientation and minimal impairment of conscious state, as opposed to total loss of consciousness frequently seen in nonsports concussion [15]. The underreporting of sports concussions may be related, in part, to a lack of appreciation that altered consciousness of *any* degree warrants the diagnosis. Sports-related concussions are not restricted to intercollegiate and professional athletes. A recent study by Lincoln and colleagues [16] of high-school concussions found a dramatic (over 400%) increase in reported sports-related concussion over the past 11 years.

In 2011, over 62 000 youth athletes were reported to have sustained a concussion during participation in sporting events. The sports with the highest number of concussions were boys' American football and girls' soccer. This significant increase in reported cases could be the result of a number of factors, including better recognition and reporting by trainers and coaches, along with an actual increased incidence of concussions. A number of factors are being considered to explain increasing numbers of actual sports concussions in youth athletes. These include poor fitting equipment (especially football helmets), bigger, faster athletes, increased intensity of participation (more full contact practices, less time off), and inadequate coaching on "brain-safe" playing techniques. A 2012 survey of parents of youth athletes, conducted by an independent research firm from 21 countries, reported that 90% relied on their children's coaches for safety, while only 52% of coaches felt they were knowledgeable about head safety. Virtually all of the coaches polled worldwide reported needing more training, but had no access to it.

PREVENTION OF CONCUSSION

The concern for safety in sports equipment is not new. In 1969, the National Operating Committee on Standards for Athletic Equipment (NOCSAE) was formed in the United States. Since its inception, the organization has focused on baseball, softball, ice hockey, and soccer equipment. As a result of the recent focus on concussion in youth sports, the organization has contributed more than 5 million U.S. dollars to support clinical research to better understand this growing concern. On June 15, 2012, NOCSAE issued a warning to youth athletes and their parents and trainers to help them understand the extent of protection provided by, and not provided by, athletic equipment, and the consequences of sports concussion. As a result of this and other warnings, Pop Warner football (the largest youth sports organization for American football) has mandated limitations in the amount of contact permitted in practice and established strict limitations on any head-to-head contact. Other contact sports are very likely to follow their lead in establishing prevention strategies to help avoid concussions on the practice field and during competition. These efforts, along with improved training of trainers, coaches, and parents on recognition of concussion symptoms in athletes, are intended to result in a significant reduction in the prevalence of this potential serious injury. Its impact has extended beyond the world of sport, with the September 2012 release of a Hollywood documentary focused on the potential adverse consequences of head trauma in youth sports.

Brain injury resulting from motorcycle accidents was first reported in the *British Medical Journal* by Cairns and Holbourn in 1943 [17]. They examined the role of wearing a helmet on the extent of concussion. As a result of their research, they concluded that concussion was caused by a change in rotational velocity of the head. They observed that wearing a helmet was somewhat protective and resulted in milder concussion. This research played an important role in the growth of the use of helmets in collision sports. Unfortunately, sports helmets do not fully protect from rotational or angular acceleration forces of the brain resulting in neuronal shearing. Furthermore, for futbol players worldwide, helmets are not used as a preventive strategy.

POST-CONCUSSION SYNDROME

Post-concussion syndrome (PCS) is the term used to describe a group of neuropsychiatric symptoms that may continue for weeks to years as a consequence of concussion. These symptoms include headache, dizziness, fatigue, irritability, labile mood, anxiety, depression, insomnia, decreased concentration and memory, and light and noise sensitivity. It is estimated that 38–80% of patients who suffer a mTBI will develop PCS, making it one of the most commonly diagnosed clinical entities following head trauma. As defined in the literature, symptoms must persist for more than 3 months following the concussion, but frequently appear within a few days of the initial trauma.

The original description was "shell shock," and included physical and psychological symptoms. In fact, the proposed etiology included physical head trauma and psychological stress. To date, the exact etiology is not known, but ongoing research in neuroimaging and with animal models is advancing in the field.

PCS does not require multiple concussions and typically results from a single incident. Athletes often present initially with headaches and sleep disturbances. Changes in psychiatric functioning develop later. What determines those at risk for PCS after head trauma is unknown. Unlike chronic traumatic encephalopathy (CTE, see following text), which is thought to be associated with β-amyloid plaques and tau body formation, PCS has been linked to a reduction in glucose utilization in the brain and fMRI changes within a week of the concussion. There is no definitive diagnostic test.

Treatment of PCS includes rest and decreasing sound and light stimulation. Analgesic medication should be used conservatively in low doses and for short periods of time. More research is needed to determine the role of psychotropic medications.

The prognosis of PCS is generally excellent, with full remission of symptoms in most patients. However, for those athletes experiencing ongoing symptoms for a year, full recovery is less likely. Athletes experiencing ongoing PCS are at an increased risk for second impact syndrome (SIS, see following text) and should take special precautions to avoid additional brain injury.

SECOND IMPACT SYNDROME

SIS is a serious (sometimes fatal) syndrome that results from cerebral edema following a second head trauma before symptoms of an initial concussion resolve. It is most common in younger athletes and likely results from a cerebrovascular autoregulatory mismatch following additional head trauma that occurs during the incomplete resolution phase of an initial concussion. The initial concussion need not be severe. Schneider (1973) first reported on the death of two young athletes following minor head trauma incurred after an initial low-grade sports concussion [18]. In 1984, Saunders and Harbaug coined the term "second impact syndrome" [19], reporting on the death of a 19-year-old American football player who returned to play after a brief loss of consciousness during a game. He sustained a minor second head trauma, reported a headache, and collapsed and died 4 days later. Autopsy results demonstrated massive cerebral edema without significant evidence of hematoma. This is considered the hallmark of SIS. The syndrome apparently occurs preferentially in younger concussion victims due to a predisposition to failure of cerebrovascular autoregulation, and the inability of the young brain arterial tree to compensate for acute hypertension following a posttraumatic catecholamine surge. The elevated blood pressure results in a rapid increase in intracranial pressure and increased cerebral blood volume expansion. This cascade of events results in malignant cerebral edema, the primary etiology of the subsequent morbidity and mortality [20, 21]. The risk of SIS is a primary reason to develop side-line return-to-play criteria for all athletes, especially young ones.

CHRONIC TRAUMATIC ENCEPHALOPATHY

Within the last few decades, the topic of concussion in athletes has gained an enormous amount of attention. Much of this attention has focused on the potential late effects of repeated concussions and subconcussive hits to the head. Once thought to occur only within the sport of boxing, CTE is a delayed presentation of an irreversible, degenerative brain disease that affects athletes (and nonathletes) who have sustained repeated concussions and/or repeated subconcussive hits to the head. Symptoms of CTE may mimic those of Alzheimer's disease, Parkinson's disease, or frontotemporal dementia, although mood symptoms, especially depression, suicidality, poor impulse control, irritability, and aggressive or violent behavior, often characterize the disease [5–7, 22].

History

The idea that sustaining repeated hits to the head can lead to long-term degenerative brain changes in athletes was first reported in the medical literature in 1928 by the American pathologist, Dr. Harrison Martland [23]. Dr. Martland had studied the brains of deceased boxers who exhibited a common spectrum of symptoms said to occur in up to half of all career boxers at the time. Symptoms included slowed movement, tremors, confusion, and speech problems. Dr. Martland concluded that these common symptoms were the direct result of sustaining repeated head injuries and the brain damage induced by such events. Martland described these fighters as being "Punch Drunk."

Several years later, Millspaugh coined the term "dementia pugilistica," emphasizing the severe cognitive deficits typical of the disease and its propensity to affect only boxers [24]. By the 1960s, the disease had been identified in a handful of nonathletes. This necessitated a new name for the disease, hence the inception of the current term "chronic traumatic encephalopathy." Interestingly, this term did not catch on at the time, and has only recently resurfaced. The disease had remained predominantly associated with the sport of boxing up until the last few decades.

In the years that followed, dementia pugilistica remained a poorly characterized and enigmatic disease, receiving little attention among the medical and sports communities. Nonetheless, research continued, albeit slowly. In 1973, Corsellis *et al.* reported their research findings on the affected brains of several deceased boxers [25]. These findings would go on to characterize the disease and distinguish it from other neurodegenerative disorders.

In 2005, Omalu published the first study identifying CTE in a professional American football player [26]. Soon after, CTE was confirmed in several more American football players and athletes within the sports of hockey, soccer, and wrestling [11, 27, 28]. These recent research findings have ignited grave concerns among the worldwide medical, sports, and legal communities in revealing that CTE is more widespread and prevalent among athletes than previously assumed.

Epidemiology

The prevalence of CTE among athletes is unknown, as there have been no randomized neuropathological studies of CTE in deceased athletes to date. The number of neuropathologically confirmed cases of CTE is limited by the number of athletes' brains donated to CTE research, which has thus far been limited due to the long-standing assumption that the disease only affects boxers. By 2009, there were only 51 neuropathologically confirmed cases of CTE. Forty-six of these cases involved athletes, and 39 of these were boxers [9].

CTE can potentially affect athletes of any sport in which a hit to the head is possible. This includes but is not limited to boxing, sparring, martial arts, football, rugby, lacrosse, soccer, hockey, baseball, professional wrestling, horseback riding, parachuting, car and motorcycle racing, and skiing [9].

The risk appears to be correlated with the frequency and severity of head injuries, and likely varies from sport to sport and by position within each sport. Several nonsevere hits to the head may be as dangerous as a single concussive injury [9]. The linemen in football fall under this category, as they sustain thousands of subconcussive hits to the head over the course of a single season. Often, these hits are not associated with any acute symptoms.

Child and adolescent athletes are potentially at risk as well. CTE was recently identified in the brain of a deceased 18-year-old multisport athlete, who suffered multiple concussions playing high-school football [29].

Clinical presentation

The clinical signs and symptoms of CTE are insidious and do not usually manifest until years or decades after exposure to repeated head trauma. Typically, onset occurs in midlife, much earlier than symptom onset in sporadic Alzheimer's disease, and often earlier than symptom onset in frontotemporal dementia [16]. In a 2009 review by McKee *et al.*, the average age of symptom onset among 33 documented and neuropathologically confirmed cases of CTE was 42 years. Ages of onset ranged from 25 to 76 years [5].

The initial symptoms are variable among athletes. The most common early manifestations of CTE include short-term memory problems, executive dysfunction (often involving planning, organization, and multitasking), depression, apathy, suicidality, irritability, emotional instability, poor impulse control (including outbursts of angry or violent behavior, or having a short fuse), confusion, unsteadiness, gait abnormalities, parkinsonism, dysarthria, and headaches [8].

Symptom progression is often slow and gradual, and there may be a period of years or even decades between initial symptom presentation and symptomatic progression [5, 8]. There have been an alarming number of cases, however, in which the athlete went on to experience a tragic death, for example, by suicide.

Memory loss in CTE can be similar to the early memory loss in Alzheimer's disease, involving deterioration of short-term and episodic memory [30]. The family of one affected athlete reported that the individual would repeatedly ask the same questions over and over.

He did not recall why he went to the store unless he had a list, and he would ask to rent a movie that he had already seen. Another athlete was reported to frequently forget what he was talking about while holding conversations, and he frequently forgot where he kept his wallet, checkbook, and keys [30].

Major depressive disorder, parasuicide, and suicide are disproportionately common in CTE [7].

Diagnosis

Currently, the only way to differentiate CTE from other neurodegenerative diseases is by postmortem examination of the brain. More specifically, CTE is defined by a characteristic distribution of abnormal tau proteins. More research is needed in this area. Utilization of radiologic imaging modalities or blood or cerebrospinal fluid biomarkers may prove to be of diagnostic utility.

Diagnosing CTE in a living individual poses a diagnostic challenge and is at best an educated guess. As mentioned, the symptoms of CTE often resemble those of early Alzheimer's or Parkinson's disease. Furthermore, it has been demonstrated that previous brain injury places an individual at increased risk for Alzheimer's disease [31].

Neuropathology

CTE belongs to a class of neuropathologically defined degenerative diseases known as tauopathies. Tauopathies are characterized by the abnormal accumulation of tau protein within the brain. Under normal circumstances, tau protein plays a role in microtubule stabilization within neurons, astrocytes, and oligodendricites. In other words, normally functioning tau plays a role in stabilizing the physical framework of neurons and neuron-supporting cells in the brain. In tauopathies, tau proteins become hyperphosphorylated, rendering them chemically unstable. In order to become more stable, the hyperphosphorylated tau undergoes a change in shape. This change in shape subsequently renders the previously soluble tau protein insoluble. The insoublized tau then accumulates over time. These insoluble aggregates are known as paired helical fragments (PHF). Although it has been postulated that these aggregates play a direct causative role in neurodegeneration in tauopathies, damaging all nearby neurons and neuron-supporting cells, the exact mechanism of disease has yet to be confirmed [5].

The most well-known tauopathy is Alzheimer's disease, characterized by abnormally phosphorylated tau proteins (neurofibrillary tangles) as well as β-amyloid peptide deposits, called amyloid plaques. CTE is easily differentiated from other tauopathies by postmortem examination of the brain. Unlike patients with Alzheimer's disease, only about half of all CTE patients are found to have β-amyloid deposits. Furthermore, the pattern of distribution of abnormal tau aggregates is distinct and unique to CTE. Neuropil neurites and glial tangles are found in the frontal and temporal cortices in a characteristic patchy, irregular distribution [5]. Abnormal tau accumulates preferentially within the depths of sulci, around blood vessels, and in the superficial cortical layers. Abnormal tau is often distributed in the limbic and paralimbic regions, diencephalon, brain stem, and subcortical white matter [9].

Other neuropathological abnormalities are found in CTE. These include abnormalities in β-amyloid and TAR DNA-binding protein (TDP-43). β-amyloid deposits, which characterize amyloid plaques in the brains of patients with Alzheimer's disease, have been found in 40–45% of individuals with confirmed CTE. Aβ deposits have been observed most frequently in CTE in the form of widespread diffuse plaques, although β-amyloid has also been found in the form of neuritic plaques and amyloid angiopathy. TDP-43 is the major disease protein found in the brains of patients with an uncommon form of frontotemporal dementia (frontotemporal lobar dementia with ubiquitin or FTLD-U, now referred to as FTLD-TDP). TDP-43 has been found in the brains and spinal cords of the majority of amyotrophic lateral sclerosis (ALS) patients, and the accumulation of it has now been found in the brains of over 80% of currently confirmed cases of CTE. Furthermore, it has been discovered in the anterior horns of the spinal cords of three athletes with CTE who developed progressive motor neuron disease several years prior to death. This suggests that some individuals with CTE, who acquire TDP-43 proteinopathy that extends into the spinal cord, may present with a motor neuron disease that mimics the symptoms of ALS.

A number of nonspecific gross brain findings are common in CTE. These include brain atrophy and reduction of brain weight, thinning of the corpus callosum, cavum septum pellucidum with fenestrations, enlargement of the lateral and third ventricles, and scarring of the cerebellar tonsils. Atrophy is common in the frontal and temporal cortices, the medial temporal lobe, parietal lobe, and, infrequently, the occipital lobe. Other common gross brain findings include hippocampal sclerosis, atrophy of the hypothalamic floor, shrinkage of the mammillary bodies, and pallor of the substantia nigra [3].

Risk factors

CTE is the only neurodegenerative dementia with a known cause: head trauma. Head trauma is the largest risk factor for CTE. Preventing the occurrence and recurrence of head trauma will have the greatest effect in preventing CTE. Risk conferred by other variables is not yet known. For example, it is unknown whether a single hit to the head can lead to CTE, or what severity of trauma is sufficient to activate the disease. Furthermore, it is unknown whether numerous subconcussive head injuries confer the same risk as a few severe concussive blows.

Other variables related to head trauma may also play a role. For instance, it is unknown if sustaining a concussion prior to resolution of a previous concussion is intrinsically a risk factor. An indirect risk is conferred, because this would place the player at greater risk of subsequent concussion. Likewise, the sport played and position played within each sport may be relevant, as type and severity of head trauma varies within each of these categories [3].

It is unknown what role intrinsic risk factors play. For example, it is unknown what role age plays. There is also the issue of genetic susceptibility. Not every athlete to sustain repeated head trauma acquires CTE. Some studies investigated the role of ApoE alleles, which are known to play a role in Alzheimer's disease [32]. It is unknown which genes are protective and which confer greater risk. An individual's state of health and lifestyle at the time of injury or post injury may play a role. It is unknown what role comorbid medical or psychiatric illnesses might play. Likewise, a large proportion of athletes with neuropathologically documented CTE were known to heavily abuse substances either before, during, or after disease onset. It is unknown whether this was a contributing factor for CTE versus more of a consequence of the disease. Finally, "cognitive reserve" may also play a role in the onset and course of CTE.

FUTURE RESEARCH

The need for ongoing, prospective clinical trials cannot be overstated. The extant literature consists largely of case reports, animal studies, and clinical observations. As the culture of sports continues to evolve and to acknowledge the risks associated with head trauma to athletes, better longitudinal data should be available to identify risk factors and biomarkers to help determine when it is safe for a brain-injured athlete to return to play (versus when they should consider noncontact sports participation). Advanced neuroimaging, such as diffusion tensor imaging, offers hope of an expanded understanding of core etiology, and needs to be more widely employed. Finally, possibly the most important future need is to continue to develop and globally distribute high-quality, innovative educational material to everyone involved in sports on brain safe participation. The goal of sports psychiatrists from around the world should not be to fundamentally change, or eliminate, sports participation, but rather to make the game safer for participants. To achieve this goal, a collaborative effort between basic scientists, clinical researchers, clinicians, trainers, coaches, and athletes will be required.

Case Study

A 17-year-old woman soccer player attempts to head a ball and gets elbowed in the right temple. She is temporarily dazed, but stays in the match. During half-time, she experiences vertigo, mild confusion, and cannot remember her position on the field. She does not report her symptoms to the coach, but her teammates notice a change in her behavior. She starts the second half, but is slow to react and is out of position. Despite being the high scorer on the team, the coach substitutes for her after 8 min of play. The player initially protests being substituted, but realizes she is not able to perform.

Comment: Despite not losing consciousness, this player sustained a concussion, not from the header, but from the elbow to her head. Concussions in soccer typically result from head-to-head contact, elbow or shoulder to the side of the head, being kicked in the head, or hitting the head on the pitch. In this case, the athlete did not want to come out of the match and did not inform her teammates or coach of her symptoms. It was fortunate she was taken out of the match, as she was at risk for SIS from even a minor second head trauma. Current rule changes in many contact sports now require a player to be cleared medically before returning to play. Furthermore, these rule changes are increasingly backed up by laws both requiring removal from play for symptoms of concussion and medical clearance before return to play. These changes should help prevent the occurrence of SIS. To be maximally effective, coaches and players need to be knowledgeable about the initial signs and symptoms of concussion, especially in players who sustain contact to the head or neck during play. A bruised brain is not the same as a bruised ankle.

REFERENCES

1. Google Alerts. Head trauma and concussion in athletes 2012. www.google.com/alerts. Accessed on 18 January 2013.
2. Google.com, Sports concussion 2012. www.google.com. Accessed on 18 January 2013.
3. Khurana VG, Kaye AH. An overview of concussion in sport. *Journal of Clinical Neuroscience* 2012;19: 1–11.
4. Meehan WP, Bachur RG. Sport-related concussion. *Pediatrics* 2009;123:114–123.

5. McKee AC, Cantu RC, Nowinski CJ, Hedley-Whyte ET, Gavett BE, Budson AE, Santini VE, Lee HS, Kubilus CA, Stern RA. Chronic traumatic encephalopathy in athletes: progressive tauopathy after repetitive head injury. *Journal of Neuropathology & Experimental Neurology* 2009;68:709–735.

6. Gavett BE, Stern RA, McKee AC. Chronic traumatic encephalopathy: a potential late effect of sport-related concussive and subconcussive head trauma. *Clinics in Sports Medicine* 2011;30:179–188.

7. Jorge RE, Robinson RG, Moser D, Tateno A, Crespo-Facorro B, Arndt S. Major depression following traumatic brain injury. *Archives of General Psychiatry* 2004;61:42–50.

8. Stern RA, Riley DO, Daneshvar DH, Nowinski CJ, Cantu RC, McKee AC. Long-term consequences of repetitive brain trauma: chronic traumatic encephalopathy. *Physical Medicine and Rehabilitation* 2011;3(10S2):S460–S467.

9. Victoroff J, Baron D. Diagnosis and treatment of sports-related traumatic brain injury. *Psychiatric Annals* 2012;42(10):365–370.

10. Cantu RC. Chronic traumatic encephalopathy in the National Football League. *Neurosurgery* 2007;61(2):223–225.

11. McKee AC, Gavett BE, Stern RA, Nowinski CJ, Cantu RC, Kowall NW, Perl DP, Hedley-Whyte ET, Price B, Sullivan C, Morin P, Kubilus CA, Daneshvar DH, Wulff M, Budson AE. TDP-43 proteinopathy and motor neuron disease in chronic traumatic encephalopathy. *Journal of Neuropathology & Experimental Neurology* 2010;60(9):918–929.

12. Overview and features of the ImPACT test 2012. www.impacttest.com/about/background. Accessed on 18 January 2013.

13. McCrea M, Guskiewicz K, Randolph C, Barr WB, Hammeke TA, Marshall SW, Kelly JP. Effects of symptom-free waiting period on clinical outcome and risk of reinjury after sport-related concussion. *Neurosurgery* 2009;65:876–883.

14. Miller H. Mental after-effects of head injury. *Proceedings of the Royal Society of Medicine* 1966;59(3):257–261.

15. Ellemberg D, Henry LC, Macciocchi SN. Advances in sport concussion assessment. *Neurotrauma* 2009;26:2365–2382.

16. Lincoln AE, Caswell SV, Almquist JL, Dunn RE, Norris JB, Hinton RY. Trends in concussion incidence in high school sports: a prospective 11 year study. *American Journal of Sports Medicine* 2011;39:958–963.

17. Cairns H, Holbourn H. Head injuries in motor-cyclists: with special reference to crash helmets. *British Medical Journal* 1943;1:591–598.

18. Wetjen NM, Pichelmann MA, Atkinson JLD. Second impact syndrome: concussion and second injury brain complications. *Journal of American College of Surgeons* 2010;211:553–557.

19. Saunders R, Harbaugh R. The second impact in catastrophic contact-sports head trauma. *The Journal of the American Medical Association* 1984;252:538–539.

20. Cantu RC. Second impact syndrome. *Clinics in Sports Medicine* 1998;17:37–44.

21. Mori T, Katayama Y, Kawamata T. Acute hemispheric swelling associated with thin subdural hematomas: pathophysiology of repetitive head injury in sports. *Acta Neurochirurgica* 2006;96(Suppl.): 40–43.

22. Gavett BE, Cantu RC, Shenton M, Lin AP, Nowinski CJ, McKee AC, Stern RA. Clinical appraisal of chronic traumatic encephalopathy: current perspectives and future directions. *Current Opinion in Neurology* 2011;24:525–531.

23. Martland HS. Punch drunk. *The Journal of the American Medical Association* 1928;91:1103–1107.

24. Millspaugh JA. Dementia Pugilistica. *US Naval Medicine Bulletin* 1937;35:297–303.

25. Corsellis JA, Bruton CJ, Freeman-Browne D. The aftermath of boxing. *Psychological Medicine* 1973;3:270–303.

26. Omalu BI, DeKosky ST, Minster RL, Kamboh MI, Hamilton RO, Wecht CH. Chronic traumatic encephalopathy in a National Football League player. *Neurosurgery* 2005;57(1):128–134; discussion 128–134.

27. Guskiewics KM, Marshall SW, Bailes J, Cantu RC, Randolph C, Jordan BD. Association between recurrent concussion and late-life cognitive impairment in retired professional football players. *Neurosurgery* 2005;57(4):719–726.

28. Schwarz A. (2011). "Hockey Brawler Paid Price, With Brain Trauma". *The New York Times,* March 3, p. A1.

29. "18 year old high school football player". Case Studies. Center for the Study of Chronic Traumatic Encephalopathy. July 2012. http://www.bu.edu/cste/case-studies/18-year-old/. Accessed on 12 December 2012.

30. Mcrea M, Kelly JP, Randolph C, Cisler R, Berger L. Immediate neurocognitive effects of concussion. *Neurosurgery* 2002;50:1032–1040, discussion 1040–2.

31. Costanza A, Weber K, Gandy S, Bouras C, Hof PR, Giannakopoulos P, Canuto A. Review: contact sport-related chronic traumatic encephalopathy in the elderly: clinical expression and structural substrates. *Neuropathology and Applied Neurobiology* 2011;37(6):570–584.

32. Verghese PB, Castellano JM, Holtzman DM. Apolipoprotein E in Alzheimer's disease and other neurologic disorders. *Lancet Neurology* 2011;10:241–252.

10 Posttraumatic Stress in Athletes

Thomas Wenzel[1] and Li Jing Zhu[1,2]

[1] Division of Social Psychiatry, Medical University of Vienna, Austria
[2] Physical Education College, Zheng Zhou University, Peoples Republic of China

KEY POINTS

- Athletes may be exposed to traumatic events that can lead to long-term psychological and psychosomatic suffering.
- After an athlete experiences a traumatic event, sequelae may include posttraumatic stress disorder (PTSD), but also other reactions, especially culture-specific patterns of symptoms and comorbidities such as depression. Comorbid substance abuse can hide unrecognized PTSD.
- Posttraumatic symptoms in athletes interfere with rehabilitation and performance.
- Support and treatment of posttraumatic symptoms in athletes require specialized care. Ethical dilemmas can develop, especially when traumatic stress is resulting from abuse, from events related to overtraining, or from inadequate care or violence within teams.

GENERAL ASPECTS

While stress and special challenges are common in the life of athletes, "out of the ordinary" sport-specific adverse events such as severe sport injuries, lethal accidents, or suicide as well as events encountered in life "outside of sport" can lead to long-lasting reactive symptoms or suffering, a process commonly described as traumatization. On a diagnostic level, traumatization can be reflected in nonspecific disorders such as depression, but attention has been increasingly drawn to more specific disorders such as posttraumatic stress disorder (PTSD), which usually develops only after severe stressors. By now, PTSD has become a well-understood problem that has come a long way since its inclusion in the Diagnostic and Statistical Manual of Mental Disorders (DSM) III and later the International Classification of Diseases (ICD) 10. The awareness that severely distressful life events lead to clinically relevant and at times long-lasting psychological reactions had previously not been a generally accepted paradigm [1] and is still not easily applied in sport. Since its first description after the Vietnam War, the initially narrow list of events that could potentially trigger PTSD, as reflected in the DSM criterion A (Box 10.1), has been extended to include such diverse "everyday" events as child birth and traffic accidents [2]. In recent years, PTSD has become

Clinical Sports Psychiatry: An International Perspective, First Edition. Edited by David A. Baron, Claudia L. Reardon and Steven H. Baron.
© 2013 John Wiley & Sons, Ltd. Published 2013 by John Wiley & Sons, Ltd.

one of the most frequent subjects of psychiatric research and has been identified as a crucial public health problem in, for example, postconflict zones. However, only a limited number of studies (as discussed later in this chapter) have addressed the problem in athletes. The previous bias of perceiving healthy athletes as either protected from or less prone to more severe mental health problems has changed to an increasing awareness that a number of specific psychiatric diagnoses, such as eating disorders [3], are even more frequent than in the general population. Moreover, there is an increasing number of reported athlete suicides [4] linked to sport-related stressors and to the interaction with other factors inherent in the setting of especially competitive sports.

Box 10.1   DSM IV criteria for posttraumatic stress disorder [5]

Criterion A: stressor

The person has been exposed to a traumatic event in which both of the following have been present:

1. The person has experienced, witnessed, or been confronted with an event or events that involve actual or threatened death or serious injury, or a threat to the physical integrity of oneself or others.
2. The person's response involved intense fear, helplessness, or horror. *Note*: In children, it may be expressed instead by disorganized or agitated behavior.

Criterion B: intrusive recollection

The traumatic event is persistently reexperienced in at least one of the following ways:

1. Recurrent and intrusive distressing recollections of the event, including images, thoughts, or perceptions. Note: in young children, repetitive play may occur in which themes or aspects of the trauma are expressed.
2. Recurrent distressing dreams of the event. Note: in children, there may be frightening dreams without recognizable content.
3. Acting or feeling as if the traumatic event were recurring (includes a sense of reliving the experience, illusions, hallucinations, and dissociative flashback episodes, including those that occur upon awakening or when intoxicated). *Note*: In children, trauma-specific reenactment may occur.
4. Intense psychological distress at exposure to internal or external cues that symbolize or resemble an aspect of the traumatic event.
5. Physiologic reactivity upon exposure to internal or external cues that symbolize or resemble an aspect of the traumatic event.

Criterion C: avoidance/numbing

Persistent avoidance of stimuli associated with the trauma and numbing of general responsiveness (not present before the trauma), as indicated by at least three of the following:

1. Efforts to avoid thoughts, feelings, or conversations associated with the trauma
2. Efforts to avoid activities, places, or people that arouse recollections of the trauma
3. Inability to recall an important aspect of the trauma
4. Markedly diminished interest or participation in significant activities
5. Feeling of detachment or estrangement from others
6. Restricted range of affect (e.g., unable to have loving feelings)
7. Sense of foreshortened future (e.g., does not expect to have a career, marriage, children, or a normal life span)

Criterion D: hyperarousal

Persistent symptoms of increasing arousal (not present before the trauma), indicated by at least two of the following:

1. Difficulty falling or staying asleep
2. Irritability or outbursts of anger
3. Difficulty concentrating
4. Hypervigilance
5. Exaggerated startle response

Criterion E: duration

Duration of the disturbance (symptoms in B, C, and D) is more than 1 month.

Criterion F: functional significance

The disturbance causes clinically significant distress or impairment in social, occupational, or other important areas of functioning.

Specify if:
Acute: if duration of symptoms is less than 3 months
Chronic: if duration of symptoms is 3 months or more

Specify if:
With or without delayed onset: Onset of symptoms at least 6 months after the stressor

For the present discussion, posttraumatic reactions in athletes will be considered. However, such reactions can also become a problem for other exposed team members such as trainers and coaches or for sport audiences and family members.

Types of traumatic experiences suffered by athletes, or anyone else with PTSD, may include:

- Being the actual threatened or injured party in a trauma
- Being an observer of a trauma experienced by another person, either while being present, through live or recorded media, or in some cases by emotionally sharing with immediate victims (indirect traumatization)

Case Study

Ben, an Olympic ski athlete and frequent participant in world cup races, observed a fatal accident of a close friend during especially bad track conditions. He had protested against the continuation of the competition because of the dismal weather and track conditions, but had withdrawn his objections in the face of psychological pressure from coaches and officials. After the accident, he was frequently distracted by vivid memories of it, suffered anxiety when weather conditions worsened, experienced impaired concentration, awoke during the night from nightmares in which he lost control in dangerous ski situations, and ruminated with feelings of guilt because of a growing conviction that the accident would not have happened if he had persisted in his protests. He became increasingly anxious in training situations, avoiding difficult weather conditions and suffering from declining performance. Psychotherapy identified significant feelings of guilt and anger, and he gradually recovered his prior self-confidence.

RISK FACTORS

Conditions that may determine whether an event leads to lasting posttraumatic symptoms include the following:

Preexisting factors

Preexisting factors include aspects of the athlete that may increase the likelihood that he will develop PTSD from a given trauma [6]. Trait-based coping and more general factors such as genetic [7] and gender factors are only partially predictive of later development of posttraumatic stress. While athletes are frequently seen as more resilient than the general population to common stressors, few actual data are available to determine if this is the case in extreme and unexpected situations. Recent models indicate that coping consists of a complex set of state and trait characteristics that can change dynamically with the situation [8]. Coping strategies that might protect against disruptive stress in potentially traumatic events (such as observing lethal accidents) might not necessarily be the ones that make an athlete successful in sport. Additionally, trait coping strategies utilized by athletes after injuries in sport (potentially traumatic experiences) might differ among different sports and cultures [9].

Aspects of the event

Severe or unusual violence such as sexual abuse or torture can be expected to lead to reactions and potentially PTSD in most people exposed [10]. However, the meaning and overall disruptive quality of an event, regardless of how severe, will vary among people experiencing the same type of event. Situational, emotional, and neurobiological factors associated with the trauma help to determine its impact [11–13].

Events in the case of sport could be classified as those that are frequent and somewhat expected, such as common injuries, and those unrelated to or uncharacteristic of the training and competitive environments. Earlier research in sports psychology had focused mainly on the sequelae of sport injuries and indicated a considerable impact even of minor injuries, and an even more severe impact of "catastrophic" injuries (see also Heil [14] for an overview). Even in these earlier publications, the meaning of an event in the specific setting of sport had been observed to be an important factor determining psychological impact [15, 16] in addition to physical impact [17]. Threat to physical integrity [18] – a factor that has been demonstrated to be of major relevance [19] – is not surprisingly of special importance to athletes, who have invested much into perfecting their bodies and physical performance. The impact of an injury includes immediate and long-term physical sequelae, including pain and physical limitations as well as psychological, economic, and social sequelae. An athlete's social identity and long-term life plan are often dependent on health and integrity. Events that are highly distressing for athletes might not be objectively life threatening, but nonetheless can have a devastating impact on a career. Furthermore, the events can include "catastrophic" injuries to self-esteem and social expectations, as seen, for example, with the loss of a crucial game or with public recognition as a "doper." These latter types of "injuries" might be especially devastating to competitive athletes whose life and identity can depend on their sport career. Some authors have discussed athletic retirement as a potential cause of PTSD [8]. However, it is the authors' opinion that retirement should be seen as neither sport-specific nor fitting into present PTSD models. However, it can obviously be a major stressor and lead to mood disorders or other indicators of failing adaptation to a changing environment.

Until a first severe injury is experienced, athletes may view themselves as "invincible" and part of a perfect world, and, consequently, even in a situation in which an incurred injury is not severe, this image of a consistent and safe world might be shattered. Complex psychodynamic models of trauma address these aspects, including the possibility of narcissistic injury and increased importance given to the impact of an event based on its emotional meaning [20].

Responsibility and identity in this context can be strongly influenced by culture. The meaning of an event may be different in "universalistic cultures," wherein identity is more strongly group based, and "particularistic cultures," with a strong focus on individual identity. Failing – and accidents with loss of capacity can be seen as that – in a universalistic society can mean also failing the group and an end to the athlete's "social life" as it was perceived before the event.

Besides accidents and injuries, some potentially traumatic experiences receive heightened attention in sport. Sexual abuse, a common problem in any type of "closed" environment with attendant increased risk of abuse of dependency and transference, is an important possible factor in the development of PTSD and related disorders, including eating disorders [21]. As discussed in Chapter 16, sexual abuse has recently become a more frequently reported issue in sport [22], and published cases indicate that the close relationship between athletes and coaches carries a special risk. Prevention and early recognition should be implemented by sports organizations, as sexual abuse needs to be seen as comparable to eating disorders and doping in being potential severe challenges to sport as a healthy environment.

As discussed in Chapter 8, suicide among athletes is an event more common than previously realized [4]. Team members, including coaches, as well as family members, need special attention as "suicide survivors" vulnerable to posttraumatic symptoms. "Psychological autopsy" studies on the impact of suicide on such survivors, as well as on events leading to suicide in athletes, are still largely missing.

In addition to potentially traumatic events directly related to sport, athletes can obviously be exposed to the same "ordinary" potentially traumatic events as the general population. Such events include accidents or violence against themselves or family members. Private life cannot be disregarded in work with athletes.

Coping and the social environment after the event

Finally, recent research has demonstrated that social factors, such as the reaction of those in the athlete's social environment, can influence interpretation and later coping with an event. Recent studies show that positive social support is a key factor in the determination of whether a distressing event leads to more permanent psychological injury [23]. Blaming the victim for "irresponsible" behavior leading to the injury or accident (best studied in sexual abuse) might contribute to a negative or catastrophic evaluation of the event or of the victim, thereby impacting self-esteem and interfering with normal recovery [24]. This can reinforce the well-documented tendency of victims to develop self-blaming [24, 25].

The still-limited data on PTSD in athletes indicate the importance of all three of the previously mentioned categories of factors impacting development of posttraumatic stress symptoms.

OTHER RESEARCH ON DIAGNOSIS OF POSTTRAUMATIC STRESS SYMPTOMS IN ATHLETES

Studies as far back as the 1970s [26] demonstrated posttraumatic stress in sport, for example, by showing a comparable incidence of posttraumatic stress reactions in work-injured and ski-accident groups. In early publications, the issue of litigation as a driver of PTSD symptoms in athletes was much discussed. For example, Teff and others [27, 28] explored compensation for "nervous shock" in the context of the "Hillsborough football disaster." However, more recently, litigation has not been an issue in the discussion of posttraumatic stress reactions in sport.

The general impact of sport injuries independent from posttraumatic stress symptoms has been explored by a number of authors [14], but will not be discussed in this chapter per se.

Mountain climbing accidents [29] have been an obvious focus of research because of the dangers and relatively high mortality, which can be associated with posttraumatic stress and affective symptoms in survivors. However, rates of such symptoms might be lower than expected [30] in the case of mountain guides (2.7%), whose role might best be compared to coaches due to their special responsibilities. Sommer observed a high sense of coherence as a possible explanation and protective factor against PTSD development in general (though not limited to mountain accidents as primary events). This relative protection against PTSD symptoms may be related to extreme situation training designed to develop resilience, which may translate to other settings.

FURTHER SPECIFIC REACTIONS TO EXTREME STRESS IN SPORT

PTSD has a well-demonstrated severe impact on functioning, quality of life, and even physical health. However, it is only one of a number of possible sequelae of severe life events that should be considered [31, 32].

Complex PTSD

The conflict between the original conceptualization of PTSD and the present broader understanding reflects both the importance of the subjective evaluation of events and an integrative model that includes a primary neuropsychological fight/flight response pattern at the core of the PTSD symptomatology. Socio-psychological symptoms such as the aforementioned feelings of shame and guilt, which are common after extreme life events even when no sufficient objective reason for feeling that way can be identified, as well as loss of trust and withdrawal, are seen as part of the extended "complex" PTSD model [33].

Acute stress disorder

Acute stress disorder (ASD) is a transient phenomenon (again reflecting aspects of an increased fight/flight response) that consists of symptoms similar to PTSD and by definition lasts less than 1 month after exposure to a stressful event. It might not require immediate treatment, since it very well could resolve on its own, though some studies indicate that the development of ASD might indicate a higher probability of later developing PTSD [34].

Posttraumatic embitterment disorder

Posttraumatic embitterment disorder (PED) is a new model describing generalization of negative expectations and beliefs [35], though data on athletes besides anecdotal observations are still missing.

Culture-specific symptoms and disorders

Following recent developments in the understanding of posttraumatic stress, cultural and social factors should be given special consideration. Culture has been observed to shape not only sensitivities and conflicts but also characteristic reactions to stressful or traumatic events. The concept of culture-specific "idioms of distress" (IoDs) has been proposed in this context [36]. IoDs describe reactive cognitive and behavioral patterns common in certain cultures in stressful situations or events and are usually recognized as a sign of distress or call for help by members of the same culture. In earlier times, the well-known "faint" in embarrassing situations could be seen as such an idiom. IoDs reflect health belief models prevalent in a culture and that shape the interpretation and presentation of symptoms. They can also reflect stigma of mental health symptoms through a focus on perceived "physical" symptoms rather than acknowledgement of psychiatric ones. Examples in Chinese athletes include disorders such as "kidney-type depression" or "acute shock wind" that are experienced as somatic processes triggered by external physical events. Physical symptoms associated with these conditions might well be of more concern to those affected than would be the more classic PTSD symptoms, which are more likely to draw the attention of mental health professionals. Athletes firmly anchored in their own culture must be supported based on a solid understanding of culture, or else important indicators of distress will be missed.

The meaning of events in the subculture of especially competitive athletes was discussed earlier in this chapter. In the recent, more open concept of posttraumatic stress spectrum disorders, it may be justified to include less apparently "severe" traumas. However, the recent postulation of a specific "sport PTSD" need not necessarily replace a more evidence-based and general, though "sport culture"-sensitive, approach.

Chronic pain

Recent studies have demonstrated possible interactions between PTSD and processing of pain related to physical injuries. The interactions appear to be more complex than explained by simple comorbidity [37–39]. Somatoform disorders – impairment and suffering exceeding what can be explained by existing injuries – might reflect these interactions on a diagnostic level, though not as a sufficient model to explain the complex reactive pattern involved [39].

Nonspecific disorders not limited to severe life events

Depression is quite frequently associated with PTSD. In exposed populations, it can develop either as a complication of PTSD or as a separate or alternative reactive pattern [40]. Other possible reactions include related reactions such as adjustment disorders that are characterized by symptoms of depression and/or anxiety in what may be unusually severe reactions to more common or less dangerous events. Some disorders common in athletes, especially eating disorders, have also been demonstrated to be frequently related to earlier trauma, especially sexual violence experienced in childhood or early adulthood independent of sport [21].

Bereavement

Bereavement-related reactions and complex grief after accidents in sport or in private life can lead to adjustment disorders [41], though the line between normal and atypical or persisting reactions indicating interrupted processes and inhibited coping is fluid. Cultural expectations can influence what is seen as an adequate reaction or period of mourning.

RELEVANCE

PTSD and other mental health problems related to stressful events can be relevant both as disorders to be recognized and treated as in any other setting and as underlying factors in achievement stagnation directly interfering with performance.

Impact and complications in sport

Development of PTSD has been demonstrated to be accompanied by reduction in prior sport and exercise activities, while concrete symptoms can be expected to interfere with performance and rehabilitation, especially if the event occurred during sport activities. At present, data do not give sufficient information on the influence of PTSD on the risk of first or repeated injuries, but life stress in general can increase sport injury risk [42], and characteristic PTSD symptoms or posttraumatic reactive high risk seeking could be expected to increase injury risk.

Especially if the traumatic event occurred in the sport setting, avoidance, as one of the most common symptoms of PTSD, can lead to avoidance of crucial or challenging activities within sport. Dissociation (a "blanking out" of the present perception of environment, frequently experienced as short amnestic episodes) can be part of the cognitive aspect of an avoidance pattern. The "intrusive recollection" symptom cluster can lead to generally or situation-dependent increased anxiety, flashbacks with distraction or even partial disorientation, or ruminations about the traumatic event. Reexposure to the original setting in training or in competition or even in indirectly related situations such as watching of the sport in media or in physical therapy after injuries might increase this cluster significantly. Nightmares and hypervigilance can contribute to disturbed sleep, which is potentially one of the most severe problems that should be addressed early in treatment. Disturbed sleep patterns interfere not only with performance [43], but, if chronic, also with general health. Hypervigilance can lead to an increased startle response or inadequate or premature action, as well as to increased irritability, distraction, and conflicts in the training and family environment. Besides interfering with performance, PTSD can also interfere with recovery and physical therapy after injuries, especially via its propensity to cause avoidance and feelings of shame or guilt. Mobilization and pain might increase intrusive symptoms and flashbacks, thereby leading to avoidance of participation in rehabilitation.

Complications

Secondary complications such as alcohol and substance abuse, common in other PTSD patient groups when used to "cope" with symptoms [44], should also be expected but could be overlooked in athletes. Alcohol is frequently used by untreated victims in an attempt to self-medicate disordered sleep, flashbacks, and anxiety, but only serves to further interfere with recovery of healthy sleep patterns. Tranquilizers such as benzodiazepines may be habit-forming and might interfere with "healthy" coping (see more information later in this chapter). Abuse and dependency patterns developing after stressful events should, therefore, be identified early in treatment.

Suicide risk is increased in some PTSD patients groups [45], and traumatic experiences have been suspected as a factor in some recent athletes' suicides.

CLINICAL CONSIDERATIONS AND INTERVENTIONS

While many people exposed to traumatic events recover well, especially if conditions are supportive, the potential severe impact of PTSD and associated disorders including possible interference with rehabilitation [46] should be considered, especially after events that challenge the athlete's basic self-confidence and perception of the world.

Data on early event-related interventions, for example, critical incident debriefing after a potentially high-impact event such as the death of a team member, confirm a potentially positive effect if applied by professionals but caution against unqualified interventions [47, 48]. Interventions might be offered to the team, or at least to those members most affected by the incident, by competent outside expert providers.

A setting integrating evidence-based standard strategies with sport- and culture-specific models should be created in treatment [31, 49, 50]. In the initial session, providers should stress the essentially normal neurophysiological nature of stress responses, for example, the role of fight/flight activation in PTSD. Psychoeducation should be provided to the athlete regarding the common misconception that early fight/flight symptoms are signs of "weakness" or signs of being "mentally disturbed." Countertransference [49] in the form of hesitancy to address difficult issues with athletes might interfere with early recognition and treatment. Care must be taken to address comorbid problems such as depression and suicidal ideation, and complications such as adverse coping strategies including harmful behavior, self-blaming, increased risk seeking, and substance abuse. Blunt brain trauma [51, 52] (discussed in Chapter 9) should be considered, as symptoms in post-concussion syndrome, such as irritability or concentration difficulty, partly overlap with or can mimic typical PTSD symptoms. Moreover, unrecognized brain trauma appears to be common. As in chronic pain, complex models are under development to describe interactions between PTSD and brain trauma [52].

Diagnosis of PTSD as part of a comprehensive approach can usually be based on clinical assessment, though standard questionnaires such as the Posttraumatic Stress Diagnostic Scale (PDS) [53] might be used for screening for the disorder. As part of a culturally sensitive approach, possible psychosocial conflicts interacting with posttraumatic stress, IoDs, culture-based coping, and health belief models should be recognized and respected.

In treatment, psychotherapy should be prioritized, both because of potential medication side effects and because of potential conflicts with doping regulations. Cognitive behavioral therapy (CBT) with a focus on concrete "here-and-now" problems in PTSD could be considered the first choice among psychotherapies in competitive settings. CBT and its special adaptation, trauma-focused CBT, have been well established as evidence-based, reliable, and efficient treatments that might be particularly well-suited for athletes (see also Chapter 11) [54]. Adjunctive tools such as eye movement desensitization and reprocessing (EMDR) [54] can be used to address specific problems such as intrusive imagery. In more complex psychodynamic reactions that might interact with earlier trauma or other mental health problems, time-limited psychodynamic psychotherapy should be considered, even if it might be more time-consuming and demanding. It has been demonstrated to be potentially effective, for example, in college athletes [55]. Regardless of the type of psychotherapy chosen, individual assessment and intervention addressing culture-based IoDs and modifying factors such as team expectations, expected coping, and support models should be a guiding principle. The long-term benefits to general health should be given priority over short-term functioning because of the already-mentioned impact and complications of insufficiently treated PTSD. If medications are considered [56], low-dose trazodone [57] can address sleep regulation, and decisions should be based on state-of-the-art guidelines and doping regulations. Selective serotonin reuptake inhibitors (SSRIs) for general symptoms might be the first choice, considering both physical side effect profiles and possible cytochrome factors associated with many medications, especially as plasma levels can be influenced considerably by ethnic-genetic background [58]. Benzodiazepines should usually be avoided due to the significant risk of dependency, potential conflicts with developing doping regimes, and, finally, general cautions in PTSD [59] that indicate they might interfere with posttraumatic recovery.

Sport in itself and as resilience training conversely has been observed to be either protective or supportive in recovery from PTSD through a sense of renewed mastery [60, 61]. The special situation of athletes developing PTSD or related disorders related to training or competition requires special consideration. After primary interventions and under careful observation, training might actually contribute to the recovery process. However, use of physical training as treatment should be employed with care, as unguided reexposure can lead to reactivation of memories and increased symptoms. Exposure steps may need to follow psychotherapeutic models in an integrated setting coordinated between physical therapy and physiotherapy, team members, the coach, and mental health expert(s). Social support by the team or coach can be an important adjunct to treatment.

CONCLUSIONS

Reactions to unusually severe events that include considerable threats to physical integrity, life, and social identity need special consideration in athletes, not only because of possible interference with performance but also because of the potential significant impact on long-term well-being and functioning. The classic reaction to such events is PTSD, but many other psychiatric symptoms and disorders may result as well. Special models of treatment and support, such as those seen with eating disorders in athletes [62], might be necessary to address the specific complexity of the athlete's particular situation and environment after a traumatic incident.

REFERENCES

1. Lowe B, Henningsen P, Herzog W. (2006) Post-traumatic stress disorder: history of a politically unwanted diagnosis. *Psychotherapie, Psychosomatik, medizinische Psychologie* **56**, 182–187.
2. Easton S. (2003) Psychological effects of road traffic accidents: issues, research and complexities for expert reports. *The Medico-Legal Journal* **71**, 130–137.
3. Sundgot-Borgen J, Torstveit MK. (2010) Aspects of disordered eating continuum in elite high-intensity sports. *Scandinavian Journal of Medicine & Science in Sports* **20**(Suppl. 2), 112–121.
4. Baum AL. (2005) Suicide in athletes: a review and commentary. *Clinics in Sports Medicine* **24**, 853–869, ix.

5. American Psychiatric Association (2000) *Diagnostic and Statistical Manual of Mental Disorders: DSM-IV-TR*. American Psychiatric Publishing, Inc., Washington, DC.

6. Udwin O, Boyle S, Yule W, Bolton D, O'Ryan D. (2000) Risk factors for long-term psychological effects of a disaster experienced in adolescence: predictors of post traumatic stress disorder. *Journal of Child Psychology and Psychiatry, and Allied Disciplines* **41**, 969–979.

7. Mellman TA, Alim T, Brown DD, Gorodetsky E, Buzas B, Lawson WB, *et al.* (2009) Serotonin polymorphisms and posttraumatic stress disorder in a trauma exposed African American population. *Depression and Anxiety* **26**, 993–997.

8. Melissa D. (2012) Coping with trauma in sport. In: Thatcher J, Jones Marc LD (eds.) *Coping and Emotions in Sport*. Routledge, Abingdon.

9. Rider SP, Hicks RA. (1995) Stress, coping, and injuries in male and female high school basketball players. *Perceptual and Motor Skills* **81**, 499–503.

10. Wenzel T. (2007) Torture. *Current Opinion in Psychiatry* **20**, 491–496.

11. van Zuiden M, Geuze E, Willemen HL, Vermetten E, Maas M, Amarouchi K, *et al.* (2012) Glucocorticoid receptor pathway components predict posttraumatic stress disorder symptom development: a prospective study. *Biological Psychiatry* **71**, 309–316.

12. Adams RE, Boscarino JA. (2006) Predictors of PTSD and delayed PTSD after disaster: the impact of exposure and psychosocial resources. *The Journal of Nervous and Mental Disease* **194**, 485–493.

13. Kazantzis N, Kennedy-Moffat J, Flett RA, Petrik AM, Long NR, Castell B. (2012) Predictors of chronic trauma-related symptoms in a community sample of New Zealand motor vehicle accident survivors. *Culture, Medicine and Psychiatry* **36**(3), 442–464.

14. Heil J. (1993) *Psychology of Sport Injury*. Human Kinetics Publishers, Champaign.

15. Hardy L. (1992) Psychological stress, performance, and injury in sport. *British Medical Bulletin* **48**, 615–629.

16. Brewer BW. (1993) Self-identity and specific vulnerability to depressed mood. *Journal of Personality* **61**, 343–364.

17. Smith AM, Stuart MJ, Wiese-Bjornstal DM, Milliner EK, O'Fallon WM, Crowson CS. (1993) Competitive athletes: preinjury and postinjury mood state and self-esteem. *Mayo Clinic Proceedings* **68**, 939–947.

18. Carlier IV, Lamberts RD, Gersons BP. (2000) The dimensionality of trauma: a multidimensional scaling comparison of police officers with and without posttraumatic stress disorder. *Psychiatry Research* **97**, 29–39.

19. Fontana A, Rosenheck R. (1999) A model of war zone stressors and posttraumatic stress disorder. *Journal of Traumatic Stress* **12**, 111–126.

20. Herman JL. (1997) *Trauma and Recovery* (Revised edition). Basic Books, New York.

21. Jonas S, Bebbington P, McManus S, Meltzer H, Jenkins R, Kuipers E, *et al.* (2011) Sexual abuse and psychiatric disorder in England: results from the 2007 Adult Psychiatric Morbidity Survey. *Psychological Medicine* **41**, 709–719.

22. Marks S, Mountjoy M, Marcus M. (2011) Sexual harassment and abuse in sport: the role of the team doctor. *British Journal of Sports Medicine* **46**, 905–908.

23. Meyer EC, Zimering R, Daly E, Knight J, Kamholz BW, Gulliver SB. (2012) Predictors of posttraumatic stress disorder and other psychological symptoms in trauma-exposed firefighters. *Psychological Services* **9**, 1–15.

24. Canton-Cortes D, Canton J, Cortes MR. (2012) The interactive effect of blame attribution with characteristics of child sexual abuse on posttraumatic stress disorder. *The Journal of Nervous and Mental Disease* **200**, 329–335.

25. Hendin H, Haas AP. (1991) Suicide and guilt as manifestations of PTSD in Vietnam combat veterans. *The American Journal of Psychiatry* **148**, 586–591.

26. Braverman M. (1977) Validity of psychotraumatic reactions. *Journal of Forensic Sciences* **22**, 654–662.

27. Teff H. (1992) The Hillsborough football disaster and claims for 'nervous shock' *Medicine, Science, and the Law* **32**, 251–254.

28. Kent GG, Kunkler AJ. (1992) Medical student involvement in a major disaster. *Medical Education* **26**, 87–91.

29. Peck DF, Robertson A, Zeffert S. (1996) Psychological sequelae of mountain accidents: a preliminary study. *Journal of Psychosomatic Research* **41**, 55–63.

30. Sommer I, Ehlert U. (2004) Adjustment to trauma exposure: prevalence and predictors of posttraumatic stress disorder symptoms in mountain guides. *Journal of Psychosomatic Research* **57**, 329–335.

31. Shearer DA, Mellalieu SD, Shearer CR. (2011) Posttraumatic stress disorder: a case study of an elite rifle shooter. *Journal of Clinical Sport Psychology* **5**, 134–147.

32. Belleville G, Guay S, Marchand A. (2009) Impact of sleep disturbances on PTSD symptoms and perceived health. *The Journal of Nervous and Mental Disease* **197**, 126–132.

33. Ide N, Paez A. (2000) Complex PTSD: a review of current issues. *International Journal of Emergency Mental Health* **2**, 43–49.

34. Birmes P, Brunet A, Carreras D, Ducasse JL, Charlet JP, Lauque D, *et al.* (2003) The predictive power of peritraumatic dissociation and acute stress symptoms for posttraumatic stress symptoms: a three-month prospective study. *The American Journal of Psychiatry* **160**, 1337–1339.

35. Linden M, Baumann K, Rotter M, Schippan B. (2007) The psychopathology of posttraumatic embitterment disorders. *Psychopathology* **40**, 159–165.

36. Hollan D. (2004) Self systems, cultural idioms of distress, and the psycho-bodily consequences of childhood suffering. *Transcultural Psychiatry* **41**, 62–79.

37. Alschuler KN, Otis JD. (2012) Coping strategies and beliefs about pain in veterans with comorbid chronic pain and significant levels of posttraumatic stress disorder symptoms. *European Journal of Pain* **16**, 312–319.

38. Asmundson GJ, Coons MJ, Taylor S, Katz J. (2002) PTSD and the experience of pain: research and clinical implications of shared vulnerability and mutual maintenance models. *Canadian Journal of Psychiatry (Revue canadienne de psychiatrie)* **47**, 930–937.

39. Basser DS. (2012) Chronic pain: a neuroscientific understanding. *Medical Hypotheses* **78**, 79–85.

40. Tural U, Onder E, Aker T. (2012) Effect of depression on recovery from PTSD. *Community Mental Health Journal* **48**, 161–166.

41. Kristensen P, Weisaeth L, Heir T. (2012) Bereavement and mental health after sudden and violent losses: a review. *Psychiatry* **75**, 76–97.

42. Kolt G, Kirkby R. (1996) Injury in Australian female competitive gymnasts: a psychological perspective. *The Australian Journal of Physiotherapy* **42**, 121–126.

43. Taheri M, Arabameri E. (2012) The effect of sleep deprivation on choice reaction time and anaerobic power of college student athletes. *Asian Journal of Sports Medicine* **3**, 15–20.

44. Subica AM, Claypoole KH, Wylie AM. (2012) PTSD'S mediation of the relationships between trauma, depression, substance abuse, mental health, and physical health in individuals with severe mental illness: evaluating a comprehensive model. *Schizophrenia Research* **136**, 104–109.

45. Tarrier N, Gregg L. (2004) Suicide risk in civilian PTSD patients – predictors of suicidal ideation, planning and attempts. *Social Psychiatry and Psychiatric Epidemiology* **39**, 655–661.

46. Taylor AH, May S. (1996) Threat and coping appraisal as determinants of compliance with sports injury rehabilitation: an application of protection motivation theory. *Journal of Sports Sciences* **14**, 471–482.

47. Zohar J, Juven-Wetzler A, Sonnino R, Cwikel-Hamzany S, Balaban E, Cohen H. (2011) New insights into secondary prevention in post-traumatic stress disorder. *Dialogues in Clinical Neuroscience* **13**, 301–309.

48. Hawker DM, Durkin J, Hawker DS. (2011) To debrief or not to debrief our heroes: that is the question. *Clinical Psychology & Psychotherapy* **18**, 453–463.

49. Glick ID, Horsfall JL. (2005) Diagnosis and psychiatric treatment of athletes. *Clinics in Sports Medicine* **24**, 771–781.

50. Kamm RL. (2005) Interviewing principles for the psychiatrically aware sports medicine physician. *Clinics in Sports Medicine* **24**, 745–769.

51. Wilk JE, Herrell RK, Wynn GH, Riviere LA, Hoge CW. (2012) Mild traumatic brain injury (concussion), posttraumatic stress disorder, and depression in U.S. soldiers involved in combat deployments: association with postdeployment symptoms. *Psychosomatic Medicine* **74**, 249–257.

52. Simmons AN, Matthews SC. (2012) Neural circuitry of PTSD with or without mild traumatic brain injury: a meta-analysis. *Neuropharmacology* **62**, 598–606.

53. Adkins JW, Weathers FW, McDevitt-Murphy M, Daniels JB. (2008) Psychometric properties of seven self-report measures of posttraumatic stress disorder in college students with mixed civilian trauma exposure. *Journal of Anxiety Disorders* **22**, 1393–1402.

54. Bisson J, Andrew M. (2007) Psychological treatment of post-traumatic stress disorder (PTSD). *Cochrane Database of Systematic Review* **2007**, CD003388.

55. Barnette V. (2001) Resolving PTSD through time limited dynamic psychotherapy. *Journal of College Student Psychotherapy* **16**, 27–41.

56. Reardon CL, Factor RM. (2010) Sport psychiatry: a systematic review of diagnosis and medical treatment of mental illness in athletes. *Sports Medicine* **40**, 961–980.
57. Maher MJ, Rego SA, Asnis GM. (2006) Sleep disturbances in patients with post-traumatic stress disorder: epidemiology, impact and approaches to management. *CNS Drugs* **20**, 567–590.
58. Lin KM, Tsou HH, Tsai IJ, Hsiao MC, Hsiao CF, Liu CY, *et al.* (2010) CYP1A2 genetic polymorphisms are associated with treatment response to the antidepressant paroxetine. *Pharmacogenomics* **11**, 1535–1543.
59. Bernardy NC, Lund BC, Alexander B, Friedman MJ. (2012) Prescribing trends in veterans with posttraumatic stress disorder. *The Journal of Clinical Psychiatry* **73**, 297–319.
60. Hammermeister J, Pickering M, McGraw L, Ohlson C. (2012) The relationship between sport related psychological skills and indicators of PTSD among Stryker Brigade soldiers: the mediating effects of perceived psychological resilience. *Journal of Sport Behavior* **35**, 40–60.
61. David WS, Simpson TL, Cotton AJ. (2006) Taking charge: a pilot curriculum of self-defense and personal safety training for female veterans with PTSD because of military sexual trauma. *Journal of Interpersonal Violence* **21**, 555–565.
62. Ranby KW, Aiken LS, MacKinnon DP, Elliot DL, Moe EL, McGinnis W, *et al.* (2009) A mediation analysis of the ATHENA intervention for female athletes: prevention of athletic-enhancing substance use and unhealthy weight loss behaviors. *Journal of Pediatric Psychology* **34**, 1069–1083.

Part Two
Treatment Approaches and Therapeutic Issues with Athletes

11 Psychotherapeutic Treatment of Athletes and Their Significant Others

Mark A. Stillman,[1] Eva C. Ritvo,[2] and Ira D. Glick[3]

[1] Department of Psychology, School of Liberal Arts, Georgia Gwinnett College, USA
[2] Department of Psychiatry and Behavioral Sciences, University of Miami School of Medicine, USA
[3] Psychiatry and Behavioral Sciences, Stanford University School of Medicine, USA

KEY POINTS

- The sports psychiatrist must possess a unique set of psychotherapeutic skills when working with athletes.
- Entitlement issues, narcissism, and aggression are shared by many athletes, making psychotherapeutic interventions more challenging.
- Various modalities of psychotherapy, including individual therapy, marital and family therapy, and group interventions, may be useful for athletes in particular contexts.

INTRODUCTION

Providing psychotherapy to professional athletes involves unique challenges. Certain characteristics, specifically entitlement issues, narcissism, and aggression, are shared by many athletes, making psychotherapeutic interventions more challenging. This chapter focuses on these special issues in the provision of individual, marital/family, and group psychotherapy with this population.

Previous publications have delineated both the pharmacological treatment of athletes with mental illness and the delivery of psychoeducation after the initial evaluation. For instance, Reardon and Factor discussed findings related to the use of psychopharmacological agents and their effects on and relationship to athletic performance, safety, and anti-doping guidelines [1]. Moreover, Glick *et al.* stressed the importance of providing education to the athlete and his or her family regarding the specific diagnosis, the treatment plan, and the prognosis (with and without treatment) as an essential part of treatment in sports psychiatry [2].

This chapter focuses specifically on the use of psychotherapy as a treatment in sports psychiatry, the various modalities used, and unique challenges often encountered with this population.

Clinical Sports Psychiatry: An International Perspective, First Edition. Edited by David A. Baron, Claudia L. Reardon and Steven H. Baron.

THE ATHLETE-PATIENT

Diagnosis

Athletes have an equal if not greater risk for the development of psychiatric illness (especially eating disorders and substance abuse) than the general population. More specifically, depression is equally common among athletes and nonathletes, although, in athletes, it can be triggered by unique factors, such as overtraining, poor performance, and retirement [1, 3]. Furthermore, significant mood disturbances, such as elevations in depression, tension, and anger, have been found in seriously injured athletes [4]. Although athletes have been found to have normal levels of "state anxiety," they tend to experience higher rates of performance anxiety and jet-lag-induced insomnia [3, 5].

Eating disorders and substance abuse appear to be the most common problems among athletes [1, 3]. Up to 60% of female athletes in particular sports, such as distance running, figure skating, and gymnastics, suffer from eating disorders [3]. Substance abuse disorders also appear to be somewhat common among athletes, with alcohol being more abused than any other substance [1].

Despite the prevalence of psychiatric illness in this population, athletes generally do not seek out or make contact with sports psychiatric providers to receive appropriate treatment [6]. This is likely due to the social stigma regarding psychiatric illness, and the notion that mental health treatment represents weakness to athletes and coaches [6, 7].

As a result, the sports psychiatrist must possess a unique set of skills when working with athletes, particularly in the context of psychotherapy. Given the athlete's probable reluctance to use psychiatric treatment, as noted earlier, the clinician may need to reframe psychiatric treatment as "performance help" to encourage participation in the therapeutic process [8]. The following case illustrates the difficulty many clinicians face in encouraging athletes to follow treatment recommendations, as well as the importance of engaging collateral support systems to ensure the enforcement of said recommendations:

Case Study

A 32-year-old Italian professional soccer player with no history of depression until his late 20s presented for treatment due to symptoms of depression. In the context of some marital discord and worries about performance on his soccer team, he developed low mood, insomnia, anhedonia, and suicidal ideation. He presented for psychiatric treatment reluctantly, encouraged by his wife. His psychiatrist started him on treatment with an antidepressant and strongly recommended psychotherapy. His depressive symptoms worsened, however, following a missed goal in a crucial soccer game. Moreover, he never showed up for psychotherapy. His psychiatrist recommended an increase in his medication, but he was fearful of taking it, worried it might affect his performance. After another poor performance in a subsequent game, he became more depressed and suicidal but continued to deny that he needed psychotherapy or a change in medications. The psychiatrist, at that point, recommended hospitalization, but the patient refused to go. No contact with significant others was made. One week later, he jumped in front of a train and killed himself.

Once the athlete comes in (or is brought in) for help, the sports psychiatrist's first job is to evaluate the athlete's personality and coping mechanisms; thereafter, the signs and symptoms defining a psychiatric diagnosis should be explored in the context of the workup [6]. Denial of psychological problems and of pain is common among successful athletes [6, 9]. A clinical interview should be conducted with the athlete and significant others (including family, agents, teammates, and others important in the athlete's life), during which time the sports psychiatrist must exercise judgment and maintain confidentiality when contacting others [6].

Treatment

Following an extensive diagnostic workup involving the athlete and any significant others, various treatment modalities should be considered. As evident in the case example provided earlier, psychopharmacological treatment alone may not be sufficient. Further efforts to engage the athlete in psychotherapy will oftentimes be indicated to ensure best practice, provide the most empirically supported treatment approach, and to undertake motivational enhancement for adherence to medication recommendations.

Individual psychotherapy

Under many circumstances, individual psychotherapy is useful as an adjunct to medication therapy and psychoeducation [10]. In some instances, individual psychotherapy alone may be sufficient as a unilateral treatment approach for mild cases of depression, anxiety, or sports-related adjustment issues. Individual psychotherapy may be provided by the sports psychiatrist or, oftentimes, a referral is made to a psychologist or counselor who specializes in the treatment of athletes. Among the variety of individual psychotherapy approaches, cognitive-behavioral therapy has received the most empirical support for the treatment of a variety of psychiatric conditions [11]. The athlete is a particularly good candidate for this type of therapy given his or her comfort with structure, direction, and practice [12]. Moreover, athletes involved in individual sports (such as golf, tennis, swimming, and running) may respond especially well to this modality, given their familiarity with individual goal setting and self-reliance.

Marital/family psychotherapy

While individual psychotherapy is a common treatment option, the sports psychiatrist must recognize that he not only treats problems, symptoms, and/or disorders associated with the athlete, but also with the athlete's family/significant others, team, or even spectators/fans [5]. Therefore, the clinician must possess a clear understanding of the impact that an athlete's family has on the development of the athlete's mind, and the role that sports play in the family system [2].

Oftentimes, a family member or significant other is necessary in order to induce the patient into treatment and to corroborate information (see case 3 in Glick *et al*. [3]). Authors have proposed that, in certain circumstances, psychoeducation for both patient and family member(s) should be mandatory prior to starting psychotropic medication [3]. Athletes are especially unique in that oftentimes coaches, trainers, or agents, in addition to family members or other significant others, may want to be included in treatment, as they are accustomed to being involved in the athlete's day-to-day life. While inclusion of these individuals can be intrusive, they can also provide a critical component to the treatment process by providing supplementary information and supporting adherence with treatment recommendations [3].

The following case published by Glick *et al.* [3] provides a common example of an instance where the psychiatric issues and symptoms were primarily related to the couple or family, and highlights the importance of the athlete-patient attending sessions regularly and cooperating with the family therapy format for treatment to be successful:

Case Study

The young wife of a high-profile athlete and mother of a toddler presented with a chief complaint of marital dissatisfaction. She felt overwhelmed with the responsibilities of motherhood, and her husband was traveling for much of the season. They met in her home state, but he played for a team out of town. She had relocated to be with him, but in the process had given up her support system. She was born and raised in a close multicultural family, the other members of which remained in her home state. She temporarily returned to the area to be with her mother to seek treatment. She was anxious and tearful. She was seen individually for several months, was treated with medication and psychotherapy, and improved. During the off-season, her husband joined her in her home state and participated fairly regularly in sessions. When the season resumed, she and her husband returned to their home together to pursue treatment in that area. Despite her moving to be with him, he did not attend sessions. Months into the season, she returned to her home state, as her symptoms of depression returned. The provider now suspected that she was abusing substances. The couple separated and divorced.

As evidenced by the previous case, it is not uncommon for an athlete-patient to present for psychiatric treatment complaining of symptoms caused by or related to family issues and/or marital discord. It is essential for the sports psychiatrist to provide (or properly refer the patient for) marital/family psychotherapy in order to appropriately address these underlying issues. The case further illuminates the challenge many clinicians may face in enlisting the ongoing participation of the athlete-patient, as well as the spouse and family member(s).

Group psychotherapy

In addition to individual and family psychotherapy, there are instances in which group therapy may be the most beneficial treatment option. Like individual psychotherapy, group therapy is often indicated as an adjunct to medication treatment and can be facilitated by the sports psychiatrist or another qualified mental health professional. Most often, this modality is selected in cases of substance abuse [13]. Self-help groups, such as Alcoholics Anonymous, are popular among individuals diagnosed with substance abuse and/or substance dependence [14]. Athletes may benefit from listening to others with similar problems and from sharing their experiences involving abuse of substances, such as performance-enhancing drugs, with other athletes who can appreciate their unique perspective [14]. Moreover, athletes involved in team sports may be particularly responsive to physiatrist/psychologist-led groups, as they are accustomed to the team–coach dynamic, in which the "team" is led by the "coach." This format may easily draw upon existing strengths given athletes' comfort in this setting.

PSYCHOTHERAPY WITH THE ATHLETE-PATIENT: UNIQUE CHALLENGES

Narcissism and aggression

As a product of the praise and attention many athletes (particularly at the elite level) receive, they can provide especially unique and challenging characteristics during the provision of any of the aforementioned psychotherapeutic modalities. As documented by Glick *et al.*, many athletes are used to being the "VIP" and in charge [3]. People often give them extra attention and are solicitous of their opinions. Many have had a high degree of success at young ages and are used to being in the spotlight. As a result, they may have what Robert B. Millman has termed "acquired situational narcissism" (R. Millman, personal communication, June 2005). According to Millman, this type of narcissism can be driven by the celebrity, wealth, and fame brought on by their athletic success. These athletes may develop grandiose fantasies, demonstrate diminished ability to empathize, and respond with fury to slights, both real and imagined. Jared DeFife documented instances of "impulsive acts of rage and aggression," which he noted are not uncommon among athletes confronted with real or imagined threats to their sense of self-worth, which is oftentimes "overinflated and unstable" [15]. Many athletes who, on the surface, appear to be very confident in their skills and abilities are actually quite insecure. Athletes who have experienced the most fame and success often have the most fragile egos. While sports foster a sense of "sportsmanship," healthy competition, and cooperation, they also promote a strong sense of individualism, aggression, and pride [15]. Fans' reaction to their performances often provides much of the motivation and reinforcement for the hours spent practicing. Their intense drive to succeed is fueled by the praise of their fans, whose loyalty persists only during success. Thus, the same praise they receive when they succeed can subside quickly following a poor performance or a losing season. This can result in a significant "injury" to their ego, and some react to the perceived denunciation with impulsive and explosive rage [15].

Entitlement issues

Entitlement and control issues may emerge rapidly in treatment, especially regarding scheduling and fees [3]. Many athletes work very long hours and require continuous travel. Many enjoy significant financial success, while at the same time may *not* be used to paying for much [3]. Others in their lives often take care of daily needs and travel arrangements. Services and goods are often provided for free from their admirers (i.e., fans). Thus, setting and collecting fees for psychotherapy services may be more challenging than usual.

Confidentiality issues are particularly important, especially to high-profile athletes [3]. Many athletes are used to health care providers coming to them for treatment on the court or at practice sessions. They may expect providers to come to their home or hotel to avoid public exposure. The therapist must carefully weigh the pros and cons of providing psychotherapy for any patient outside of the usual office practice. Coaches, trainers, or agents as well as family members may try to intrude or want to be included in treatment (which certainly can be appropriate and helpful at times) as they are used to being involved in the athlete's day-to-day life; this too can create complexities regarding confidentiality.

The sports psychotherapist must balance the special needs of the athlete with the necessity of providing appropriate treatment based on the (i) patient diagnosis, (ii) circumstances of each case, and (iii) context in the sport [8]. By way of existing guidelines for the clinician, the general principle is "flexibility with appropriate boundaries" [3]. The following case published by Glick *et al.* [3] provides an illustration of this issue:

Case Study

Dr. R was called by the agent of a high-profile athlete, who was out of town competing and was involved in a car accident that led to the death of a child. The athlete was to return on a Friday evening and was requesting to be seen quickly because of severe anxiety and insomnia since the accident. The doctor agreed to see him Saturday morning to expedite the visit and avoid him being seen by other patients. At the end of the visit, he requested to pay with a credit card. Dr. R was unable to process the card, so she requested he pay at a next visit. Instead, two days later, four tickets to a game arrived with a thank you note from the agent. The monetary value of the tickets was comparable to the visit charge. The doctor called the agent to explain that it would be unethical to accept the tickets. The agent understood the concern and sent a check instead. He also insisted that the tickets be kept. The patient never returned for a second visit. It is unclear if the interaction with the agent in some way hampered the therapeutic process.

This case illustrates the need to maintain as "normal" (i.e., treatment as usual) an atmosphere as possible. Athletes may feel entitled to receive special treatment. Simple accommodations, such as seeing a patient outside of usual hours, may hamper the therapeutic process. Some flexibility in treatment may be necessary for privacy and to accommodate travel schedules, but establishing a relationship with a patient that does not follow the "usual rules" can lead to unintended boundary violations. The case was further complicated by the involvement of the agent. In treatment, it is oftentimes necessary to deal with significant others who are close to the identified patient. In this case, the agent was involved with the physician for scheduling and dealing with payment, and that prevented the doctor from getting information directly from the patient.

Coaches, trainers, or agents, as well as family members, may try to intrude or want to be included in treatment, as they are used to being involved in the athlete's day-to-day life. While it depends on the particular situation, for the purposes of providing the most effective treatment to this special population, it is recommended to err on the side of including these significant others.

CONCLUSION

Overall, athletes are driven, ambitious, and competitive. These traits may make it difficult for them to seek or accept the type of assistance provided in psychotherapy. Many are used to having agents, family, and coaches giving them advice, and they may develop a rapid and powerful transference reaction to the doctor [3].

It is important to note, however, that athletes come to therapy with a number of strengths and capabilities as well [3]. Kate Hays documented various assets athletes possess that make them good candidates for success in psychotherapy [12]. By the nature of their work, athletes typically have a very strong sense of discipline. Moreover, they are used to responding to instruction and practicing new skills. Also, though physical and not necessarily psychological, they possess the unique ability to focus internally in order to effect change [12]. These are essential qualities that can increase compliance with therapeutic suggestion and direction, particularly with homework assignments. In fact, the degree of participation and compliance may be considerably higher than when working with nonathletes who may be less focused therapy patients [12].

REFERENCES

1. Reardon CL, Factor RM. (2010) Sport psychiatry: a systematic review of diagnosis and medical treatment of mental illness in athletes. *Sports Medicine* **40**(11), 961–980.
2. Glick ID, Kamm R, Morse E. (2009) The evolution of sport psychiatry, Circa 2009. *Sports Medicine* **39**, 607–613.
3. Glick ID, Stillman MA, Reardon CL, Ritvo E. (2012) Managing psychiatric issues in elite athletes. *Journal of Clinical Psychiatry* **73**(5), 640–644.
4. Quinn AM, Fallon BJ. (1999) The changes in psychological characteristics and reactions of elite athletes from injury onset until full recovery. *Journal of Applied Sport Psychology* **11**, 210–229.
5. Glick ID, Morse E, Reardon CL, Newmark T (2010) Sport psychiatry – a new frontier in a challenging world. *Die Psychiatrie* **7**, 249–253.
6. Glick ID, Horsfall JL. (2005) Diagnosis and psychiatric treatment of athletes. *Clinics in Sports Medicine* **24**, 771–781.
7. Linder D, Brewer B, Van Raalte J, *et al.* (1991) A negative halo for athletes who consult sport psychologists: replication and extension. *Journal of Sport and Exercise Psychology* **13**, 133–148.
8. Glick ID, Horsfall JL. (2001) Psychiatric conditions in sports: diagnosis, treatment, and quality of life. *The Physician and Sportsmedicine* **29**, 45–55.
9. Pavelski R, Kryden A, Steiner H, *et al.* (1998) Adaptive styles in elite collegiate athletes [abstract]. Presented at the 45th Annual Meeting of The American Academy of Child and Adolescent Psychiatry, November, Anaheim.
10. Davidson JR. (2010) Major depressive disorder treatment guidelines in America and Europe. *Journal of Clinical Psychiatry* **71**(Suppl E1), e04.
11. Butler CA, Chapman JE, Forman EM, Beck AT. (2006) The empirical status of cognitive-behavioral therapy: a review of meta-analyses. *Clinical Psychology Review* **26**, 17–31.
12. Hays KF. (1999) *Working It Out: Using Exercise in Psychotherapy* (pp. 177–187). Washington, DC: American Psychological Association, xxi, 281 pp.
13. Weiss RD, Jaffee WB, Menil VP, Cogley CB. (2004) Group therapy for substance use disorders: what do we know? *Harvard Review of Psychiatry* **12**(6), 339–350.
14. Khantzian EJ, Mack JE. (1994) How AA works and why it's important for clinicians to understand. *Journal of Substance Abuse Treatment* **11**(2), 77–92.
15. DeFife J. (2009) Aggressive athletes: out of control and unapologetic. Why do athletes lash out? And are they really sorry? The Shrink Tank, November 19. http://www.psychologytoday.com/blog/the-shrink-tank/200911/aggressive-athletes-out-control-and-unapologetic. Accessed on 14 December 2012.

12 Mindfulness, Attention, and Flow in the Treatment of Affective Disorders in Athletes

Brandon J. Cornejo

Northwest Permanente, East Interstate Medical Office, Mental Health, USA

KEY POINTS

- Mindfulness is a state of mind focused on the present moment that has been effective in treating affective disorders.
- Mindfulness, Flow, and attentional awareness during sport may all share similar characteristics.
- Athletes may be able to exploit these characteristics to gain access to a sense of mindfulness.
- Such a mental state may prove effective in helping to treat underlying affective disorders in athletes.

INTRODUCTION

Athletes can and do suffer from psychiatric illness including mood and other disorders [1]. While many have argued that exercise has beneficial effects on mood disorders [2, 3], athletes performing at a high level may nonetheless struggle with anxiety disorders, substance use disorders [4], eating disorders [5], and depression that may have origins in both psychological and physiologic makeup [6]. With consideration to athletes' unique performance issues, both pharmacologic and psychotherapeutic management of these illnesses is warranted.

One recent development for the effective treatment of depression and anxiety is a modality known as mindfulness. Mindfulness has been defined as a nonjudgmental, present-centered awareness in which each thought, feeling, or sensation that arises is acknowledged and accepted [7, 8]. First developed to treat individuals suffering from chronic illness, practitioners and therapists have expanded its application to effectively treat anxiety and depressive disorders [9–17]. As mindfulness emphasizes a strong element of present-centered awareness, this form of therapy may be useful for athletes in particular because of many athletes' experiences of "being in the zone," or being completely focused on the sport at hand, otherwise referred to as "Flow" [18]. Like Flow, mindfulness focuses most, if not all, attentional resources on the immediate experience. However, unlike Flow, mindfulness is

Clinical Sports Psychiatry: An International Perspective, First Edition. Edited by David A. Baron,
Claudia L. Reardon and Steven H. Baron.
© 2013 John Wiley & Sons, Ltd. Published 2013 by John Wiley & Sons, Ltd.

unique in its openness to and acceptance about the present moment. As clinicians, we may be able to harness this experience of Flow in the athlete as we introduce and incorporate mindfulness into the treatment of affective disorders. Others have also postulated the potential for theoretical overlap between Flow and mindfulness [19] as they both express elements of "[shared] focus on present experience and are often associated with feelings of calmness, serenity, and mind-body unity, suggesting that the practice of mindfulness techniques may render an athlete more likely to experience Flow, and by extension, peak performance" [20]. The main goals of this chapter are to briefly introduce the concept of mindfulness as it relates to the treatment of affective disorders and attempt to bridge conceptual gaps of mindfulness, attention, and Flow. We will also attempt to provide a framework for using mindfulness in treatment of athletes.

Case Study

SK is a 28-year-old former collegiate swimmer who presents to the clinic with a complaint of worsening depression. On exam, she is well-groomed and casually dressed but appears mildly slowed and makes poor eye contact. She is tearful and reports that she feels her life has "gone downhill" following recent struggles at work. She is completing a PhD in neuroscience but feels unsupported by her mentors and thesis committee. She feels like she is unable to make progress on her project, explaining "I am not sure I even enjoy it anymore. I just feel stuck, like I will never finish." She is married and has no children. However, they would like to start a family as soon as she finishes her PhD and gets a job. The tension between her work and their desire for a family has created interpersonal stress within the marriage. She has also stopped exercising and has gained 10 pounds over the past 6 months. The lack of exercise is unusual for her, as she has typically competed in triathlons on an annual basis. She states that her interest in completing triathlons shortly before stopping exercise had morphed into "just something I do…to know that I can check that off a list." Her mood is "low." She often feels guilty for not exercising and feels as though she is powerless to finish her thesis. Importantly, she is not suicidal. She had previously experienced episodes of depression and now was diagnosed with major depressive disorder, recurrent. She was started on a selective serotonin reuptake inhibitor (SSRI) and experienced minimal side effects. Her treatment was augmented with mindfulness classes. Over a period of 8 months, she began to make a recovery, as her mood improved and her depressive symptoms lessened. She found herself enjoying exercise again and was able to complete and defend her thesis. She found that she was able to use mindfulness techniques effectively while engaged in longer distance triathlons. Subjectively, she felt that her performance and experience of exercise improved.

MINDFULNESS

In working with athletes, we can introduce the concept of mindfulness and relate it to the sense of Flow an athlete may have developed during sport. In turn, as we help the athlete harness mindfulness-based skillsets, we can define mindfulness in terms of Flow [21]. We may be able to use either Mindfulness-Based Cognitive Therapy (MBCT) or Mindfulness-Based

Stress Reduction (MBSR) and exploit the athlete's attentional state developed during exercise to help effectively treat affective dissonance. As has been strongly suggested by Sakyong Mipham Ripinoche, the mental states brought about by exercise and purely mindful activities such as meditation are likely not the same thing [22]. These mental states may, however, share some common elements. As such, it may be effective for the athlete to mentally bridge from the sense of Flow experienced during exercise to the practice of mindfulness. Based on Ripinoche's experience and suggestions, the athlete should treat mindfulness and exercise as separate but interrelated experiences [22]. Should an athlete need treatment for an affective disorder, that athlete should set aside regular specific time for mindfulness and meditation practice. Experts in meditation have argued that patient-athletes should engage productively in mindfulness practice alone, while physically still, before allowing mindfulness or a sense of meditative awareness to blend into physical movement [22].

Jon Kabat-Zinn [7, 8, 23] first provided a detailed description of mindfulness-based stress reduction, in which attention is selectively focused on the immediate time point. Others have defined mindfulness as "[involving] the self-regulation of attention so that it is maintained on immediate experience, thereby allowing for increased recognition of mental events in the present moment. [A] second component [of mindfulness] involves adopting a particular orientation toward one's experiences in the present moment, an orientation that is characterized by curiosity, openness, and acceptance" [24]. Kabat-Zinn has further stated that "[mindfulness] is historically a Buddhist practice; mindfulness can be considered a universal human capacity proposed to foster clear thinking and open-heartedness" [25]. Mindfulness practice, as a therapeutic approach, consists of formal daily meditation along with skill-building homework that ties the patient to the "here and now." The patient works on not judging or evaluating the present moment, but rather focuses on simply "being" present and attempts to extend this mindset to day-to-day life [7]. Mindfulness gives the patient the mental "space" between perception and response that enables her to have a reflective and not reflexive response. This may trigger an increase in metacognitive awareness that prevents depressive relapse [12, 16]. MBCT, a form of therapy that combines elements of mindfulness with cognitive-based approaches to treatment, can be an effective approach for the treatment of anxiety [12] or depressive disorders [26–28]. It is believed that mindfulness, a distinct philosophical underpinning of MBCT, may enhance mood as well as help eliminate negative cognitions associated with depressive and anxious states [12, 29, 30]. It stands to reason that just such an approach would also be effective in athletes. Moreover, athletes may have a particular advantage when developing mindfulness-based skillsets.

FLOW

Athletes, when seeking to be mindful, may have experienced just such a state while engaged in their sport of choice [31]. The vernacular to describe this mental state has not traditionally been associated with mindfulness. Many athletes have described it as being "in the zone" or "in a groove." Each of these descriptors conveys the sense that the athlete is completely absorbed in his activity; in short, he is only aware of the activity at hand and is completely absorbed in sport. We may be able to capture the athlete's experience of complete absorption in sports, i.e., Flow [18], and translate it to the practice of mindfulness. In turn, the athlete may be able to draw upon this experience to better access a mindful state.

Mihaly Csikszentmihalyi introduced the idea of Flow to describe the sense of complete involvement in an activity [18]. This sense of Flow represents a harnessing of emotional resources in the complete immersion of an activity such as a sport. In many regards, exercise can focus the mind in an unselfconscious awareness during an intrinsically rewarding activity with immediate feedback. These conditions are characteristic of Csikszentmihalyi's Flow state [18, 32]. It may be that mindfulness and Flow have similar properties that overlap and may prove beneficial to mental health; that is, both induce a mental state wherein there is balance between skill, specific objective, and immediate feedback [18, 33, 34]. If so, this may help explain why physical movement, such as yoga or running, has been shown to have positive benefits for individuals suffering from affective and thought disorders [35]. It also suggests that athletes may be able to tap into inner resources unconsciously sought out during exercise as they develop a mindfulness practice.

In fact, some have sought out to explore this exact relationship between Flow, mindfulness, and improved performance [36]. Results have suggested that mindfulness may be helpful in improving the athletic performance of distance runners as shown by a significant improvement in mile times following mindfulness training combined with significant correlations with trait variables associated with mindfulness [20]. This may result from a reduction in the athlete's sense of task-related worries and task-irrelevant thoughts [20].

To be in a Flow state, the task at hand must be equally matched with the skill level of the practitioner [33]. If the task is too difficult or the skill level is too low, anxiety and worry will prevail and Flow will not be achieved [18, 33, 34]. In much the same manner, early in the practice of meditation and development of mindfulness, there may be difficulties for the individual as she learns to quiet her mind and focus on her breath. As the skill of the meditator increases, her sense of tranquility, oneness with self, and unselfconscious awareness of the present moment improves. In essence, her ability to attain a Flow state while meditating improves as her meditating skill improves.

Like many beginning practitioners of meditation and mindfulness, athletes may likely have difficulty staying in the present moment, for example, by focusing on their breathing; that is, their skill and the task of meditating will be unmatched. Practice of staying with the breath during meditation will improve a present-centered awareness. It may be useful to remind the athlete that the sense of mindfulness may be similar to "being in the zone" while engaged in sport. Sport and mindfulness may be psychologically similar in that both may require development of a skillset that leads to an open awareness [18, 22] and sense of "presentness" within the activity itself. As the athlete grows in his practice of mindfulness and meditation, hopefully his ability to attain a sense of Flow in the present moment will also improve.

ATTENTION IN SPORTS

While there has been little to specifically address mindfulness in exercise with some exceptions [10, 37], there has been devotion to the concepts of attention and disassociation during exercise. Specifically, sports psychologists have investigated the role of attention in exercise and have described various modalities of focus while engaging in physical activities [21]. Disassociation and associative strategies have long been accepted as two elementary cognitive strategies to coping with exercise [38, 39]. Association has been suggested to allow an individual to engage her attention on a particular activity [38]. In contrast, dissociative techniques may be more effective as distraction – thus enabling an athlete to complete an event (e.g., marathon runners reporting entering a state where their awareness of the present moment is lacking).

Attention and focus have been defined in various manners in the literature; however, the common theme among the various definitions is a task-related cognitive strategy to keep one's mental energies engaged with the task at hand [39]. Initially, attentional focus was defined as a cognitive strategy characterized by focused awareness of bodily states during exercise [40, 41]. However, further exploration of attention during exercise suggests that it can be either narrowly focused (e.g., cognitions targeted at sensations of exercise), broadly focused (e.g., thoughts or ideations of the gestalt of the sport at hand), or can have a directionality (internalization vs. externalization) [42, 43]. These thoughts have been further classified into task-relevant and task-irrelevant [42]. Interestingly, there have been conflicting views on the use of association and disassociation on performance; some studies have suggested that the direction and relevancy of cognitive strategies may be related to subjective experience in endurance sports [44]. In contrast, other studies have found no relationship between perceived experience of endurance sports and cognitive strategies employed [45].

Attentional focus may have elements in common with both Flow and mindfulness. As mentioned earlier in the chapter, attention can be either narrowly or broadly focused on a specific task in the present moment. Likewise, complete unselfconscious focus on the present moment can be an important element of both Flow and mindfulness. There are data to substantiate performance enhancement related to attentional focus [21, 44], depending on both technique and sport. It may be that athletes unknowingly use elements of mindfulness or Flow in exercise as a sort of attentional strategy. If so, they may be able to bring this attentional practice to bear when engaging in mindfulness practice.

MINDFULNESS, EXERCISE, AND MENTAL HEALTH

Independent of mindfulness, we know that aerobic and non-aerobic exercise may be effective in treating depressed mood [46]. Both forms of exercise allow for a form of mindful movement wherein the practitioner attempts to stay present while engaged in physical activity. There are also data to suggest that those with schizophrenia and bipolar disorder benefit from improved mood and a sense of well-being from physical exercise [35]. Yet, there have been few studies that examine a synergistic effect of physical movement and mindfulness on psychiatric populations; despite this paucity, those available studies have focused on yoga or tai chi [37, 46, 47]. Overall, these studies suggest a beneficial effect of mindfulness-based movement on mood, affect, and cognitive distortions in patients with depressive mood [46]. Thus, we should encourage athletes to continue exercising despite struggling with psychiatric illness.

BRIDGING THE GAP BETWEEN FLOW AND MINDFULNESS – DEVELOPING A TREATMENT APPROACH

If mindfulness, exercise, and mindful movement enhance mood and improve cognitive distortions, it stands to reason that athletes should continue in their sport of choice while simultaneously seeking treatment for affective disorders. As suggested earlier, the development of a mindfulness skillset may also enhance performance for endurance athletes, such that mindfulness as a form of treatment for athletes makes sense in many ways [20].

Should an athlete seek out adjunctive treatment in the form of mindfulness, practitioners of meditation, exercise, and mindfulness encourage the development of the mental skillset separately from exercise [22]. Thus, in the treatment of affective disorders, formalized MBSR or MBCT may be a separate allotment of time and energy from exercise. As a corollary, engaging in sport in a mindful manner may not be a complete substitution for the use of MBSR or MBCT to treat cognitive distortions associated with affective dysfunction. The athlete may be best served by setting aside time to address underlying depressive or anxiety states. As with nonathlete populations, this time may include specific mindfulness-based practices as a component of mindfulness-based therapy.

For example, the athlete would learn to focus on the breath and adapt to dealing with mental chatter and negative emotion that influence behavior in a nonproductive fashion. Awareness of the bodily state can keep the athlete from being on "automatic pilot" wherein he acts and reacts without conscious awareness. By learning to stay present, the athlete can gain an awareness of and accept events, such as discomfort, as a temporary state. Furthermore, labeling thoughts may allow the individual to gain insight into his cognitive and emotional states that limit his ability [48]. This dynamic skillset could then be carefully transitioned to mindfulness practice while engaged in exercise. For example, remaining mindful while walking is a common meditation practice; the athlete could extrapolate this moving practice to her sport of interest. That is, she would attempt to retain an open awareness during sport so as to keep a present-centered awareness of her actions.

As alluded to earlier, mindfulness-based techniques are not only effective for psychiatric illness, but recent work also suggests that mindfulness can enhance sport-specific performance [19, 20]. Mindfulness can make an athlete more immediately aware of his body through a sharpening of focus on the present moment. Much as mindfulness can act as a treatment for anxiety disorders [14], it may improve sport-related worry and perfectionism in long-distance runners [36]. In essence, by placing the concept and practices of mindfulness in the vernacular of both Flow and sports psychology, we may be able to develop effective armament in the treatment of affective disorders in athletes.

CONCLUSIONS

Athletes may find the use of mindfulness an effective adjunctive treatment for affective disorders. MBCT and MBSR have been shown to be effective treatments for both anxiety and depression [12, 29, 30]. These treatments could be adapted in athletes and extrapolated to their sport of choice. The rationale for this possibility is that the inherent experience of "being in the zone" or being in a Flow state shares attentional components with mindfulness and meditation. As a consequence, it may be useful for the athlete struggling with a psychiatric diagnosis to develop a mindfulness practice that is effective. Then, this might be transferable to the athlete's sport, potentially resulting in both improved performance and improved mood state.

REFERENCES

1. Schaal K, Tafflet M, Nassif H, *et al.* (2011) Psychological balance in high level athletes: gender-based differences and sport-specific patterns. *PloS One* 6:e19007.
2. Wipfli BM, Rethorst CD (2008) The anxiolytic effects of exercise: a meta-analysis of randomized trials and dose-response analysis. *Journal of Sport and Exercise Psychology* **30**:392–410.

3. Lawlor DA (2001) The effectiveness of exercise as an intervention in the management of depression: systematic review and meta-regression analysis of randomised controlled trials. *British Medical Journal* **322**:763–767.

4. Kondo W (2003) Athletes' "designer steroid" leads to widening scandal. *Lancet* **362**:1466.

5. Byrne S, McLean N (2002) Elite athletes: effects of the pressure to be thin. *Journal of Science and Medicine in Sport/Sports Medicine Australia* **5**:80–94.

6. Lucía A, Morán M, Zihong HRJ (2010) Elite athletes: are the genes the champions? *International Journal of Sports Physiology and Performance* **5**:98–102.

7. Kabat-Zinn J, Massion AO, Kristeller J, *et al.* (1998) Effectiveness of a meditation-based stress reduction program in the treatment of anxiety disorders. *American Journal of Psychiatry* **149**:936–943.

8. Kabat-Zinn J (2011) *Mindfulness for Beginners: Reclaiming the Present Moment – And Your Life*. Boulder: Sounds True.

9. Smith BW, Ortiz JA, Steffen LE, *et al.* (2011) Mindfulness is associated with fewer PTSD symptoms, depressive symptoms, physical symptoms, and alcohol problems in urban firefighters. *Journal of Consulting and Clinical Psychology* **79**:613–617.

10. Robert McComb JJ, Tacon A, Randolph P, *et al.* (2004) A pilot study to examine the effects of a mindfulness-based stress-reduction and relaxation program on levels of stress hormones, physical functioning, and submaximal exercise responses. *Journal of Alternative and Complementary Medicine* **10**:819–827.

11. Eisendrath SJ, Delucchi K, Bitner R, *et al.* (2008) Mindfulness-based cognitive therapy for treatment-resistant depression: a pilot study. *Psychotherapy and Psychosomatics* **77**:319–320.

12. Evans S, Ferrando S, Findler M, *et al.* (2008) Mindfulness-based cognitive therapy for generalized anxiety disorder. *Journal of Anxiety Disorders* **22**:716–721.

13. Witkiewitz K, Bowen S (2010) Depression, craving, and substance use following a randomized trial of mindfulness-based relapse prevention. *Journal of Consulting and Clinical Psychology* **78**:362–374.

14. Kim YW, Lee SH, Choi TK, *et al.* (2009) Effectiveness of mindfulness-based cognitive therapy as an adjuvant to pharmacotherapy in patients with panic disorder or generalized anxiety disorder. *Depression and Anxiety* **26**:601–606.

15. Finucane A, Mercer SW (2006) An exploratory mixed methods study of the acceptability and effectiveness of mindfulness-based cognitive therapy for patients with active depression and anxiety in primary care. *BMC Psychiatry* **6**:14.

16. Kuyken W, Byford S, Taylor RS, *et al.* (2008) Mindfulness-based cognitive therapy to prevent relapse in recurrent depression. *Journal of Consulting and Clinical Psychology* **76**:966–978.

17. Segal ZV, Bieling P, Young T, *et al.* (2010) Antidepressant monotherapy vs sequential pharmacotherapy and mindfulness-based cognitive therapy, or placebo, for relapse prophylaxis in recurrent depression. *Archives of General Psychiatry* **67**:1256–1264.

18. Csikszentmihalyi M (2008) *Flow: The Psychology of Optimal Experience*. New York: Harper-Collins.

19. Moore ZE (2009) Theoretical and empirical developments of the mindfulness-acceptance-commitment (MAC) approach to performance enhancement. *Journal of Clinical Sport Psychology* **3**(4):291–302.

20. Thompson RW, Kaufman KA, Petrillo LAD, *et al.* (2011) One year follow-up of mindful sport performance enhancement (MSPE) with archers, golfers, and runners. *Journal of Clinical Sport Psychology* **5**(2):99–116.

21. Lind E, Welch AS, Ekkekakis P (2009) Do "Mind over Muscle" strategies work? Examining the effects of attentional association and responses to exercise. *Sports Medicine* **39**:743–764.

22. Rinpoche SM (2012) *Running with the Mind of Meditation: Lessons for Training Body and Mind*. New York: Harmony.

23. Kabat-Zinn J (1982) An outpatient program in behavioral medicine for chronic pain patients based on the practice of mindfulness meditation: theoretical considerations and preliminary results. *General Hospital Psychiatry* **4**:33–47.

24. Bishop SR, Lau M, Shapiro S, *et al.* (2006) Mindfulness: a proposed operational definition. *Clinical Psychology: Science and Practice* **11**:230–241.

25. Ludwig DS, Kabat-Zinn J (2008) Mindfulness in medicine. *The Journal of the American Medical Association* **300**:1350–1352.

26. Teasdale JD, Segal ZV, Williams JM, *et al.* (2000) Prevention of relapse/recurrence in major depression by mindfulness-based cognitive therapy. *Journal of Consulting and Clinical Psychology* **68**:615–623.

27. Ma SH, Teasdale JD (2004) Mindfulness-based cognitive therapy for depression: replication and exploration of differential relapse prevention effects. *Journal of Consulting and Clinical Psychology* **72**:31–40.

28. Teasdale JD, Moore RG, Hayhurst H, *et al.* (2002) Metacognitive awareness and prevention of relapse in depression: empirical evidence. *Journal of Consulting and Clinical Psychology* **70**:275–287.

29. Evans S (2010) Review: mindfulness-based therapies effective for anxiety and depression. *Evidence-Based Mental Health* **13**:116.

30. Anonymous (2011) Mindfulness may rival medication at preventing depression relapse. *The Harvard Mental Health Letter* **27**:7.

31. Wanner B, Ladouceur R, Auclair AV, *et al.* (2006) Flow and dissociation: examination of mean levels, cross-links, and links to emotional well-being across sports and recreational and pathological gambling. *Journal of Gambling Studies* **22**:289–304.

32. Satterfield JM, Csikszentmihalyi M (2000) Positive psychology: an introduction. *The American Psychologist* **55**:5–14.

33. Abuhamdeh S, Csikszentmihalyi M (2012) The importance of challenge for the enjoyment of intrinsically motivated, goal-directed activities. *Personality & Social Psychology Bulletin* **38**:317–330.

34. Moneta GB, Csikszentmihalyi M (1996) The effect of perceived challenges and skills on the quality of subjective experience. *Journal of Personality* **64**:275–310.

35. Martinsen EW, Stephens T (2004) Exercise and mental health in clinical and free-living populations. In: Dickman R (ed.) *Advances in Exercise Adherence*. Champaign: Human Kinetics, 55–72.

36. De Petrillo LA, Kaufman KA, Glass CR, Arnkoff D (2009) Mindfulness for long-distance runners: an open trial using mindful sport. *Journal of Clinical Sport Psychology* **4**: 357–376.

37. Netz Y, Lidor R (2003) Mood alterations in mindful versus aerobic exercise modes. *Journal of Psychology* **137**:405–419.

38. Schomer HH (1986) Mental strategies and the perception of effort of marathon runners. *International Journal of Sport Psychology* **17**:41–59.

39. Nideffer RM (1981) *The Ethics and Practice of Applied Sport Psychology*. New York: Movement Publications.

40. St. Clair Gibson A, Foster C (2007) The role of self-talk in the awareness of physiological state and physical performance. *Sports Medicine* **37**:1029–1044.

41. Weinberg RS, Smith J, Jackson A, *et al.* (1984) Effect of association, dissociation and positive self-talk strategies on endurance performance. *Canadian Journal of Applied Sport Sciences* **9**:25–32.

42. Stevinson CD (1998) Cognitive orientations in marathon running and "hitting the wall." *British Journal of Sports Medicine* **32**:229–235.

43. Stevinson CD (1999) Cognitive strategies in running: a response to Masters and Ogles. *Sport Psychology* **13**:235–236.

44. Summers JJ, Machin VJ, Sargent G (1983) Psychosocial factors related to marathon running. *Journal of Sport Psychology* **5**:314–331.

45. Buman MP, Brewer BW, Cornelius AE, *et al.* (2008) Hitting the wall in the marathon: phenomenological characteristics and associations with expectancy, gender, and running history. *Psychology of Sport and Exercise* **9**:177–190.

46. Uebelacker LA, Epstein-Lubow G, Gaudiano BA, *et al.* (2010) Hatha yoga for depression: critical review of the evidence for efficacy, plausible mechanisms of action, and directions for future research. *Journal of Psychiatric Practice* 2010 **16**:22–33.

47. Wall RB (2005) Tai Chi and mindfulness-based stress reduction in a Boston Public Middle School. *Journal of Pediatric Health Care* **19**:230–237.

48. Hathaway CM (2011) *Mindfulness and Sport Psychology for Athletes: Consider Awareness Your Most Important Mental Tool*. Madison, WI: Innergy.

13 Performance Enhancement and the Sports Psychiatrist

Michael T. Lardon[1] and Michael W. Fitzgerald[2]

[1] Department of Psychiatry, School of Medicine, University of California, San Diego, USA
[2] Warrior Behavioral Health, U.S. Army Health Center, Schofield Barracks, USA

KEY POINTS

- The aim of both the sports psychiatrist and the sports psychologist is to enhance performance and maximize healthy cognition in athletes.
- Sports psychiatrists are ideally suited for helping the elite athlete achieve peak performance.
- Motivational theory and goal setting are fundamental components for elite athletic performance.
- Cognitive behavioral therapy techniques are utilized to manage negative thoughts and emotions.
- Other mental practices such as meditation, breathing techniques, heart rate variability (HRV) training, biofeedback, self-hypnosis, and pre-competitive routines are useful in helping the athlete maintain emotional and autonomic control in the competitive environment.
- Building self-confidence with athletes utilizing Bandura's self-efficacy model is effective in integrating these techniques into a coherent, successful performance.

INTRODUCTION

What is performance enhancement? Who practices it? What are the principles taught and what is the science behind them? These are the important questions that this chapter will address.

Performance enhancement consists of simply but thoughtfully using fundamental concepts from neurobiology and psychology, in particular from the burgeoning field of positive psychology, and applying them to the domain of sport with the goal of enhancing performance.

In North America, The Association for Applied Sport Psychology (AASP) is the only professional association that offers certification in this field of practice to its members. AASP defines performance enhancement consultants as "professionals trained in sport but are not licensed psychologists or counselors" [1]. When a sports psychologist has dual training and expertise in both clinical psychology and performance enhancement, these

Clinical Sports Psychiatry: An International Perspective, First Edition. Edited by David A. Baron, Claudia L. Reardon and Steven H. Baron.
© 2013 John Wiley & Sons, Ltd. Published 2013 by John Wiley & Sons, Ltd.

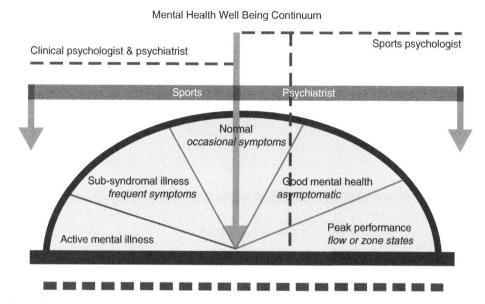

Fig. 13.1 The mental health well-being continuum, which ranges from active mental illness at one extreme to flow or zone states at the other. © Michael Lardon, MD

practitioners are at a clear advantage over a solely trained performance enhancement consultant. Mental health is a continuum, not a discreet fixed state of mind or mood where an athlete spends his entire life (Fig. 13.1). Athletes are human and not immune to mental issues. The literature supports that athletes may be at higher risk of developing various mental illnesses, including eating disorders and substance abuse [2]. Athletes may at one time be mentally healthy and at a later time suffer from panic attacks, mood disorders, substance abuse, marital conflicts, or any other mental health issue. Most mental disorders have a strong biological basis, and therefore the sports psychiatrist with performance enhancement expertise as well as medical and psychiatric training is optimally suited to address the entire spectrum of psychological issues facing athletes throughout their careers.

Performance enhancement skills and techniques have been elucidated by studying elite athletes. We will address four of these key techniques:

1. Motivation and goal setting
2. Managing cognition and emotion in the competitive environment
3. Attentional focus and mental imagery
4. Positive psychology, peak performance, and the athletic zone

MOTIVATION AND GOAL SETTING

Motivation

Motivation is the cognitive-affective process that initiates, directs, and maintains goal-oriented behavior. It is well understood in motivational theory that a living organism's *primary motivation* is survival. The concept of a *secondary motivational drive* is fueled by our innate affinity to seek reward and avoid punishment [3]. Dr. Harry Harlow, a pioneer in

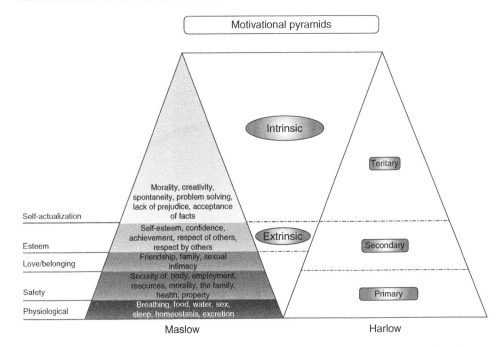

Fig. 13.2 Comparison of Maslow's and Harlow's conceptualizations of motivation. © Michael Lardon, MD

motivational research, demonstrated with primates that there is still a higher drive, a drive that supersedes reward and punishment. In his lab, primates not only solved puzzles without incentivization via reward/punishment, but performed better in their absence, leading him to theorize that "performance of the task provided intrinsic reward" [4]. This phenomenon is called *tertiary motivation* or intrinsic motivation. Self-determination theorists propose that competency, autonomy and psychological relatedness are three universal needs that drive intrinsic motivation [5]. In the case of the athlete, intrinsic love for the sport (or *autotelic*, meaning done for the sake of itself) [6] often quiets the experience of fear and doubt.

In contrast to *intrinsic motivation*, *extrinsic motivation* is derived from the external environment (*secondary motivation*). Examples include praise and financial reward. This idea of extrinsic and intrinsic motivation dovetails nicely with the work of Abraham Maslow, whose framework establishes psychological needs in a hierarchical structure, setting forth a paradigm that positions self-actualization as the most sophisticated goal of human motivation (Fig. 13.2).

Elite athlete Dr. Eric Heiden, winner of five individual gold medals in the 1980 Olympic games in the sport of speed skating and winner of the 1985 U.S. Professional Cycling Championship [7], exemplifies intrinsic motivation when he speaks of his own experience as follows:

> I have found myself to be a person who does not necessarily use the praise of others as the fuel for the pursuit of a goal. Instead, it is the hard work and the desire to discover my limitations that drives me toward realizing my dreams. I have been able to incorporate this philosophy into many other endeavors, which include professional cycling, education, and sports commentating. Although I have not always been as successful at some things as with skating, I still find tremendous satisfaction in knowing that I have given 100% in pursuing a goal. By giving 100%

no one, including yourself, can ever be considered a failure. By giving your all you understand your limits and you have grown in self-knowledge [8].

© Eric Heiden

An all-too-common destructive cycle seen with professional athletes occurs when the levels of motivations move in reverse from tertiary to secondary or primary. The elite athlete typically plays the sport initially because of the love of the game (intrinsic motivation), and it is this type of intrinsic motivation that drives him to greatness. However, when he reaches a pinnacle of success, the athlete often falls into the seductive trap of focusing on fame, adoration of fans, and financial rewards; these rewards and goals are extrinsic, or external, to him. Too often, athletes then begin to find themselves overly concerned with their public image, rather than being concerned with the meticulous training that led them to success. Their lifestyles and training regimens can lose vigor as their motivation moves from intrinsic to extrinsic. This lower order of motivation often does not provide the psychic energy needed to motivate them to train at their previous level, thereby resulting in compromised perfor-mance. Additionally, if the athlete has not been careful financially, she is left playing for her survival (a primary drive that is often accompanied by heightened anxiety), and the inherent fun in competition dwindles.

Mike Tyson, a former Undisputed World Heavyweight Champion in boxing, is one of the more notorious examples of an athlete who reached a pinnacle of greatness, only to be undone by the trappings of wealth and fame. His well-chronicled excesses in extrinsically derived reward (fame, celebrity, drugs, and women) eroded any intrinsic motivation and enjoyment he had previously derived from training and competing, ultimately leading to imprisonment for rape, bankruptcy, and appearances in World Wrestling Entertainment (WWE) and various other media merely to repay his debts.

Goal setting

Goal setting runs in tandem with motivation. Without clear, specific goals, intrinsic motivation is easily eroded. Goals should include those that are process-oriented and those that are result-oriented. They should be broken down temporally into immediate feedback (daily training) goals, intermediate (weekly or monthly) goals, and long-term (yearly) goals. The goals should be specific and achievable, but not easy. Goals should create a sense of struggle, which, when achieved provide a sense of accomplishment and self-mastery [9].

An example of a process-oriented goal for a runner might be to complete a particular workout on a given day, or a weekly mileage goal, whereas a result-oriented goal might be to surpass a personal best time or to win a race. "Winning" may also be defined in terms of one's own assessment of a given performance, and not necessarily finishing first. For example, one may have a personal best time in a race, shoot a personal best low round in golf, or merely realize he has played or done his absolute best in competition even if bettered by his opponent. When athletes utilize process-oriented goals, losses are not necessarily experienced as failures or diminishments of competence. Instead, the athlete who frames his goals in terms of process understands shortfalls or losses as information to help him do better next time. In Pete Sampras's autobiography, he states, "It wasn't about winning. It was about playing the right way" [10].

In summary, goals must be clearly defined, and of even greater importance is that the athlete holds himself accountable for meeting his personal goals. This is best accomplished by breaking goals into broad categories of result- and process-oriented ones while making them specific and measurable. Most importantly, the athlete must record her own progress (Fig. 13.3).

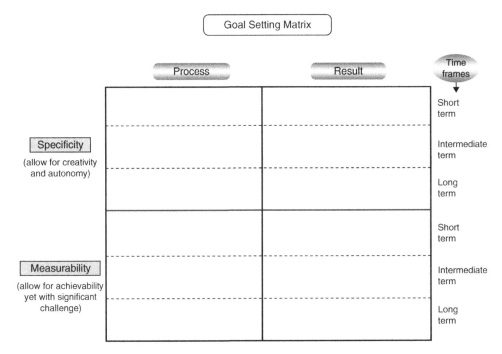

Fig. 13.3 Goal-setting matrix, including room for both process- and result-oriented goals that are specific and measurable. © Michael Lardon, MD

MAXIMIZING COGNITION AND EMOTION IN COMPETITIVE ENVIRONMENTS

It is essential that athletes learn to manage emotions and cognitions while engaged in competition. The same fundamentals of cognitive behavioral therapy (CBT) apply in the athletic realm as in general clinical practice. Common CBT examples are challenging all-or-nothing thinking (e.g., "I lost, therefore I failed today"), catastrophic thinking (e.g., "if I don't win this match, my career is over"), and negating the positive (e.g., "I hit the shot I wanted but lost the point"). Pre-competition positive self-talk has been employed for as long as sport has existed. Witness the calm, reassuring coach giving a pregame motivational speech, full of positive thoughts, images, and exhortations to his team. Teaching an athlete to manage thoughts during competition can involve reframing strategies (e.g., replacing frustration with curiosity), anchoring thoughts and emotions to positive past experiences (e.g., "I've been in this situation before and had success"), and blocking out unwanted or unhelpful thoughts (e.g., replacing the golfer's "I better avoid that water" with "I want to hit that target"). In addition to employing cognitive regulation and strategies, learning to monitor and modulate autonomic arousal is another essential task for competition. The anxiety performance curve proposed by the author demonstrates that there is a peak level of autonomic arousal at which performance is maximized, and as arousal levels move either up (over aroused or anxious) or down (under aroused), that performance levels decrease [11] (Fig. 13.4). This relationship between anxiety and performance is consistent with the Csikszentmihalyi Flow model, which will follow later in the chapter.

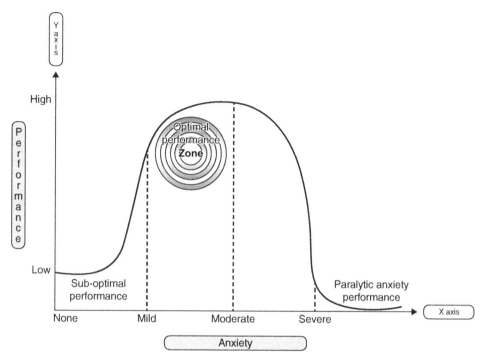

Fig. 13.4 Anxiety performance curve, illustrating that there is a certain level of anxiety at which performance is optimized. © Michael Lardon, MD

Models of ways to maximize cognition and emotion in competitive environments include the following:

- Sports psychologist Dr. Yuri Hanin developed a descriptive emotional model of performance suggesting that athletes perform better when experiencing helpful emotions. He suggests that an athlete can try to become aware of her emotions when performing at a high level and later try to recreate these emotions during future competitions. This model is called The Individual Zones of Optimal Functioning (IZOF) [12].
- Mental practices have proven beneficial both in terms of motor skill acquisition and overall performance [13]. There are many techniques that help athletes reduce stress and have better control of autonomic function and attentional control. Techniques include meditation, breathing techniques, HRV training, and self-hypnosis.
- Meditation trains the brain to be quiet and focus, thus enhancing the mental aspect of performance. Meditation not only may enhance concentration and focus, but also allows one to develop an observing ego, a sort of internal "coach," which allows an athlete to distance himself from potentially disruptive thoughts and emotions. fMRI studies comparing expert meditators to novice meditators found that experts have greater activation of brain regions involved in sustained attention [14]. Attention and control of the autonomic nervous system are vital components of peak performance in sport. Meditation practices have been shown to activate neural structures that regulate these processes [15]. See Chapter 12 for more information on this topic.

- Diaphragmatic breathing techniques have been used by Yogis for centuries to restore energy in preparation for activity. These techniques stimulate the vagal efferent pathways and induce parasympathetic reduction in heart rate and lead to reductions in the experience of stress. There are a number of breathing techniques that are utilized in competitive athletics that are effective. One technique commonly employed is referred to as a *clearing breath*. An individual does this by clearing all the air out of the mouth until a small knot is felt around the navel area. This is followed by a smooth inhalation through the *nose* until the lungs are completely filled after he slowly (via a count of 8–10) exhales through the *mouth*. This technique is particularly useful in critical moments such as when a soccer player needs to make a penalty kick or a football placekicker needs to make a field goal.

- HRV training shares many of the benefits of diaphragmatic breathing techniques. HRV is a physiological phenomenon in which the time interval between heart beats varies. It is measured by the variation in the beat-to-beat interval. Reduced HRV has been shown to be associated with chronic illness [16] and is a predictor of mortality after myocardial infarction [17]. Conversely, evidence suggests that HRV training (increasing HRV) may improve sport performance by helping athletes diffuse stress [18]. Biofeedback training can increase HRV, and there are a number of companies with easy to use, fun commercial software products such as Heartmath, Biocom, and Stresseraser. These software products may be attractive for training the athlete who enjoys the experience of playing a video game but is unlikely to meditate.

- Hypnotic susceptibility along with low neuroticism has long been thought to be an important component of the elite athlete's personality profile. Event-related potentials (ERPs) are measures of the brain response to thought or perception. In the experimental setting, highly hypnotizable individuals show significant decreases in various ERP parameters (P100 and P300 waveform) during a hypnotic hallucination that blocked perception of the stimulus. When hypnosis was used to intensify attention to the stimulus, there was an increase in P100 amplitude [19]. This phenomenon suggests that altered states of consciousness strongly influence our biologic ability to block out certain stimuli and enhance the cognitive processing of others. The great baseball hitter, Ted Williams, is well known to have said that when he was at bat about to hit, he saw nothing except the rotation of the baseball being thrown at him. Hypnosis and self-hypnosis are powerful techniques to enhance neurologic processing of stimuli, for which there is biological evidence. The corresponding author often assesses a client's hypnotizability using the Hypnotic Induction Profile (HIP) [20], and if the client scores relatively high, self-hypnosis techniques are taught.

- Pre-competitive routines help prepare the athlete to minimize distraction and keep the task at hand in focus. Athletes often have ritualistic behaviors that start the day of competition (pre-competitive routine) and more structured ritualistic behavior prior to performance (pre-performance routine) that provide a psychology "bubble," making the context of the sporting event around them less relevant and simultaneously keeping them focused at the task at hand. For example, Olympic Swimming Champion Michael Phelps is almost always seen just prior to his races listening to his iPod and going through his ritualistic pre-race routine. In the sport of competitive golf, pre-shot routines are perceived as just as important as developing a sound technical swing. The pre-shot routine feels laborious in practice, but when the competition is at a very high intensity, there is nothing more comforting for the golfer to focus on than following of her automated routine.

ATTENTIONAL FOCUS AND MENTAL IMAGERY

The role of attention and performance

Attention demands focused concentration of one's consciousness on a specific task. Autonomic arousal influences attentional processes. Robert Nideffer's *Theory of Attentional and Interpersonal Style (TAIS)* [21] has been very useful for sports psychology and military training. His theory proposes two dimensions, External–Internal and Broad–Narrow, to yield four domains of attentional focus that individuals utilize. The External–Internal distinction refers to the allocation of attention to either the external (outside of the athlete such as teammates and competitors, the field/court, etc.) or internal (inside the athlete's mind/body, such as kinesthetic movement), whereas the Broad–Narrow distinction refers to allocation of attention mainly to a wide focus (e.g., the entire playing field) or a narrow, singular focus (e.g., returning a serve in tennis).

Nideffer theorizes that each individual has a predominant style, but that each sport has its own unique attentional demands that are met best by various attentional styles. For example, in basketball, the point-guard position demands attention in the *Broad–External* domain while moving the ball down the court looking to pass. The *Broad–Internal* domain is needed to analyze external information with internal attention to one's own body in freestyle rock climbing. The *Narrow–Internal* domain, in which one mentally rehearses his performance, would be exemplified by gymnastics or diving. Lastly, *Narrow–External* attentional focus would be optimal for returning a tennis serve (Fig. 13.5).

The athlete who can seamlessly transition between attentional styles is more likely to perform at her optimal best. Nideffer also hypothesizes that "athletic zone states" occur

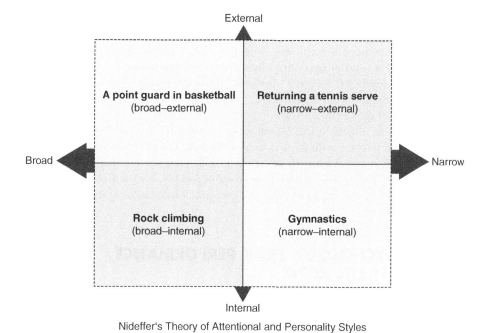

Nideffer's Theory of Attentional and Personality Styles

Fig. 13.5 Robert Nideffer's *Theory of Attentional and Interpersonal Style*, illustrating the two dimensions of External–Internal and Broad–Narrow. © Michael Lardon, MD

when attention is focused almost exclusively on the external environment (Broad–External) and conversely theorizes that "choking" is characterized by the athlete losing the ability to transition attentional styles and focusing exclusively on the internal experience (Narrow–Internal). Nideffer's theory is consistent with Easterbrook's cue utilization theory, predicting that high levels of arousal will lead to attention narrowing [22]. Sian Beilock at the University of Chicago suggests that too much attention (overthinking) paid to task control leads to a decrement in performance. Her work supports the notion that when athletes choke, they lose their capacity to access implicit learned motor programs. Thus, they start to overthink and rely on explicit (conscious) learned models, resulting in acute performance failure [23, 24]. In layperson terms, the Italian proverb that translates to "Learn how to do it and then forget you know how" encapsulates this idea.

Mental imagery

> I never hit a golf shot, not even in practice, without having a very sharp, in-focus picture of it in my head. It's like a color movie. First I see the ball where I want it to finish, nice and white and sitting up high on the bright green grass. Then the scene quickly changes and I see the ball going there: its path, trajectory, and shape, even its behavior on landing. Then there is a fadeout, and the next scene shows me making the kind of swing that will turn the previous image into reality [25].

This quote by golfer-great Jack Nicklaus is echoed by the 1984 Winter Olympics Alpine Slalom gold medalist Phil Mahre, who introduced to the world his use of mental imagery. Before each of his races, Mahre described closing his eyes and visualizing the course ahead. In the experimental setting, the effective use of mental imagery to support optimal performance has been demonstrated by George Grouios, who showed that divers benefit from mental practice [26]. In addition, functional magnetic resonance imaging (fMRI) studies have shown that motor and mental training recruit similar motor and visual systems [27], lending neurobiologic support to the use of imagery. Mental imagery has been a main stay of athletic peak performance for many years. Four variations of mental imagery are often used. Golf lends itself well to illustration of the *four fundamental imagery* domains: Internal-Visual, Internal-Kinesthetic, External-Visual, and External-Kinesthetic. A simple graph illustrates these four mental imagery domains (Fig. 13.6).

When teaching an athlete to use mental imagery, the clinician must also integrate the individual's gift for imagery with the demands of the task. The athlete may be better at kinesthetic imagery than visual imagery or better at imagining her internal experience than external experience. The goal is for the athlete to see or feel the shot (or dive, run, jump, etc.) prior to actual execution in the most clear and powerful way, similar to the Jack Nicklaus example given earlier.

POSITIVE PSYCHOLOGY, PEAK PERFORMANCE, AND THE ATHLETIC ZONE

Self-confidence

The use of mental imagery, in addition to optimizing motivation, goal setting, cognition, attention, and emotional stability, are all important components in the development of self-confidence. A very useful model to understand the science of self-confidence is Albert

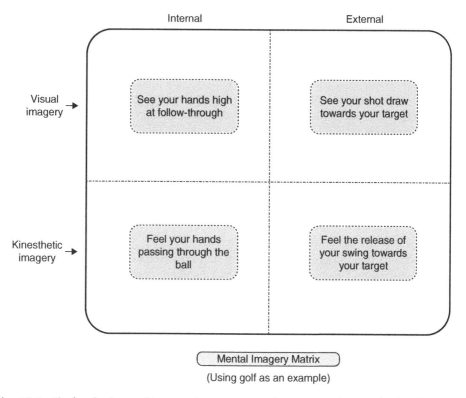

Fig. 13.6 The four fundamental imagery domains using golf as an example. © Michael Lardon, MD

Bandura's model of self-efficacy. The term "self-efficacy" [28] refers to an individual's belief in his or her ability to succeed in a particular situation. Bandura described a model for self-efficacy with four essential components that facilitate the development of self-confidence. The strongest such component he calls "mastery experiences," wherein one has previously experienced success in a particular task. The second component he describes as "modeling behavior," in which an athlete is inspired by someone who succeeds. "Vicarious learning" is self-confidence derived through witnessing peers or familiar colleagues succeed. Finally, the concept of "social persuasion" is characterized by an individual being convinced by others that he can accomplish the task.

Self-affirmations are commonly employed and often helpful, but these authors caution their use. If the self-affirmation is realistic, it leads to a positive mind set, but if the self-affirmation is unrealistic, it may set an athlete up for a false sense of confidence (arrogance). Excessive ego and arrogance add another layer of self-imposed pressure that, at an elite level, complicates an already delicate balance of humility and confidence.

Positive psychology and the zone

Competition, from the Latin *competere*, means to strive together. Often, competition is misconstrued as the practice of conquering or outperforming one's opponent, and when this happens, the inherent joy that comes from full engagement and from one's intrinsic motivation in the activity is lost. A contemporary case that exemplifies the way in which embracing competition positively elevates both the players and the sport is the competition at the top of the men's Association of Tennis Professionals rankings. Novak Djokovic, Rafael Nadal, and Roger Federer have rotated atop the men's rankings for the past several years. While they battle each other fiercely each time they take the court, their post-match embraces and comments indicate that they recognize that the synergy of their competition elevates each other's performances, and in so doing, has collectively elevated their sport.

Psychologist and former American Psychological Association president, Martin Seligman, made it the platform of his term in the 1990s to rededicate the field of psychology "not to just fixing what is wrong, but also building what is right" [29]. The athletic arena is one in which the principles of Positive Psychology are clearly espoused. Virtues such as courage, optimism, honesty, perseverance, and the search for purpose are fundamental tenants of Positive Psychology. Athletes and their coaches are perhaps already accomplished Positive Psychologists. For the most part, elite athletes focus on their strengths and abilities and seek to realize their potential. They do not expend mental and physical resources on their perceived inabilities, weaknesses, or shortcomings. Athletes are among the unwitting pioneers in this pursuit to define the limits of human capacity. For any athlete who has ever experienced what is commonly referred to as being in "The Zone," a state of peak concentration and performance, it is perhaps toward this experience that all effort is directed, consciously or otherwise. The Zone may be considered the pinnacle of sporting experience. One athlete describes being in The Zone as, "it feels like nobody's out there, you're playing by yourself." Another states, "it's like an out of body experience, like you're watching yourself. You almost feel like you don't even see the defense... every move you make…you're going by people…you don't even hear the regular noise you hear" [30]. It is the intense focus, at the exclusion of all distraction that leads to this dissociative state.

Susan Jackson [31] along with Mihaly Csikszentmihalyi, a psychologist who coined the term "flow" for the psychological state one experiences when completely immersed in any multitude of activities, cites nine essential elements required for achievement of the flow (or The Zone) state:

- Action-awareness merging
- Clear goals
- Unambiguous feedback
- Concentration on the task at hand
- Sense of control
- Loss of self-consciousness
- Transformation of time
- Autotelic experience (done for the sake of itself)
- Challenge–skills balance (see Fig. 13.7)

The Zone cannot be called upon by demand; one can merely understand how to optimize conditions that give rise to it and then dedicate himself with full commitment to the task at hand. Rarely but spontaneously will he then experience this ephemeral and ideal state. See also Chapter 12.

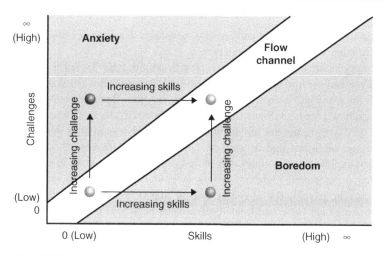

Fig. 13.7   Plot of skill level present in a given athlete versus level of challenge a given task requires, and where the intersection of those two variables is most likely to produce The Zone ("Flow Channel" on this diagram). © Michael Lardon, MD

Case Study

Athlete "TA" reached a pinnacle of success in his sport. Huge money, fortune, and fame accompanied his success. TA reported developing terrifying episodes of intense fear, overwhelming autonomic arousal, and worry. These anxiety attacks (as he called them) happened in all domains of his life but mostly while competing on the national stage. His career faltered, and he consulted one of the country's most renowned sports psychologists, who did not recognize what TA was experiencing and was unable to help him. His attacks became more severe, and he became increasingly depressed and started to withdraw from the world of sport. After almost 1 year of being fully symptomatic while trying to continue to compete, TA was finally referred to a clinical psychologist, who encouraged him to see a psychiatrist. The corresponding author was soon thereafter contacted by TA to set up an initial evaluation.

When the author first evaluated TA, he was so incapacitated by his symptoms that he had stopped competing and was on the verge of completely quitting his sport. After his initial assessment was done, it was noted that TA had a history of social anxiety but never reported any problems in his competitive sport environment. It was clear that his precipitous fall from the top of his sport coincided with his family doctor placing him on bupropion, a dopamine–norepinephrine reuptake inhibitor, for the purpose of tobacco cessation. It was at this time that TA reported first developing panic symptoms. The author's first intervention was to discontinue the bupropion and start TA on a selective serotonin reuptake inhibitor (SSRI). Within several months, TA's panic and depressive symptoms vastly improved, and he decided to return to his sport. However, he returned only to find his confidence eroded and that he was unable to compete at the level of his peers. This ignited criticism from the media. Searching for the answer, TA engaged a number of new coaches and teachers. Psychiatrically, he continued to improve and stabilize in terms of depressive and anxiety symptoms, but a new problem was born in the form of intense performance anxiety.

From a psychoeducational perspective, it was essential that TA learn why he lost his form and was buying into the media's rhetoric that he was "all washed up." He worked hard with the psychiatrist on understanding that his poor form and loss of confidence was the result of a medical illness that had now improved, and that there was no reason that he could not regain his top form again. TA had a hard time buying into this argument and often felt that he was not good anymore (that he "had lost it"). His psychiatrist explained many times to him that if he had been forced to compete with a broken leg or untreated diabetes, he also would have played poorly and lost his confidence. The psychiatrist also emphasized that if he would have been promptly placed on a medical leave and treated effectively, he would not have had to compete while fighting a full blown anxious depression. The doctor explained that no one would be able to play well while suffering through a depressive episode. As time moved on, TA started to rewrite his own narrative fragment. He began to see that maybe it was not his fault that he "lost his game" and that there was in fact no real reason why he could not make a successful comeback. The psychiatrist encouraged TA to return to his original coaches, and from there he started to show small signs of regaining his from.

TA continued to experience significant performance anxiety in very big competitions. Major depression and panic disorder were now in remission, but TA had a full-blown performance anxiety syndrome. This prompted the introduction of diaphragmatic breathing techniques, HRV training, basic CBT principles, mental imagery techniques, and other tools that the psychiatrist thought would be useful for him. As time moved on, he started to show signs of regaining his form. TA and his psychiatrist spent a great deal of time defining process-oriented goals, thereby allowing him to find positives even when he competed poorly. He learned that scores and stats do not tell the whole story, and that he was consistently making gains in small ways. He relearned that it was hard work focused on achieving process-oriented goals that would determine if he would reach his result-oriented goals. He slowly built trust in his own ability and became less focused on the results, which was not easy because of his relationship with the media. As his understanding of what happened to him became less neurotic and more accurate, he became less critical of himself, and his attitude in turn improved. TA was once asked by the media what function sports psych docs performed, and his response was that his sports psychiatrist helped him "remember who he was." Small gains were made each successive year, and he is currently competing at a very high level and once again making his living in professional sports.

This case example shows a real-life situation of an elite athlete who became afflicted with a mental disorder that was not recognized or diagnosed for almost 2 years. He competed through much of that time and in turn lost his confidence and almost quit competing in his sport. Cognitive therapy was done weekly over years, coupled with teaching of a variety of mental tools including breathing techniques, mental imagery, HRV training, and confidence building techniques (primarily utilizing Bandura's self-efficacy model). TA and his psychiatrist looked at past mastery experiences. TA saw his peers do well, and he vicariously felt that he could do well too. He looked at other elite athletes and modeled much of their behavior. The team of people constantly verbalized the positive and thus created a positive environment. The psychiatrist spoke with him at length about how his gift was dispositional, something in his DNA, and if he continued to work hard that there would be no reason why he could not find his form.

The story of TA is not yet over, but he is back competing, making a very good living in the professional sport that he almost quit. As illustrated by this case, the sports psychiatrist is ideally positioned and qualified to properly diagnose and successfully treat an athlete's illness and seamlessly transition the focus from treatment of psychiatric illness to development of self-confidence and enhancement of performance.

SUMMARY

Sport performance enhancement is in many ways an extension of the tools clinical psychologists/psychiatrists already use, applied to the athletic realm. In addition, the sports psychiatrist is an educator, trainer, and facilitator. She must learn through trial, error, and experimentation what psychological tools and techniques are most useful for her athletes. Essential to this process is development of a trusting therapeutic alliance with the athlete, and relating to the athlete both as a clinician and as one who is experienced in the realm of sport. An ideal sports psychiatrist seeks to understand the unique personality and biologic constitution of each athlete as well as the particular parameters and demands of the athlete's sport. Often those athletes who have successful athletic and post-athletic careers, as well as the most fulfilling lives, have become so because they have applied these concepts not only to sport but to other aspects of their lives, and have flourished as physicians (Eric Heiden), businessmen (Hall of Famers Magic Johnson and Roger Staubach), and in many other enterprises.

> Sport may not only be an end in itself, but the beginning of an unfoldment that will eventually extend the boundaries in all areas of life [32].

REFERENCES

1. Association for Applied Sport Psychology. Ethical code. http://www.appliedsportpsych.org/About/Ethics.htlm. Accessed on 14 April 2012.
2. Reardon CL, Factor RM. (2010) Sport psychiatry: a systematic review of diagnosis and medical treatment of mental illness in athletes. *Sports Medicine* **40**(11), 961–980.
3. Hull CL. (1935) The conflicting psychologies of learning: a way out. *Psychological Review* 42, 491–516.
4. Harlow H, Mears C. (1971) *The Human Model: Primate Perspectives*. VH Winston & Sons (Halstead Press), Washington, DC, p. 85.
5. Deci E, Ryan R. (Eds.) (2002) *Handbook of Self-Determination Research*. University of Rochester Press, Rochester, NY.
6. Csikszentmihalyi M. (1990) *Flow: The Psychology of Optimal Experience*. Harper Collins Publishers, New York.
7. Eric Heiden. (2012) http://en.wikipedia.org/wiki/Eric_Heiden. Accessed on 14 April 2012.
8. Heiden E. (2012) An excellent example of a process-oriented athlete. http://www.drlardon.com/resources.php. Accessed on 14 April 2012.
9. Bandura A. (1977) Self-efficacy: toward a unifying theory of behavioral change. *Psychological Review* **84**(2), 191–215.
10. Sampras P. (2008) *A Champion's Mind: Lessons from a Life in Tennis*. Crown Archetype, New York, p. 25.
11. Lardon M. (2008) *Finding Your Zone – Ten Core Lessons for Achieving Peak Performance in Sports and Life*. Perigee Penguin Group, New York, p. 23.
12. Hanin T. (2002) Individual zone of optimal functioning (IZOF): a probabilistic estimation. *Journal of Sport and Exercise Psychology* **24**(2), 189–208.

13. Feltz DL, Landers DM. (1983) The effects of mental practice on motor skill learning and performance: a meta-analysis. *Journal of Sports Psychology* 5, 25–57.
14. Baron E. (2007) Regional brain activation during meditation shows time and practice effects: an exploratory fMRI study. *Advance Access Publication* 27, 2, 4, 5.
15. Lazar S. (2000) Functional brain mapping of the relaxation response and meditation. *Neuroreport* **11**(7), 1581–1585.
16. Carney R. (1995) Association of depression with reduced heart rate variability in coronary artery disease. *American Journal of Cardiology* 76(8), 562–564.
17. Kleiger RE, Miller JP, Bigger JT Jr., Moss AJ. (1987) Decreased heart rate variability and its association with increased mortality after acute myocardial infarction. *American Journal of Cardiology* 59(4), 256–262.
18. Lagos L, Vaschillo E, Vaschillo B, Lehrer P. (2011) Virtual reality-assisted heart rate variability biofeedback as a strategy to improve golf performance: a case study. *Biofeedback* **39**(1), 15–20.
19. Spiegel D. (1989) Hypnotic alteration of somatosensory perception. *The American Journal of Psychiatry* 146(6), 749–754.
20. Speigel H. (1976) Psychometric analysis of the hypnotic induction profile. *International Journal of Clinical and Experimental Hypnosis* **24**(3–4), 300–315.
21. Nideffer R. (1981) *The Ethics and Practice of Applied Sport Psychology.* Mouvement Publications, Ithaca, NY.
22. Easterbrook JA. (1959) The effects of emotion on cue utilization and the organization of behavior. *Psychological Review* **66**, 183–201.
23. Beilock SL, Gonso S. (2008) Putting in the mind vs. putting on the green: expertise, performance time, and the linking of imagery and action. *The Quarterly Journal of Experimental Psychology: Human Experimental Psychology* **61**, 920–932.
24. Beilock SL, Carr TH, MacMahon C. (2002) When paying attention becomes counterproductive: impact of divided versus skill-focused attention on novice and experienced performance of sensorimotor skills. *Journal of Experimental Psychology: Applied* **8**(1), 6–16.
25. Nicklaus J. (1974) *Golf My Way.* Simon & Schuster, New York.
26. Grouios G. (1992) The effect of mental practice on diving performance. *International Journal of Sport Psychology* **23**(1), 60–69.
27. Olsson C, Jonsson B, Nyberg L. (2008) Learning by doing and learning by thinking: an fMRI study of combining motor and mental training. *Frontiers in Human Neuroscience* **2**, 5.
28. Bandura A. (2007) *Self-Efficacy: The Exercise of Control.* Worth Publishers, New York.
29. Snyder CR, Lopez S. (2002) *Handbook of Positive Psychology.* Oxford University Press, New York.
30. Kennedy K. (2005) SI players: how it feels to be on fire. *Sports Illustrated*, February 21.
31. Jackson SA, Csikszentmihalyi M. (1999) *Flow in Sports: The Keys to Optimal Experiences and Performances.* Human Kinetics Publishing, Champaign, IL, pp. 15–31.
32. Murphy M. (1992) *The Future of the Body: Explorations into the Further Evolution of Human Nature.* Jeremy Tarcher, Inc. Publications, Los Angeles, CA.

14 Applied Sports Psychology in Worldwide Sport: Table Tennis and Tennis

Kathy Toon,[1] Dora Kurimay,[2] and Tamás Kurimay[3]

[1] GlamSlam Tennis, USA
[2] SPiN New York, USA
[3] Department of Psychiatry and Psychiatric Rehabilitation, Saint John Hospital, Hungary

KEY POINTS

- The between-point times in tennis and table tennis, and probably many other sports, are crucial to competitive success.
- Between-point management is rarely taught to athletes.
- Athletes should use a personalized mental toughness routine between points and a customized holistic mental toughness training program to optimize their performance.
- Mental toughness can increase athletes' focus and improve their stress management, both on and off the playing field.

INTRODUCTION

As has been discussed earlier in this book, sports psychology commonly addresses performance enhancement techniques, where sports psychiatrists treat psychiatric symptoms and syndromes in athletes. This chapter blurs those boundaries and presents a novel approach to mental toughness in tennis and table tennis. The reader is encouraged to determine how this might apply to their care of athletes. Mental toughness is affected by a number of psychiatric syndromes, including depression and anxiety. A depressed athlete, for example, will have difficulty achieving mental toughness. Athletes who experience problems with "toughness," particularly if they were successful in the past, should be evaluated for underlying mood and anxiety symptoms. For some athletes, this may be an initial symptom of an emerging mood disorder. It may be easier for an athlete to discuss issues with their lack of toughness, rather than admit to themselves or others that this is the tip of the iceberg regarding an underlying psychiatric illness.

Within the realm of sports psychology, applied sports psychology focuses on understanding and applying psychological theories to increase athletes' performance and personal growth. It has grown tremendously in recent years, as more and more coaches and athletes realize the benefit of this special field [1]. Mental preparation plays a key role in athletes' performance. It differentiates the best athletes from the less successful ones. Most athletes spend 90% of their time in physical preparation, and the value of mental preparation is still usually underestimated [2].

Clinical Sports Psychiatry: An International Perspective, First Edition. Edited by David A. Baron, Claudia L. Reardon and Steven H. Baron.
© 2013 John Wiley & Sons, Ltd. Published 2013 by John Wiley & Sons, Ltd.

TENNIS AND TABLE TENNIS: EXAMPLES OF WORLDWIDE SPORTS

James Loehr studied the performance of great tennis players. His research brought a surprising observation: top tennis players used the time *between points* (plays) to "achieve the emotional balance and stable physiology needed for high performance" [3]. The mentally tough tennis players consistently followed distinct steps between points, whereas poor competitors failed to perform one or more of these activities.

> I spent years studying footage of top players – it was nearly impossible to determine a player's mental toughness by simply observing how they perform during points. The between-point time reveals what is really happening in terms of mental toughness. From my studies over several years I discovered that the top mentally tough competitors consistently completed four rather distinct patterns of activity between points. Players with competitive problems however failed to complete one or more of these activities. From this understanding I developed a between-point training sequence of mental and physical activity modeled by the top tennis players [4, p. 80].

Loehr [3, 4] found that the top tennis players consistently applied four distinct steps in between points and that this crucial time reveals what is really happening in terms of mental competency and consistency. Mental toughness is a learned disposition, and, therefore, it can be improved [5–7].

The main focus in sports psychology has been on pre-performance emotions, and there has been less emphasis on the emotion state that occurs during the task execution. An exploratory study showed initial empirical support for the notion of bidirectionality in emotion–performance relationships with table tennis athletes [8]. There has been little research undertaken on how distraction affects table tennis athletes' performance during competitions. However, task-irrelevant cognitions manifested by table tennis athletes engaged in competition may interfere with the course of an ongoing contest [9]. There has not been any standardized research yet on how in-between time affects table tennis athletes' performance in competition.

James Loehr dramatically changed the approach and method of elite and professional tennis players' mental preparation. As in tennis and table tennis, the time between breaks and points are crucial in other sports as well such as in American football, baseball, basketball, and volleyball. Some sports allow longer breaks between points than others. For example, there are 25 s between the points in tennis, but only a couple of seconds in table tennis. Regardless of the length of time, these breaks between points are crucial regarding athletes' mental preparation. Using routines between points helps athletes to handle stress better and to increase the level of their concentration and confidence.

Every athlete has an optimal energy level for performing at his or her highest level. Anxiety has a considerable impact on performance. The optimal functioning model [10, 11] explains that athletes have a zone of optimal state anxiety, which results in their best performance. Outside of this zone, their performance decreases. The optimal performance state, usually called Flow [12] or "the zone," is considered a universal phenomenon in sports. Flow is a state of concentration. It suggests that the athlete is fully focused on the activity and experiences joy while performing a task. People who experience Flow recognize its characteristics: feelings of strength, alertness, effortless control, unselfconsciousness, and peaking of abilities. Both a sense of time and emotional problems seem to disappear (see more information on Flow in Chapter 12).

Toon [2] named one manifestation of the phenomenon of Flow as "Game Face." "Getting into the zone" is described as a product of faithfully following one's Game Face Routine. This routine is an "on-the-playing-field" tool designed to assist athletes in handling the pressures of competition. It consists of four steps that are repeated during the course of competition. The specifics and sequencing of the pattern of activity will vary by sport; however, the steps are universal and can be applied to any sport. The four steps are collectively called the Game Face Routine, or the "4 R's": Reaction, Recovery, Readiness, and Ritual. The Game Face Routine helps athletes to maximize their performance during competition. It is important to highlight that every athlete has to train his or her Game Face Routine each and every day, and must keep balance in other areas of life to be able to perform at their highest potential. The key is to create a customized Game Face Training Program that will support the 4 R's in the heat of the competition. The Game Face Training Program involves simple lifestyle choices in four categories: physiological, physical, mental preparation, and daily life. Athletes have to create their routine between points and train it every day while simultaneously fulfilling optimal lifestyle choices. In summary, the Game Face Training Program is a holistic program that involves both mental and physical training to maximize athletes' performance [2].

This chapter will introduce the 4 R's (The Game Face Routine) first, followed by the Game Face Training Program (specifically involving different lifestyle choices).

THE GAME FACE ROUTINE

Reaction

Step one is Reaction. If an athlete wants to maintain his Game Face during competition, he must learn to control his reaction the instant the action stops. An athlete's goal is to keep his Game Face even in the face of adversity.

Top competitors learn to control their reaction so that they keep their Game Face on, no matter what happens on the playing field. An athlete's reaction appears in his physical response, body language, and self-talk. There are two pathways to controlling one's reaction to stimuli or stressors. One pathway is to control thoughts, and the other is to monitor body language.

How we perceive something triggers our thoughts about it. The moment the action stops, an athlete has some feelings or thoughts about it. An athlete's mind reacts long before his body does. Consequently, athletes' thoughts directly impact how their bodies respond. As soon as one is faced with a stimulus (or stressor), it is filtered through his values and beliefs. His values and beliefs then determine his perception of the stimulus as a challenge or a problem.

Top competitors perceive stressors as challenges and believe that they can cope with them. Their inner voice says, "Bring it on!" or "I can do this" or "This is tough, but I am tougher." In contrast, poor performers see stressors as problems. They struggle with limiting beliefs about their abilities. Their inner voice often says, "I can't" or "This is too hard" or "I'm not sure" or "This sucks."

Here's a really important point: Beliefs often become self-fulfilling [13]. Athletes' beliefs and perceptions can be changed if they are negative and diminish their performance. One's belief system is comprised of habitual thought patterns. Continuously thinking about the same thing over and over again will eventually make it an attitude or belief. The key component is to stay on the "High Road" in the face of stressors and train "High Road" thought patterns. In a calm, non-stressful situation, the athlete should consciously choose how he would like to think about the stressors he faces in his life. Another tool is to write (positive/ constructive) thoughts down and repeat them over and over again.

It is critical to train the way one's body reacts to stressors as well. Dr. Loehr found that top tennis players learned to control their emotions by projecting a strong, fighting, and positive physical image as soon as a point was over. He highlighted the importance of watching top performers in action and observing what their bodies project between plays. For example, the top tennis player Roger Federer quickly turns around, places the racket in the nondominant hand, and holds the racket head up as he walks energetically to take his position for the next point.

Step one is in the Game Face Routine, then, is about controlling one's reaction as soon as the action stops. The Reaction step involves the following components:

1. Standing strong and confidently
2. If a mistake has been made, using a mistake ritual to deal with it
3. Saying or thinking something positive or challenging to yourself

Recovery

The second step in the Game Face Routine during competition is to take a moment to recover as much as possible physically, mentally, and emotionally during play. Lack of a proper Recovery step often brings quick, nervous movements and thoughts between plays. This can cause problems with concentration, negative thinking, and anxiety during competition.

Less successful athletes often rush between points or plays. In tennis, poor performers will walk hastily to retrieve the ball and plunge right into the next point. Rushing between points prevents the peace of mind necessary to perform at their highest level.

In contrast, top athletes use a variety of physical strategies to recover energy and minimize anxiety between plays, including the following:

1. Deep breathing
2. Keeping eyes focused on one thing
3. Walking at a comfortable pace
4. Stretching and shaking out their hands, arms, or legs

Between points during a match, tennis star James Blake walks over to the ball person, quickly wipes himself off with his towel, and occasionally grabs a drink from his water bottle.

Actually refueling during competition is another way to recover energy. Top performers look for opportunities to grab quick bites of food, or small drinks of water or sports drinks, during pauses in the action as well as during intermissions.

Readiness

The third step in the Game Face Routine is Readiness. The purpose of this step is to ensure that athletes are mentally prepared for the action to resume. They can achieve mental readiness by becoming aware of the particular situation and knowing their plan for the upcoming action.

Readiness begins as soon as one is *near* his restart position. This step is often initiated by a signal that the action is about to start. Upon detecting the signal, such as the opponent bouncing the ball on the floor/tennis court, athletes pause momentarily, assume a strong posture, and reflect briefly on the following two questions:

1. What's the situation?
2. What's my job?

Athletes have to quickly assess what is happening on the tennis court and at the table tennis table, e.g., the score, the weather conditions, the condition of the facility, etc., and then decide what their objective is for the upcoming action. They prepare themselves mentally before they physically act.

Ritual

Ritual is the final step in the Game Face routine, and it is all about physical preparation. The purpose of this step is to deepen athletes' concentration and help them adjust their energy levels. Ritual begins as soon as athletes *take* their final position just before the action resumes.

Visually, a ritual is the way athletes position themselves just prior to the action – how they set their feet and their hands, where they look, and the position they take.

Athletes have much to think about when they are performing well. What rituals do they use between points? How do they ensure that their body is positioned for action? Do they bounce the ball two or three times before serving? Do they have a ritual for ensuring they adopt the correct stance? These seemingly "mindless" rituals are all about being physically prepared to perform at the highest level. At this point, they should only be thinking about and visualizing the action right in front of them. This step does not include thoughts about technique or tactics. The goal is to execute instinctively and automatically, and rituals are designed to make it happen. Of importance, these types of athlete rituals do *not* represent obsessive compulsive disorder, as they are adaptive and do not extend to the rest of the athlete's life.

Case Study 1

Amy was a 21-year-old elite college tennis player who used this systematic approach, with dramatic improvement in her game. These four steps helped Amy win three national championships.

Reaction

Amy's Reaction step would start as soon as a point ends. No matter what had just happened, she trained herself to react in a very consistent manner. She had the first few seconds following the point to herself. It was key that she portrayed a strong, powerful, and confident image, no matter what the previous events had been. When she and her doubles partner win the point, Amy would usually give a small fist pump and do a small hop-step to turn around. If they lose the point (especially if she missed the shot), Amy faced a bigger challenge. She worked hard to eliminate anger from her repertoire. The use of deep breathing and disciplined posture in those first 3 s made all the difference in the world in dealing with anger. She also worked hard on controlling what came out of her mouth right after the point, moving from words of anger and disgust to words of challenge such as "Right back!" and "Come On!"

Recovery

The key to maintaining one's intensity for an entire competition is to balance the energy spent during the action with the energy recovered between plays. The purpose of the Recovery step was to allow Amy's body, mind, and emotions to recover from the point. Amy would walk in the direction of her partner with her racket in her nondominant hand and maintain a pace that allowed her to recover yet not lose her intensity. Once Amy met up with her partner, they would walk side by side to the area of the court behind the baseline. The intent was to recover energy and connect as a team at the same time. The conversation was minimal and always encouraging.

Readiness

The Readiness step occurred behind the baseline. This was the time when Amy would get mentally ready for the point. She and her partner would stand behind the baseline and discuss their strategy for the next point. They would discuss any pertinent information: What is the score? What are the weather conditions? What are the opponent's tendencies? Then they would decide what their objective was for the upcoming point: "Serve up the middle and look to poach," "Attack a second serve and come in," "Take the return up the line," or otherwise. They would always maintain a strong and confident posture during their discussion.

Ritual

Amy's final step in maintaining her Game Face was physical preparation just prior to the next point. This is often referred to as Ritual. Rituals helped to deepen Amy's concentration and help her adjust her energy levels just prior to the action.

When it was her turn to serve, Amy's ritual started a bit behind the baseline. She wanted to approach the line with some energy. After a quick check of her body, was she feeling flat or tight? Amy would use her breathing to create the feeling of challenge. She would set her left foot as close to the baseline as she could and bounce the ball three times with her weight just on her left leg. She would then pick one technical piece of her serve to think about, such as "Keep my left side up" or "Quads be explosive." This technique kept her focused on the process of serving rather than the outcome. Finally, Amy would mentally see where she wanted to serve as well as feel and hear the contact she wanted to make.

When Amy's side was returning the serve, her ritual was somewhat different. She would turn her back to the court and keep her eyes on the strings of her racket. Again she would do a quick check-in with herself: was she tight, flat, loose, fired up? At this point, she wants to keep her focus internal and on her own game. When Amy was ready, she would turn around to face the court and move to the baseline with energy. She would always keep her racket in her left hand while shaking out her right hand. Then she would gently touch her right leg with her right hand to connect with her body. Mentally, Amy would focus on one technical cue that would help her hit the selected return, such as "Let the ball come in a bit" or "Stay low." She would visualize and mentally feel the contact she wanted to make and her first step. Physically, Amy would crouch into a solid athletic stance, her weight on her toes and her left foot forward. Just as the opponent's toss goes up, she would split step and be ready to move forward into her return.

Case Study 2

Peter was a 13-year-old competitive table tennis athlete. He had a hard time controlling his anger during his matches, and it greatly held him back from his best performance. With it not being uncommon that psychiatric and psychological functioning on the playing field also impacts the athlete off the field, his anger management problem and frustration affected his close family as well. After he went through the program, his mental game and his performance, as well as his family relationships, improved dramatically.

Reaction
Peter's first step would be to create a ritual routine after missed points, centered around a confident body posture. He would learn how to maintain a consistent game face manner after every missed point. His mistake ritual would be turning away from the table so as not to stare at the place where his mistake had occurred, which is what he had done previously. The other aspect of his mistake ritual would be to focus on a spot away from the table, for example, the banner on the left side of the hall or another point in the distance. This routine would help him clear his mind and think about the next point. Furthermore, he would replace his negative self-talk with a positive one.

Recovery
Peter had a very energetic character, and he would bounce on his feet between points and focus on his deep breathing. He would also use his towel after every six points (athletes can use their towel only after every six points in table tennis). He would wipe the table after points.

Readiness
His readiness routine consisted of bouncing the ball on the floor while he was behind the table and looking at the opponent as he answered the following questions in his mind: What kind of serve do I want to use, and where do I want to place it? What tactics do I want to play? He would learn to analyze the situation and make a strategic plan for the next point while exuding a strong, confident body posture.

Ritual
He would bounce the ball three times on the floor and take a deep breath before his serve. When he got into his ready serve position, he would touch the table with his racket. Before every serve receive, he would get into his serve receive body position and take a deep breath.

THE GAME FACE PYRAMID

To be able to perform their 4 R's routine between points, when they need it the most, athletes must create a customized training program that helps them to balance their life. The Game Face Training Program includes four different lifestyle aspects: physiological, physical, mental preparation, and daily life. These four basic needs are called the Game Face Pyramid (Fig. 14.1).

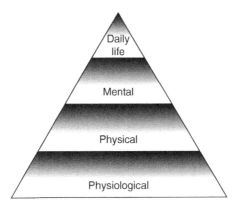

Fig. 14.1 Game Face Pyramid.

Within these four categories, there are 14 key performance areas that form the foundation of athletes' Game Face Program:

Physiological:

1. Nutrition
2. Hydration
3. Sleep

Physical:

1. Conditioning
2. Practice
3. Rehearsal

Mental:

1. Self-talk
2. Focus
3. Visualization

Daily life:

1. Time management
2. Academics
3. Fun
4. Relationships
5. Environment

Physiology is the foundation of the Game Face Training Program. The dictionary defines physiology as "the functions and vital processes of living organisms." These vital processes include nerves, muscles, circulation, breathing, and immune system. All are key to peak performance. Without a solid physiological base, athletes will not be able to derive the energy needed to train physically and mentally or attend to the requirements of their daily life. Food, drink, and sleep choices have a huge impact on these vital functions. For this reason, athletes' Game Face Training Program must address these basic areas. For example, Amy and Peter had to eat essential nutrients including carbohydrates, proteins, fats, vitamins, minerals, and water. Proper breakfast was crucial in the morning. They needed 8 h of sleep every day to be able to perform their best.

Physical training is the next level in the pyramid. Athletes' physical training determines their sport performance. The Game Face Training Program encompasses the quantity and quality of athletes' conditioning and practice sessions. For example, Peter and Amy both had personalized specific training programs designed for them by their coaches.

Most athletes know that the mental aspect of performance is hugely important. It is commonplace that the mental part of a sport is often what separates the "chokers" from the heroes. Yet, most athletes spend 95% of their time on physical training instead of devoting substantial time to their mental training program customized to the demands of their sport. Amy and Peter had mental training sessions every week, and they practiced their personalized Game Face routine along with the techniques of visualization during their training. Both of their coaches helped to create their personalized routines.

The top of the pyramid is daily life. It includes school, family, friends, environment, and time management. All these areas of athletes' lives affect their performance.

Amy and Peter regularly spent time with their friends and were good students in school despite their very tight training programs.

RECOMMENDATIONS AND CONCLUSIONS

Mental toughness is learned, not inherited, and therefore it can be improved [5–7]. This chapter highlighted how elite and professional tennis and table tennis athletes use their time between points to minimize the effect of negative attitudes and to achieve a balance between mind and muscle. The in-between time includes four steps: Reaction, Recovery, Readiness, and Ritual. Additionally, athletes have to balance other areas of their lives as well. Balancing includes four different lifestyle issues: physiological, physical, mental preparation, and daily life. The Game Face program has been specifically applied to tennis [2] and table tennis [14] in this chapter, but the principles almost certainly apply to other sports as well. This chapter illustrates how factors including motivation [15, 16] and individualized programs for athletes are crucial and cannot be ignored in any performance enhancement program. Mental toughness may improve psychological functioning both on and off the playing field. Likewise, new-onset problems with mental toughness may warrant evaluation for psychiatric disorders such as depression and anxiety outside of sport.

Recommendations for future studies include the following:

- Develop a longitudinal study with college athletic teams and individuals using the Game Face Program in different sports. Use specific criteria to measure how in-between rituals can help to reduce stress-related mental challenges.
- Create a long-distance (online) Game Face program specifically tailored to different sports and study its effectiveness on performance.
- Study the relationship between sport-related mental toughness and psychiatric disorders.

REFERENCES

1. Williams, J. M., William, F. S. (2006). Sport psychology: Past, present, future. In J. M. Williams (Ed.), *Applied Sport Psychology: Personal Grows to Peak Performance* (pp. 1–14). McGraw-Hill, New York.
2. Toon, K. (2009). *Get Your Game Face On!* Good Sports Productions, Inc., Berkeley, CA.
3. Loehr, J. E. (1994). *The New Toughness Training for Sports: Mental, Emotional, Physical Conditioning from One of the World's Premier Sports Psychologists*. Dutton, New York.

4. Loehr, J. E. (1988). The 16 second cure. *World Tennis*, September, p. 80.

5. Loehr, J. E. (1995). Six keys to getting and staying in the zone. *Tennis* 31(3): 36.

6. Kuehl, K., Kuehl, J., Tefertiller, C. (2005). *Mental Toughness: Baseball's Winning Edge*. Ivan R. Dee, Chicago, IL.

7. Selk, J. (2008). *10 Minute Toughness: The Mental Training Program for Winning Before the Game Begins*. McGraw-Hill, New York.

8. Séve, C., Ria, L., Poizat, G., Saury, J., Durand, M. (2007). Performance induced emotions and experienced during high-stakers table-tennis players. *Psychology of Sport and Exercise* 8: 25–46.

9. Krohne, H. W., Hindel, C. (2000). Anxiety, cognitive interference and sport performance; the cognitive interference test – Table-tennis. *Anxiety, Stress and Coping* 13(1): 27–52.

10. Hanin, Y. L. (1980). A study of anxiety in sports. In W. F. Straub (Ed.), *Sport Psychology: Analysis of Athlete Behavior* (pp. 236–249). Mouvement, Ithaca, NY.

11. Hanin, Y. L. (1986). State and trait anxiety research on sports in the USSR. In C. D. Spielberger, R. Diaz-Guerreo (Eds.), *Cross-Cultural Anxiety* (pp. 45–64). Hemisphere, Washington, DC.

12. Csikszentmihalyi, M. (1990). *Flow: The Psychology of Optimal Experience*. Harper & Row, New York.

13. Bandura, A. (1997). *Self-Efficacy: The Exercise of Control*. Freeman, New York.

14. Toon, K., Kurimay, D. (2012). *Get Your Game Face On! Table Tennis*. E-book. Good Sports Productions, Inc., Berkeley, CA.

15. Weinberg, R. (2010). *Mental Toughness for Sport, Business and Life*. Author House, Bloomington, IN.

16. Hagger, M. S., Chatzisarantis, N. L. D. (2007). *Intrinsic Motivation and Self-Determination in Exercise and Sport*. Human Kinetics, Champaign, IL.

15 The Use of Psychiatric Medication by Athletes

Claudia L. Reardon and Robert M. Factor

Department of Psychiatry, University of Wisconsin School of Medicine and Public Health, USA

KEY POINTS

- Three important issues to consider in prescribing psychotropic medications to athletes are: effects on performance, safety, and anti-doping guidelines.
- The scientific research base on psychotropic medication use by athletes is in its infancy, with only small studies of athletes to date.
- Future studies on psychotropic medication use by athletes should include sensitive performance measures, longer-term use of psychotropics, athletes who actually have the psychiatric disorder for which the medication is designed, and more women subjects.

INTRODUCTION

There are many issues to consider concerning the use of psychotropic medications by athletes. These include three important factors:

1. effects on performance (either negative or positive),
2. safety, and
3. anti-doping guidelines [1].

Reardon and Factor recently conducted a review of the literature on these topics [1] and have continued to search the literature since then. There have not been any large, systematic studies on the use of psychotropic medications in athletes. However, small studies have been reported. Physicians should be aware of the methodological limitations of these studies. Importantly, most involve administration of only one or two doses of the medication in question, which is problematic given that it takes several weeks for many psychotropic medications to exert their psychiatric effects [1]. Additionally, it is uncertain how readily one can extrapolate the performance measures used in some of these studies to the real-world athletic arena. For example, how readily do measures of grip strength and manual dexterity translate into the performance effect of a medication that one would see in an athlete's sport of choice? Thus, the literature in this area is in its infancy, but smaller, preliminary studies at

Clinical Sports Psychiatry: An International Perspective, First Edition. Edited by David A. Baron,
Claudia L. Reardon and Steven H. Baron.
© 2013 John Wiley & Sons, Ltd. Published 2013 by John Wiley & Sons, Ltd.

least can guide medical decision-making in treatment of athletes with mental illness, and this chapter will provide such guidance.

ANTIDEPRESSANTS

There have been small studies of the effects of selective serotonin reuptake inhibitors (SSRIs), bupropion, and a norepinephrine reuptake inhibitor in which participants served as their own controls. Based on preliminary data, the SSRI fluoxetine may not impact performance [2, 3]. These findings indeed are only preliminary, though, as they are based on only two small studies with fluoxetine used in ways that do not mimic its use in the clinical world. The first involved 11 college athletes who took either a single dose of fluoxetine 40 mg, fluoxetine 40 mg for 2 weeks, or placebo. Neither fluoxetine treatment impacted muscle strength, anaerobic capacity, power, or fatigue as measured by maximal voluntary isometric strength and evoked peak twitch torque, maximal cycle ergometer test, and test to fatigue on a cycle ergometer [2]. The second fluoxetine study involved eight male cyclists performing cycling time trials after taking fluoxetine 20 mg or placebo the evening before and the morning of the trials. Fluoxetine did not impact performance, though it was associated with decreased endorphin release with exercise [3].

One study shows the SSRI paroxetine to limit performance [4], while another shows no such impact [5]. The former study involved seven men bicycling to exhaustion after taking a single dose of paroxetine 20 mg or placebo [4]. Exercise time after paroxetine was significantly less than after placebo. The authors could not find any physiologic explanation for this via the parameters they measured in both groups: carbohydrate oxidized, blood glucose at exhaustion, blood lactate, plasma ammonia, and water consumption. They thus hypothesized that this supported a central component to fatigue that was mediated by the activity of serotonergic neurons, with this possible explanation for exercise fatigue previously and since then discussed in other papers as well. The second study saw eight men bicycle to exhaustion in a warm environment (temperature being the main difference from the first study) after taking one dose of paraoxetine 20 mg or placebo. Paroxetine did not impact performance. The authors were surprised by the findings, given that the paroxetine group exhibited higher core body temperature, which may be a limiting factor in exercise.

Bupropion is of particular interest because it is on the World Anti-Doping Agency's (WADA) Monitoring List, meaning WADA is monitoring for any concerning trends in inappropriate use given the possibility of performance enhancement [6]. Early data show that bupropion might be performance enhancing in hot [7] but not temperate [8] climates and especially when used acutely (just a single dose) as opposed to over longer periods of time [9]. One of these studies showed that in the heat, exercisers' core temperature and heart rate were higher after taking bupropion, though those exercisers did not perceive greater effort or thermal stress [8]. Thus, bupropion seemed to facilitate greater performance in the heat by allowing athletes to push themselves to higher temperatures and heart rates. Again, these studies involved small sample sizes (eight or nine men). Researchers have wondered whether it is the dopaminergic or noradrenergic effects of bupropion that may be performance enhancing, as bupropion is theorized to impact both of those neurotransmitters. Early evidence suggests that it is the dopaminergic properties that may be the performance-enhancing ones [10, 11], which fits with the known performance-enhancing effects of stimulants, which are also dopaminergic [12–14]. Specifically, a small study involved seven men taking the norepinephrine reuptake inhibitor reboxetine 8 mg or placebo the night before and morning of cycling time trials. Reboxetine did not seem to impact performance, with the conclusion being that noradrenergic effects are not performance enhancing, leaving dopaminergic effects as the more likely performance-enhancing ones. In fact, not only may noradrenergic psychotropic medications not enhance performance, but they may even limit it in hot conditions, as found in another small study of reboxetine [11].

Tricyclic antidepressants have been studied minimally in athletes and not in any randomized controlled trials [1]. Supraventricular and ventricular arrhythmias have been described in young and otherwise healthy people taking tricycles. However, the effects of tricyclic antidepressant-induced cardiac effects on athletic performance have not been studied [1]. One small study showed that a single dose of desipramine given to 22 children and adults did not affect exercise tolerance on a graded treadmill exercise test, though actual maximal athletic performance was not measured [15]. Additionally, a very small study of two patients taking stable, chronic doses of desipramine and amitriptyline, respectively, showed that exercise resulted in mild, transient increases in medication blood levels (10% and 14.9%, respectively), but these increases were probably not clinically significant or dangerous [16]. Moreover, levels returned to baseline within 1 h after exercise.

Researchers have not studied the use of the antidepressants venlafaxine, duloxetine, mirtazapine, nefazodone, trazodone, or vilazodone in athletes, nor of the biologic antidepressant treatments of electroconvulsive therapy or phototherapy [1].

Antidepressants may be used in athletes to treat a variety of psychiatric conditions: depression, anxiety, eating disorders, and attention deficit hyperactivity disorder (ADHD). Additionally, some researchers have recommended treatment of overtraining syndrome with antidepressants, given that there is significant symptom overlap between depression and overtraining syndrome [17]. While this might be reasonable, this use has not been studied in any rigorous manner [1]. Moreover, there are no data on whether antidepressants restore physical performance in athletes with depressive symptoms more or less effectively if symptoms are due to overtraining versus a depressive episode not associated with overtraining per se.

ANXIOLYTICS AND SEDATIVE-HYPNOTICS

Anxiolytics and sedative-hypnotics are important to consider, as athletes may suffer from performance anxiety and jet lag-induced insomnia. Beta-blockers are sometimes used for performance anxiety. They may be performance enhancing in some sports because of their ability to improve fine motor control and thus are banned at elite levels for shooting, archery, darts, diving, skeleton, and ski jumping [6]. On the other hand, they are probably performance inhibiting in endurance sports, having been shown to decrease time for a 20 km run, $VO_{2\,max}$ [18], and muscle strength [19].

Buspirone may be used for anxiety too. One small study suggested that it negatively impacted performance [20]. This study consisted of 13 men exercising after taking a single dose of buspirone 45 mg or placebo. Time to volitional fatigue was less, and perceived exertion greater, following buspar ingestion. As with the other studies, this one is very preliminary given the small sample size and dosing strategy employed. Beyond only a single dose of the medication being taken, that dose itself is higher than what would normally be taken at a single time.

Clonidine is another medication sometimes used for anxiety. One report suggested that this medication may stimulate endogenous growth hormone release, which could be performance enhancing [21]. However, this medication is not on the WADA Code of banned substance as it has not been studied in athletes.

Case Study

Billy was a 24-year-old professional track and field athlete who suffered jet lag–induced insomnia for the first several days when flying from the United States to Europe for summer competition. His physician thus prescribed clonazepam for him to use for the first week of all of his trips to Europe. Billy described experiencing "dead legs" and fatigue in his practices and competition on the days after taking the medication. He thus stopped the clonazepam and instead wanted to try a "natural" remedy for sleep, such as melatonin, but he was unsure if this would risk testing positive for banned substances. He ended up avoiding all medications, prescription or otherwise, for sleep because of concerns about impact on performance and potential doping violations. Instead, he utilized behavioral strategies to improve his insomnia.

A concern with the use of sedative-hypnotics used to help sleep in athletes is that they could cause next-day hangover sedation that might interfere with performance. Among the sleep aids, melatonin is the most widely studied in athletes, may be useful in jet lag, and, importantly, appears to have no impact on next-day performance after taking it before sleep [22, 23]. While reassuring that there do not appear to be negative performance effects of melatonin, some researchers have wondered about the opposite problem: performance-enhancing effects. Melatonin has been shown to have hypothermic properties, and studies have shown that exercise may be limited by high core body temperatures. Thus, strategies that use medications such as melatonin to attempt to reduce core body temperature prior to exercise theoretically could provide a greater margin before performance-limiting temperatures are reached. However, studies do not bear out any performance-enhancing effects of melatonin [22], and it is not on banned medication lists. Theoretical concerns for athletes taking melatonin include decreased blood pressure and reduced insulin sensitivity [24]. Additionally, melatonin is considered a supplement in some countries and thus not subject to the same stringent standards applied to other prescription medications. It is possible, then, that use of unregulated melatonin could result in unintentional exposure to banned substances. If concerned about this, an alternative may be a prescription melatonin receptor agonist, such as ramelteon. However, this medication has not been studied in athletes nor in transmeridian travel. Moreover, ramelteon has a longer half-life than melatonin such that next-day sedation could be more of a concern [24].

The non-benzodiazepine agonists zolpidem [25] and zopiclone [26, 27] appear to have less of a negative hangover effect on performance than do actual benzodiazepines [28, 29]. For example, in one small study, seven athletes were given zolpidem 10 mg or placebo on two consecutive nights. Zolpidem did not affect athletic performance as measured by a combined test of finger dexterity, a simple discriminatory reaction test, critical flicker fusion (CFF) test (a sensitive measure of arousal levels), vertical jump, and a 50 m sprint [25]. This is a potentially important finding, albeit a preliminary one, as prior studies of benzodiazepines showed that CFF in medicated groups was lower than or equal to control groups [28, 29]. Likewise, another small study involved eight male volleyball players taking the non-benzodiazpine agent zopiclone 7.5 mg or placebo on two consecutive nights. The groups showed no differences in measures of athletic performance batteries consisting of a choice reaction time test, eye–hand coordination test, CFF test, standing jump test, and running time test [26].

Though non-benzodiazepine agonists may cause less hangover effect than do actual benzodiazpines, they may cause more of a negative effect than does melatonin [23]. A study of 23 subjects used psychomotor testing prior to, and 7 h after, administration of a single dose of zaleplon 10 mg, zopiclone 7.5 mg, temazepam 15 mg, melatonin time-released 6 mg, or placebo. Zaleplon, zopiclone, and temazepam all impaired performance compared with placebo, while melatonin did not impair any task. As with some of the other studies described earlier in this chapter, though, one must extrapolate with caution the performance measures used in this study to the real-world athletic arena. In this case, performance measures utilized were serial reaction time, logical reasoning, serial subtraction, and multitask.

Long-acting benzodiazepines, especially when used multiple nights in a row, have more of a negative performance impact than do shorter-acting ones [30], which makes intuitive sense. For example, one study of 27 physical education students involved administration of nitrazepam 10 mg, temazepam 30 mg, or placebo for nine nights. Researchers made morning observations after nights 2 and 9. Nitrazepam, with a significantly longer half-life than temazepam, had a subjective hangover effect, while temazepam did not. Maximum exercise levels on a bicycle ergometer were comparable across all three groups on day 2, but were higher on temazepam and placebo than on nitrazepam by day 9 [30].

STIMULANTS

Effects on performance, safety, and anti-doping guidelines are all concerns when considering use of stimulants in athletes. Stimulants were first reported to be performance enhancing in 1959, after the American Medical Association created an *ad hoc* committee to study the use of amphetamine in sport [12]. Since 1959, further studies have replicated performance-enhancing effects consisting of increases in strength, acceleration, anaerobic capacity, time to exhaustion, and maximum heart rates [13]. As with the antidepressant bupropion described earlier in this chapter [8], there is evidence that athletes taking stimulants may be able to exercise to higher core temperatures and heart rates without perceiving greater effort or thermal stress. For example, one study involved eight men taking methylphenidate 20 mg or placebo 1 h before 60 min of cycling in temperate or warm climates immediately followed by a time trial [14]. Methylphenidate improved time trial performance in the heat but not in temperature conditions. Core body temperatures and heart rates were higher in the medicated group cycling in the heat, though they did not perceive greater effort or thermal stress. Accordingly, stimulants might not only be performance enhancing but may also be harmful in the heat since athletes might be unaware of increasing thermal stress [14].

Additionally, athletes competing in "leanness sports" may seek stimulant prescriptions for a weight loss advantage [31].

Given their reported ergogenic effects and safety concerns, prescription of stimulants to athletes is controversial. If physicians wish to prescribe stimulants to athletes, despite these concerns, they must complete Therapeutic Use Exemptions (TUEs) if the athlete is competing at the elite level of many sports [32]. Most elite athletes who compete on the international scene and whose physicians feel they should continue stimulant use will obtain a TUE from WADA or another international sports federation. However, if an athlete is going to compete in the Olympic Games, wants to take stimulants, and has not, for whatever reason, already obtained a TUE from WADA or another sports federation, then she may apply for one from the International Olympic Committee (IOC). Of note, even then WADA retains the right to overturn any IOC decision on a TUE.

Other medications sometimes used to treat ADHD include atomoxetine, bupropion (discussed earlier in this chapter), and modafinil. Atomoxetine, a norepinephrine reuptake inhibitor, has not been studied in athletes. Modafinil was added to the WADA banned list in 2004 because of concerns about performance enhancement [6].

MOOD STABILIZERS AND ANTIPSYCHOTICS

Mood stabilizers have been minimally studied, and antipsychotics not at all, in athletes. The mood stabilizer lithium is of potential concern when used by athletes because of the risk of toxicity while sweating. However, even that seemingly well-known risk has been called into question, with some evidence showing that lithium levels can actually be *reduced* during intense exercise [33, 34]. Other potential concerns associated with lithium use include tremor, which can negatively impact fine motor coordination, important in some sports [35]. Finally, it could negatively impact cardiovascular performance, though one small study showed no such negative affect [36]. There are no literature reports on the use of valproic acid or other mood stabilizers in athletes.

RECOMMENDATIONS AND CONCLUSIONS

High-level athletes suffering from depression, anxiety, insomnia, or other psychiatric symptoms often have reservations about taking medication with unknown performance and safety effects. Even the slightest effect on performance, e.g., a few hundredths of a second in a sprint race, could mean the difference between success and failure. Additionally, athletes and their physicians must be knowledgeable about which medications are prohibited in given sports. Preliminary recommendations for prescribers are listed in Table 15.1.

There are important methodological issues with the current literature on use of psychiatric medications by athletes. Recommendations for future study include the following:

- Use more real-world performance measures, such as athletes performing in their actual athletic events, after administration of the medication being studied.
- Measure effects on performance and safety after administration *for several weeks* of the medication being studied. Longer-term use of a psychotropic medication, which is how most patients who actually need these medications take them, may have different performance effects than just one-time or few-day dosing.
- Use athlete-subjects who actually have the psychiatric disorder or symptom that the medication studied is intended to treat. For example, in an athlete who suffers from severe insomnia, there might be no next-day sedation (or even improved alertness) compared with the baseline of that athlete who has chronic sleep deprivation. In contrast, studies that use athletes who do not suffer from insomnia may show next-day sedation compared with their baseline.
- Use women athlete-subjects, as most current studies only use men.
- Measure performance and safety effects of venlafaxine, duloxetine, mirtazapine, nefazodone, trazodone, valproic acid, and antipsychotics in athletes, and of the biological treatment of phototherapy. Studies of these particular treatments are lagging in the literature.
- Develop *larger* randomized controlled trials studying the performance and safety effects of psychotropic medications in athletes.

Table 15.1 Recommendations for prescribers of different classes of psychiatric medications to athletes.

Antidepressants	• Consider fluoxetine as a first-line choice for depression, as it is more studied than most antidepressants and preliminarily seems neither to enhance nor interfere with performance • Avoid paroxetine, which could cause side effects that interfere with performance • Be cautious about prescribing bupropion for athletes exercising in hot temperatures, as it could cause increased thermal stress • Check baseline and intermittent electrocardiograms and intermittent medication blood levels in athletes taking tricyclic antidepressants
Anxiolytics and sedative-hypnotics	• Avoid beta-blockers in most sports, since they may be either performance inhibiting or performance enhancing, depending on the sport, and are banned by several sports federations • Fluoxetine may be a better choice than buspirone for anxiety, based on preliminary evidence that buspirone may interfere with performance • Consider melatonin as a first-line choice for insomnia, as it seems neither to enhance nor interfere with performance. If worried about its unregulated status, consider ramelteon instead • If melatonin or ramelteon are ineffective for insomnia, consider the non-benzodiazepine agonists zolpidem and zopiclone • If benzodiazepines must be used for insomnia or anxiety, use shorter-acting agents that are more likely to "wear off" by the time of practice or performance
Stimulants	• Given concerns about performance enhancement and safety, consider trials of non-stimulant medications, e.g., atomoxetine, first for ADHD. If an athlete has comorbid depression, then bupropion may be a good first-line choice, as it could treat symptoms of both conditions • If stimulant medications must be used, try formulations and dosing regimens that allow for use of the medications during school/occupation times but not during practice or competition • Make sure that the athlete is aware of the potential for performance enhancement and safety risks associated with use of stimulants in sport so that he or she can make a fully informed decision • Complete Therapeutic Use Exemption applications if necessary for the prescription of stimulants
Mood stabilizers and antipsychotics	• Check baseline and intermittent electrocardiograms and regular medication blood levels in athletes taking lithium • Monitor for tremor, sedation, and weight gain in athletes taking lithium, valproic acid, or antipsychotics
All medications	• Check anti-doping guidelines, such as those of the World Anti-Doping Agency [6], specific national anti-doping agencies, or collegiate anti-doping guidelines (in the United States, this is the National Collegiate Athletic Association) [37], before prescribing any medications for collegiate or elite athletes

REFERENCES

1. Reardon CL, Factor RM (2010) Sport psychiatry: a systematic review of diagnosis and medical treatment of mental illness in athletes. *Sports Medicine* 40(11), 1–20.
2. Parise G, Bosman MJ, Boecker DR (2001) Selective serotonin reuptake inhibitors: their effect on high-intensity exercise performance. *Archives of Physical Medicine and Rehabilitation* 82, 867–871.
3. Meeusen R, Piacentini MF, van Den Eynde S *et al.* (2001) Exercise performance is not influenced by a 5-HT reuptake inhibitor. *International Journal of Sports Medicine* 22, 329–336.
4. Wilson WM, Maughan RJ (1992) Evidence for a possible role of 5-hydroxytryptamine in the genesis of fatigue in man: administration of paroxetine, a 5-HT re-uptake inhibitor, reduces the capacity to perform prolonged exercise. *Experimental Physiology* 77, 921–924.
5. Strachan AT, Leiper JB, Maughan RJ (2004) Paroxetine administration fails to influence human exercise capacity, perceived effort or hormone responses during prolonged exercise in a warm environment. *Experimental Physiology* 89(6), 657–664.
6. World Anti-Doping Agency (2012) List of prohibited substances and methods, January 1. http://list.wada-ama.org. Accessed on 25 March 2012.
7. Watson P, Hasegawa H, Roelands B *et al.* (2005) Acute dopamine/noradrenaline reuptake inhibition enhances human exercise performance in warm, but not temperate conditions. *The Journal of Physiology* 565(3), 873–883.
8. Piacentini MF, Meeusen R, Buyse L *et al.* (2004) Hormonal responses during prolonged exercise are influenced by a selective DA/NA reuptake inhibitor. *British Journal of Sports Medicine* 38, 129–133.
9. Roelands B, Hasegawa H, Watson P *et al.* (2009) Performance and thermoregulatory effects of chronic bupropion administration in the heat. *European Journal of Applied Physiology* 105(3), 493.
10. Piacentini MF, Meeusen R, Buyse L *et al.* (2002) No effect of a noradrenergic reuptake inhibitor on performance in trained cyclists. *Medicine and Science in Sports and Exercise* 34(7), 1189–1193.
11. Roelands B, Goekint M, Heyman E *et al.* (2008) Acute noradrenaline reuptake inhibition decreases performance in normal and high ambient temperature. *Journal of Applied Physiology* 105(1), 206–212.
12. Smith GM, Beecher HK (1959) Amphetamine sulfate and athletic performance. I: objective effects. *Journal of American Medical Association* 170, 542–557.
13. Chandler JV, Blair SN (1980) The effect of amphetamines on selected physiological components related to athletic success. *Medicine & Science in Sports & Exercise* 12(1), 65–69.
14. Roelands B, Hasegawa H, Watson P *et al.* (2008) The effects of acute dopamine reuptake inhibition on performance. *Medicine & Science in Sports & Exercise* 40(5), 879–885.
15. Waslick BD, Walsh BT, Greenhill LL *et al.* (1999) Cardiovascular effects of desipramine in children and adults during exercise testing. *Journal of the American Academy of Child and Adolescent Psychiatry* 38(2), 179–186.
16. de Zwaan M (1992) Exercise and antidepressant serum levels. *Biological Psychiatry* 32, 210–211.
17. Armstrong LE, VanHeest JL (2002). The unknown mechanism of the overtraining syndrome: clues from depression and psychoneuroimmunology. *Sports Medicine* 32, 185–209.
18. Cowan DA (1994) Drug abuse. In: Harries M, Williams C, Stanish WD *et al.* (eds.) *Oxford Textbook of Sports Medicine*. Oxford University Press, New York, pp. 314–329.
19. Wilmore JH (1988) Exercise testing, training, and beta-adrenergic blockade. *Physician and Sportsmedicine* 16, 45–50.
20. Marvin G, Sharma A, Aston W *et al.* (1997) The effects of buspirone on perceived exertion and time to fatigue in man. *Experimental Physiology* 82, 1057–1060.
21. Kennedy M (1994) Drugs and athletes: an update. *Adverse Drug Reaction Bulletin* 169, 639–642.
22. Atkinson G, Drust B, Reilly T *et al.* (2003) The relevance of melatonin to sports medicine and science. *Sports Medicine* 33(11), 809–831.
23. Paul MA, Gray G, Kenny G *et al.* (2003) Impact of melatonin, zaleplon, zopiclone, and temazepam on psychomotor performance. *Aviation, Space, and Environmental Medicine* 74(12), 1263–1270.
24. Herman D, MacKnight JM, Stromwall AE *et al.* (2011) The international athlete – advances in management of jet lag disorder and anti-doping policy. *Clinics in Sports Medicine* 30, 641–659.
25. Ito SU, Kanbayashi T, Takemura T et al. (2007) Acute effects of zolpidem on daytime alertness, psychomotor and physical performance. *Neuroscience Research* 59, 309–313.

26. Tafti M, Besset A, Billiard M (1992) Effects of zopiclone on subjective evaluation of sleep and daytime alertness and on psychomotor and physical performance tests in athletes. *Progress in Neuropsychopharmacology & Biological Psychiatry* 16, 55–63.

27. Grobler LA, Schwellnus MP, Trichard C *et al.* (2000) Comparative effects of zopiclone and loprazolam on psychomotor and physical performance in active individuals. *Clinical Journal of Sport Medicine* 10(2), 123–128.

28. Holmberg G (1982) The effects of anxiolytics on CFF. *Pharmacopsychiatry* 15(Suppl.), 49–53.

29. Maddock RJ, Casson EJ, Lott LA *et al.* (1993) Benzodiazepine effects on flicker sensitivity: role of stimulus frequency and size. *Progress in Neuropsychopharmacology & Biological Psychiatry* 17, 955–970.

30. Charles RB, Kirkham AJT, Guyatt AR *et al.* (1987) Psychomotor, pulmonary and exercise responses to sleep medication. *British Journal of Clinical Pharmacology* 24, 191–197.

31. Conant-Norville DO, Tofler IR (2005) Attention deficit/hyperactivity disorder and psychopharmacologic treatments in the athlete. *Clinics in Sports Medicine* 24, 829–843.

32. World Anti-Doping Agency (2011) Therapeutic use exemptions, December. Available from URL: http://www.wada-ama.org/en/Science-Medicine/TUE. Accessed on 25 March 2012.

33. Miller EB, Pain RW, Skripal PJ (1978) Sweat lithium in manic depression. *The British Journal of Psychiatry* 133, 477–478.

34. Jefferson JW, Greist JH, Clagnaz PJ *et al.* (1982) Effect of strenuous exercise on serum lithium level in man. *The American Journal of Psychiatry* 139(12), 1593–1595.

35. Macleod AD (1998) Sport psychiatry. *Australian and New Zealand Journal of Psychiatry* 32, 860–866.

36. Tilkian AG, Schroeder JS, Kao J *et al.* (1976) Effect of lithium on cardiovascular performance: report on extended ambulatory monitoring and exercise testing before and during lithium therapy. *American Journal of Cardiology* 38, 701–708.

37. NCAA guidelines to document ADHD treatment with banned stimulant medications (2010) Addendum to the January 2009 guidelines, July 20. http://www.ncaa.org/wps/wcm/connect/2aab920046d88461bc 4bfdac20c3c72c/ADHD+Q++A+July+2010+update.pdf?MOD=AJPERES&CACHEID=2aab920046d 88461bc4bfdac20c3c72c. Assessed on 25 March 2012.

16 Sexual Harassment and Abuse in Sport

Saul I. Marks

FINA Sports Medicine Committee, Canada
International Society for Sport Psychiatry, North York General Hospital, Canada
Department of Health and Disease, Department of Psychiatry, University of Toronto, Canada

KEY POINTS

- Sexual harassment and abuse in sport is a global issue and occurs at all levels of sport, and in all sports, with an increased risk at the elite level. There are different types of sexual harassment and abuse in sport.
- There are both physical and psychological consequences of sexual harassment and abuse in sport. This issue not only threatens the integrity of sport in general, but has significant consequences for athletes and their teams.
- Sports psychiatrists have a major role to play in the prevention of sexual harassment and abuse in sport by advocating for increased education and awareness regarding this problem. Increased awareness of the reality of this issue will allow health-care professionals to advocate for its prevention.
- Sports psychiatrists must have strategies to recognize and manage sexual harassment and abuse in sport when they suspect that such abuse is occurring in their sporting arenas.

Unfortunately, sexual harassment and abuse in sport (SHA) has been occurring in sport for decades, if not centuries. It occurs in all sports and at all levels of sport [1]. It is essential that all people in the athlete entourage have knowledge of the risk factors involved and the outcomes of SHA. Team doctors, sports medicine physicians, and sports psychiatrists are in frequent contact with athletes and therefore need to be aware of the risk factors and potential consequences of SHA.

WHAT IS SEXUAL HARASSMENT AND ABUSE IN SPORT?

There are various forms in which SHA can occur in sport and it is paramount that all forms are given equal attention. These include sexual harassment, sexual abuse, gender harassment, hazing, and homophobia. As with all forms of abuse, SHA is "based upon an abuse of power and trust and that is considered by the victim or a bystander to be unwanted or coerced." Sexual harassment is considered sexualized verbal, nonverbal, or physical

Clinical Sports Psychiatry: An International Perspective, First Edition. Edited by David A. Baron,
Claudia L. Reardon and Steven H. Baron.
© 2013 John Wiley & Sons, Ltd. Published 2013 by John Wiley & Sons, Ltd.

behavior. It can be intended or unintended, legal or illegal. It can be very obvious to subtle or completely unnoticeable. Sexual abuse occurs when there is not mutual consent, or when consent <u>cannot be</u> given or is obtained in an aggressive, exploitative, manipulative, or threatening manner [2]. In sport, with so much at stake, especially at the elite level, manipulation or entrapment of the athlete by someone in a position of power can easily be imagined. Gender harassment consists of "derogatory treatment of one gender or another that is systematic and repeated but not necessarily sexual in nature." Hazing is "any activity expected of someone joining a group that humiliates, degrades, abuses, or endangers regardless of the person's willingness to participate" [3]. Homophobia is a "form of prejudice and discrimination ranging from passive resentment to active victimization of lesbian, gay, bisexual, and transgendered people.

PREVALENCE OF SEXUAL HARASSMENT AND ABUSE IN SPORT

The scientific literature has shown that SHA occurs in all sports and at all levels, including child and youth sports [1, 4]. The studies vary widely as to the prevalence, from 2% to 48%, while the prevalence does appear to be higher as you move into the world of elite athletics [5]. This occurs because the more achievements the athlete has, the greater the power differential between the athlete and the coach or other particularly necessary personnel in the athlete entourage.

PERPETRATORS OF SEXUAL HARASSMENT AND ABUSE IN SPORT

As previously stated, perpetrators of SHA, such as the coach or other members of the athlete entourage, are in positions of power. By no means are coaches the only perpetrators of SHA. Athletes actually harass each other, for example, via hazing, more often than members of the coaching staff harass athletes [6, 7]. Males are more commonly perpetrators of SHA. However, females can also be perpetrators of SHA, just as they can be outside of sport. Males may be seen as perpetrators more often simply because there are more men in positions of power in the world of sport, especially at the elite level.

RISK FACTORS FOR SEXUAL HARASSMENT AND ABUSE IN SPORT

There are both very real risk factors for SHA and many myths about what leads to SHA. Location is a major risk factor for SHA. Areas of isolation such as the locker room, coach's car, coach's home, trips away, and other areas involving isolation from other athletes increase the risk [8, 9]. Risk is also increased at team events that may involve alcohol or power differentials, for example, as can occur at team socials, initiations and hazing, and year-end events. Other risk factors can be found in Table 16.1.

Table 16.1 Risk factors for sexual harassment and abuse in sports.

Athlete variables	Coach variables	Sport variables
• Poor and distant relationship with parents • Younger female • Low self-esteem • Strong talent • Dedication to the coach	• Male • Older • Good reputation in the sport • Trusted by the athlete's parents	• Away trips • Limited opportunity for reporting SHA

There are many myths regarding SHA. There is no evidence that revealing clothing, touching of the athlete, or type of sport are in any way risk factors for SHA [9].

Case Study (Sexual Abuse)

MR is an 18-year-old woman. She is a talented long-distance swimmer and hopes to make the Olympic team several times in the years ahead. She has been selected to move to the National Team Training center and has decided to move one thousand miles away from her family, so she can be in the city where the Training center is, and where one of the best coaches in the country, Jim, resides.

After MR moves, Jim continually praises her performances, saying that if she follows his directions, he will make all of her sporting dreams come true. It is obvious to many of the staff at the National Team Training center that Jim is very much enamored by MR, as he continues to give encouraging comments and praise to an extreme. Many of these are seen as inappropriate. However, it continues to be ignored by all of the other staff at the National Team Training center.

Initially, MR is happy with how her coaching relationship is going. Later, though, Jim's "special attention" toward MR is noticed by her teammates. Not only are her teammates making comments to her about this attention, but she begins to become isolated, as her teammates become increasingly jealous of her. Being so far away from her family, her normally "bubbly" personality becomes flat and introverted.

Additionally, MR starts underachieving at school, and one day Jim offers to tutor her in her school work after practice in his office. He drives her home after the tutoring session and buys her dinner on the way home. They are alone in the restaurant for several hours in a booth, and MR starts to feel extremely uncomfortable. After a few weeks, Jim changes the tutoring sessions from being held at his coach's office to his home in the evenings. MR wants so much to achieve in her sport she goes along with the plan despite how awkward she is now feeling.

Time goes on, and the night before her first big qualifying race to make the Olympic trials, Jim calls MR to his hotel room for a "special pre-competition talk." She walks in, and he closes the door. MR starts to have a "sinking" feeling overcome her. While sitting on the bed together, he puts his arm around her. She begins to feel uncomfortable, more than ever before, as he places his hand on her thigh. He says that if she performs special favors for him, he will ensure her success tomorrow. MR feels completely trapped and, as always, does what her mentor and coach tells her to do.

As MR leaves the room, she passes by the team manager and her teammates. Although she is visibly crying and upset, they turn around and walk away. She feels completely isolated and invisible to the world around her.

The next day, MR qualifies for the Olympic trials. Her parents have come to see the event and do not understand why she is not excited. She says nothing other than that of course she is excited and that she is well on her way to her sporting dream coming true.

Case Study (Homophobia)

MJ is a 17-year-old male who has been an up and coming gymnast in the junior ranks in his province for the last three previous seasons. As he is getting older, more and more people are predicting his future success in the sport of gymnastics. MJ comes from a conservative family, and his father was a former Olympian in boxing. While he is supportive of his son's success, he has never been happy that his son has chosen such an "unmanly" sport. While his mother and his younger sister have always been very supportive and excited about MJ's success, his father often ridicules him.

MJ's coach begins to notice that he is less "himself" at the gym and starts to become concerned that there is a problem at home, school, socially, or in some intimate interpersonal relationship that he does not know about. MJ's coach, Bob, approaches his athlete alone and privately in a corner of the gymnasium where they can be seen by the rest of the team, but not heard. Bob begins to discuss that he has noticed that MJ's normal bubbly outgoing personality seems to be somewhat guarded and that he seems less comfortable around his teammates both in the gym and out. Bob has also noticed that he seems more uncomfortable on away trips, not so much if he is in a room of two with one of his best friends, RP, but if he is in a room of four.

MJ completely denies that there is any problem. He says that he finds rooms of four difficult in terms of getting a good night of sleep, and that he is much more able to concentrate on the competition when he is a room of two with his friend. As for him not quite being himself, he discusses that his father at home has become increasingly vocal about his choice of sports and about how gymnastics is "unmanly." His coach is very understanding and says, "I have always wondered why your mother and sister come to all of your gymnastics events and your father I have only ever met once." Bob offers to discuss the problem with his father, and MJ begs him not to for fear of the repercussions this could have on him in his home life. His coach agrees to leave things alone for the time being, but that MJ should always feel free to come and talk to him about the problems he is facing. He also discusses the fact that it is important for MJ to be able to be honest with his coach if he is to continue his success into the senior ranks. Bob further explains that in the next year, because he and his friend both have been team leaders and are increasingly the most successful on the team, he is going to start introducing them into the senior ranks, and there will always only be two in a room. MJ is very excited by this and quickly tells his friend, RP. The team sees them give each other a big hug, and rumors begin to start about them being homosexual.

In fact, MJ and his friend, RP, are homosexual and have been becoming increasingly close and have discussed having a relationship just a week before. They are both scared and excited at the prospect of being together.

One night, early into the next season, after an extremely successful National Qualification meet, where MJ has made it to the Senior National Gymnastics Championships for the first time, he walks into his home with his mother and sister. They have been at the championships with him for support, and they are all excited to tell MJ's father. Immediately, all three notice that MJ's father is enraged. While they were away, MJ's father, John, has heard of the rumors of his son having a homosexual relationship. He confronts him in front of his mother and his sister. MJ's mother tries to calm John down, but John will hear nothing of it and tells them all that he is going to tell MJ's coach that his son will no longer be doing gymnastics. MJ runs to his room and locks the door to warn his now-partner RP.

John arrives at MJ's coach's house. John confronts Bob about the rumors. John tells Bob that his son will no longer be on the gymnastics team. Bob tries to reason with John, but John will hear nothing of it. MJ's father leaves the house screaming, "The entire team is talking about my son and RP as a couple! They are making jokes about my entire family. You cannot stop that so I will." MJ's father storms out of the coach's house. He arrives home and says what he has done. MJ has left, and no one knows where he is. His mother is extremely concerned, but his father says MJ is no longer welcome at home. MJ's father and mother go up to their room where she tries unsuccessfully to reason with him. MJ is not seen for the next week, and he has been reported as missing.

PHYSICAL AND PSYCHOLOGICAL CONSEQUENCES OF SEXUAL HARASSMENT AND ABUSE IN SPORT

It is extremely important for all of those who are around athletes to recognize both the physical and psychological consequences of SHA. One sees the same types of symptoms as seen in abuse victims outside of sport. However, more research needs to be done within sport to determine if there are other consequences, or if some are more common than in non-sport abuse victims [9–12]. Any of these consequences can affect an athlete's level of functioning in any aspect of her life, including work, sport performance, intimate relationships, social life, and achievement in any educational sphere.

PHYSICAL CONSEQUENCES AND MEDICAL PRESENTATIONS OF SEXUAL HARASSMENT AND ABUSE IN SPORT

The physical consequences of SHA, both in sport and outside of sport, are more easily seen than are nonphysical consequences. They can be apparent as a victim goes through his activities of daily function. Often it is the physician that is caring for the athlete that is most likely to see these consequences.

Headaches, lethargy, sleep disturbances, weight fluctuations, and poor general health are examples of how SHA in sport can manifest physically.

PSYCHOLOGICAL CONSEQUENCES OF SHA IN SPORT

Psychological consequences of SHA are far more difficult to detect than physical ones. One must be very aware that discussion of how athletes are "feeling" is extremely important to prevent SHA. Athletes are much more willing to discuss their "physical" problems than discuss them as "emotional or psychological" ones, as emotional and psychological difficulties indicate that the athlete is weak and stigmatize them just as the normal population. Table 16.2 outlines the consequences as a result of SHA both in and out of sport [13]. More easily seen psychological symptoms of SHA share some overlap with physical ones and include weight loss or weight gain, bed-wetting, and increased or decreased energy. One can also see many acting out behaviors. These include risk taking (i.e., no use of condoms), self-harm behaviors causing physical harm, and excessive dieting or binge eating [14, 15]. There can be increased social and behavioral problems, including harming of others, harming of pets, increased bullying of peers, chaotic interpersonal relationships, and

Table 16.2 Psychological consequences of SHA in sport.

	Symptoms
Physical manifestations of psychological consequences	Weight loss/weight gain
	Bed-wetting
	Fatigue/decreased energy
	Acting out behaviors causing physical harm
	Sexually transmitted infections
Self-harm behaviors	Excessive dieting or binging
	Cutting or breaking the skin
	Pulling out of hair
Harming of others	Cruelty to pets
	Bullying of peers
	Aggression with schoolmates or neighbors
	Cruelty to family
Suicide/homicide	Suicidal ideation, attempt, or completion
	Homicidal ideation, attempt, or completion
Clinical depression	Sad or irritable mood
	Loss of interest in activities (anhedonia)
	Change in appetite
	Change in sleep habits
	Decreased concentration
	Guilt
	Hopelessness
	Helplessness
	Loss of libido
	Loss of energy
Anxiety	Physical stress, muscular tension
	Nightmares
	Obsessive-compulsive behaviors/disorder
	Acute and chronic posttraumatic stress disorder
	Hypervigilance

trust and intimacy issues [16]. If the real issue behind the symptom is a psychological one, the athlete is much more reluctant to discuss it as a problem, as one often sees with disordered eating or acting out behaviors. There often will be not only reluctance to discuss the difficulty but there will be "rationalizations" and other reasons for the difficulty.

Mood and anxiety disorders are experienced at a higher rate, and the development of these and other mental health problems are a major concern. Rates of suicidal ideation, suicide attempts, and completed suicides are higher in those who have experienced SHA. Acute and chronic posttraumatic stress disorder [17, 18], which brings nightmares, hypervigilance, and obsessive-compulsive behaviors and/or disorder, is also seen at a higher rate. As previously mentioned, eating disorders, body image problems, and lowered self-esteem also occur. There are also higher rates of substance abuse and dependence as a result of SHA in sport [19, 20].

SPECIFIC PSYCHOLOGICAL CONSEQUENCES AND MEDICAL PRESENTATIONS SEEN IN SPORT IN GENERAL

Athletes tend to be risk takers in general. Without this "edge," often good athletic performance is difficult. However, when SHA causes self-harm behaviors and excessive training, physicians may start to see an increase in unresolved injuries that do not make sense to them. Athletic performance can start to drop, as can self-confidence and consistency of performance. Athletes may even unexpectedly drop out from sport. Trust becomes an issue with people in positions of authority as the athlete begins to lose confidence in not only the perpetrator, but those who are not noticing the problem, for example, others in the athlete's entourage, family, peers, and teachers. As this loss of trust grows, the athlete has an even greater likelihood of considering dropping out of sport.

PREVENTION BY UNDERSTANDING THE COACH–ATHLETE RELATIONSHIP

The better we start to know the coach–athlete relationship and how to prevent it from moving closer to SHA, the less the sporting community will need to be concerned about the development of problematic relationships. The development of sexually abusive relationships has been labeled the "grooming process" [21–23]. There are four key steps that make the athlete increasingly vulnerable to SHA, as described in Box 16.1 [24].

Box 16.1 The grooming process

1. The perpetrator targets the victim-athlete. This athlete is usually vulnerable in some way, for example, by being more isolated on the sports team, having a poor or absent relationship with parents, and/or having few friends. The relationship with the perpetrator usually begins with increasing friendship.
2. The friendship then becomes more trusting, and the athlete is made to feel special by being given special rewards or favors. This serves to increase the cooperation between the athlete and the coach.
3. The perpetrator begins to work at further isolating the athlete. This includes isolation from family, peers, and other supportive people in the athlete's life.
4. Once the abuse has begun, secrecy becomes all-important. The perpetrator will start to say things such as "you owe me" or "it is our little secret."

As the "grooming" process continues, the athlete starts to feel powerless and completely entrapped by the perpetrator. To prevent such a relationship from developing, it is extremely important that people understand the power differential in the coach–athlete relationship and in any relationship in which someone is in a position of power over the athlete. Only with this understanding can SHA be reduced or extinguished in the world of sport.

THE TEAM DOCTOR'S ROLE IN PREVENTION OF SHA

Athlete protection policy, code of conduct, and boundaries

All sport organizations should have athlete protection policy statements. All people who are involved in the world of sport need to ensure that such policies are in place. These statements need to contain statements of intent to demonstrate a complete commitment to create a respectful and mutually safe environment [5]. There also needs to be a way to evaluate if the system that has been put into place is serving the purpose for which it was created. Those in positions of power need to understand boundaries. Thus, codes of conduct in sport should include coaches, administrative staff, peers, volunteers, parents, and the athletes as well [2]. For codes of conduct to truly make a difference in the world of sport, these guidelines need to be extremely specific and include: the physicians' specific roles and responsibilities, defined relationship boundaries, and defined appropriate professional boundaries [9].

LEADERSHIP FROM THE INTERNATIONAL OLYMPIC COMMITTEE

The International Olympic Committee (IOC) has taken a leadership role on the issue of SHA in sport since its development of a consensus statement on this issue. This document serves as an educational tool for sport organizations to learn about SHA in sport. The IOC continues to show its commitment to make the "sport playing field" a safer place. At the Youth Olympic Games in 2010 in Singapore, the IOC developed an educational animation video for the youth athlete to raise awareness of the athlete's rights in the prevention of SHA. The IOC should be applauded for its continued work to raise awareness of this issue in sport. Many of the issues not fully discussed here as well as both past and present research on the issue of SHA can be accessed from the International Olympic Committee's website (www.olympic.org/sha).

CLINICAL APPROACH TO DISCLOSURE

Sexual harassment or abuse is usually accompanied by the athlete feeling immense shame, guilt, and fear [25]. Therefore, the team physician or sports psychiatrist should focus on empathic listening and psychological support of the athlete-patient. The athlete's courage for speaking out should be acknowledged. It should also be very much validated that this is not the athlete's fault. While avoiding leading questions, it is important to encourage disclosure of the SHA. The perpetrator should not be denigrated during the disclosure. Accurate record completion by the physician is paramount. Although laws vary from country to country, in some countries it is the physician's responsibility to report the abuse. Reporting can also be made according to the sport organization's policies as previously outlined. Neglecting or ignoring the abuse only serves to increase the sequelae of SHA. When this happens, it is known as the "bystanders" effect [9, 26, 27].

CONCLUSION

Team doctors, the athlete entourage, and sports psychiatrists play a major role in the early detection of SHA. Through understanding the risk factors for SHA, possible relationships in which SHA may occur, and the physical and psychological effects of SHA, health-care professionals, including sports psychiatrist, are better able to identify SHA. Hopefully this knowledge will assist in decreasing the incidence and duration of SHA. Moreover, understanding these issues should improve the likelihood that resultant health consequences of SHA will be treated more quickly and effectively.

REFERENCES

1. Brackenridge CH (1994) Fair play or fair game: Child sexual abuse in sport. *International Review for the Sociology of Sport* **29**, 287–299.
2. International Olympic Committee (2007) Consensus statement on "Sexual Harassment & Abuse in Sport." http://multimedia.olympic.org/pdf/en_report_1125.pdf. Accessed on December 6, 2012.
3. Hoover NC (1999) National survey: Initiation rites and athletics for NCAA sports teams. http://www.alfred.edu/sports_hazing/docs/hazing.pdf. Accessed on 6 December 2012.
4. Fasting K, Brackenridge CH, Sundgot-Borgen J (2003) Experiences of sexual harassment and abuse amongst Norwegian elite female athletes and non-athletes. *Research Quarterly for Exercise and Sport* **74**, 84–97.
5. Brackenridge CH (1997) "He owned me basically…" Women's experience of sexual abuse in sport. *International Review for the Sociology of Sport* **32**, 115–130.
6. Kirby SL, Wintrup G (2002) Hazing and initiation: Sexual harassment and abuse issues. *Journal of Sexual Aggression* **8**, 41–60.
7. Waldron J, Lynn Q, Krane V (2011) Duct tape, icy hot & paddles: Narratives of initiation onto US male sport teams. *Sport, Education and Society* **16**, 111–125.
8. Kirby S, Greaves L, Hankivsky O (2000) *The Dome of Silence: Sexual Harassment and Abuse in Sport.* London: Zed Books.
9. Cense M, Brackenridge CH (2001) Temporal and developmental risk factors for sexual harassment and abuse in sport. *European Physical Education Review* **7**, 61–79.
10. Irish L, Kobayashi I, Delahanty D (2010) Long-term physical health consequences of childhood sexual abuse: A meta-analytic review. *Journal of Pediatric Psychology* **35**, 450–461.
11. Wilson DR (2010) Health consequences of childhood sexual abuse. *Perspectives in Psychiatric Care* **46**, 56–64.
12. Hillberg T, Hamilton-Giachritsis C, Dixon L (2011) Review of meta-analyses on the association between child sexual abuse and adult mental health difficulties: A systematic approach. *Trauma Violence Abuse* **12**, 38–49.
13. Hornor G (2010) Child sexual abuse: Consequences and implications. *Journal of Pediatric Health Care* **24**, 358–363.
14. Marks S, Mountjoy M, Marcus M (2011) Sexual harassment and abuse in sport: The role of the team doctor. *British Journal of Sports Medicine* **46**(13), 905–908.
15. Kearney-Cooke A, Ackard DM (2000) The effects of sexual abuse on body image, self-image, and sexual activity of women. *Journal of Gender Specific Medicine* **3**, 54–60.
16. Davila GW, Bernier F, Franco J, Kopka SL (2003) Bladder dysfunction in sexual abuse survivors. *Journal of Urology* **170**, 476–479.
17. Zierler S, Feingold L, Laufer D, et al. (1991) Adult survivors of childhood sexual abuse and subsequent risk of HIV infection. *American Journal of Public Health* **81**, 572–575.

18. Jonas S, Bebbington P, McManus S, *et al.* (2011) Sexual abuse and psychiatric disorder in England: Results from the 2007 Adult Psychiatric Morbidity Survey. *Psychological Medicine* **41**, 709–719.

19. Paolucci EO, Genuis ML, Violato C (2001) A meta-analysis of the published research on the effects of child sexual abuse. *The Journal of Psychology* **135**(1), 17–36.

20. Kendler KS, Bulik CM, Silberg J, *et al.* (2000) Childhood sexual abuse and adult psychiatric and substance use disorders in women: An epidemiological and cotwin control analysis. *Archives of General Psychiatry* **57**, 953–959.

21. Wilsnack SC, Vogeltanz ND, Klassen AD, Harris TR (1997) Childhood sexual abuse and women's substance abuse: National survey findings. *Journal of Studies on Alcohol and Drugs* **58**, 264–271.

22. Fasting K, Brackenridge CH (2005) The grooming process in sport: Case studies of sexual harassment and abuse. *Auto/Biography* **13**, 33–52.

23. Grubin D (1998) Sex offending against children: Understanding the risk. Police Research Series Paper 99. London: Research, Development and Statistics Directorate, Home Office. http://library.npia.police. uk/docs/hopolicers/fprs99.pdf. Accessed on 6 December 2012.

24. Tofetgaard NJ (2001) The forbidden zone: Intimacy, sexual relations and misconduct in the relationship between coaches and athletes. *International Review for the Sociology of Sport* **36**, 165–182.

25. International Olympic Committee (2009) Olympic Movement Medical Code. http://www.olympic. org/Documents/Fight_against_doping/Rules_and_regulations/OlympicMovementMedicalCode-EN_ FR.pdf. Accessed on 6 December 2012.

26. Banyard VL, Plante EG, Moynihan MM (2004) Bystander education: Bringing a broader community perspective to sexual violence prevention. *Journal of Community Psychology* **32**, 61–79.

27. Darley JM, Latané B (1968) Bystander intervention in emergencies: Diffusion of responsibility. *Journal of Personality and Social Psychology* **8**, 377–383.

Part Three
Psychosocial Issues Affecting Athletes

17 The Role of Culture in Sport

Claudia L. Reardon,[1] David A. Baron,[2,3,4]
Steven H. Baron,[5] Bulent Coskun,[6] and Ugur Cakir[7]

[1] Department of Psychiatry, University of Wisconsin School of Medicine and Public Health, USA
[2] International Relations and Department of Psychiatry, Keck School of Medicine at the University of Southern California, USA
[3] Keck Medical Center at University of Southern California, USA
[4] Global Center for Exercise, Psychiatry, and Sports at USC, Health Sciences Campus, USA
[5] Montgomery County Community College, USA
[6] Department of Psychiatry, Community Mental Health Center, Kocaeli University, Turkey
[7] Department of Psychiatry, Derince Education and Research Hospital, Turkey

KEY POINTS

- Sports participation and viewing often play an important role in defining a country's culture.
- Cultural beliefs have a significant impact on sports participation and community support for sporting activities.
- Sports culture affects mental illness and sports injuries.

Culture can be broadly defined as the customs, arts, social institutions, and achievements of a nation, people, or social group. Few things affect the culture of many countries more profoundly than sports. The sense of pride experienced by becoming a sports champion is seen in many parts of the world. Many cities will gladly spend money, even in challenging financial times, to honor the victorious team. The response to winning a championship often far exceeds public reaction to virtually every other culturally significant event. Viewership of important sporting events, such as the Olympics, World Cup, and the Super Bowl (U.S. football's championship game), is unmatched by any other cultural event and commands the highest price for advertising. Presidents and other leaders honor world champions, and governments pay handsomely for gold medals. Walk down the street of many cities in the world, high, middle, or low income, and people will be wearing the jersey of their favorite sports team or marquee player. People simply like to feel a part of "their" team. The social psychological phenomenon of "basking in the reflected glory" appears to be almost universal. We seek to somehow feel a part of a great athlete's world.

Sport transcends political party affiliation and tends to be geographic. Major sporting events are now major cultural and sociopolitical phenomena. The Olympic Games are the best example of this. Cities around the globe compete for the opportunity to potentially lose substantial amounts of money because of the statement hosting the Games makes to the world. Many believe the spectacular opening ceremonies of the 2008 Beijing Olympic Games was a global "coming out" party for China and the Chinese culture. No expense was

Clinical Sports Psychiatry: An International Perspective, First Edition. Edited by David A. Baron,
Claudia L. Reardon and Steven H. Baron.
© 2013 John Wiley & Sons, Ltd. Published 2013 by John Wiley & Sons, Ltd.

spared, as this was *the* cultural event for the most populated country on earth. This phenomenon is not unique to the Olympics. Countries will seek a bid to host soccer's World Cup with equal fervor. Recently we have even seen countries unite in order to be given the honor of hosting a World Cup.

This is not to say, though, that there are not some countries in which sports are not as widely lauded as they are in others. For example, in some countries education is given more esteem than athletic accomplishment. In these countries, there is less systematic and disciplined training provided for promising young athletes. The relatively weak cultural value assigned to sports is "blamed" for such countries' relatively poor athletic performance on international stages. These countries devote fewer economic resources to training facilities and other requirements for the nurturance of future world champions.

Worldwide cultural beliefs allow for, and in fact encourage, behaviors not readily accepted outside of the sporting venue. Outlandish dress, alcohol consumption, and behavior otherwise deemed socially unacceptable such as screaming at players and officials who are simply trying to do their job are accepted and in fact become cultural norms. Often it is only when the behaviors cross the line of endangering personal safety that they are sanctioned.

The cultural beliefs within sports also play an important role, often exceeding the rules created in order to govern the game. The best example of this is the "culture of toughness." Until very recently, one way in which athletes showed their commitment and desire was by playing even when hurt. Injured athletes were cheered when they refused to succumb to the pain by finishing the game or not sitting out a game. Despite rules intended to protect athletes, cultural norms within the sport dictated such irrational behavior. As discussed in Chapter 9, the consequences of the culture of toughness can be severe. Rules can influence behavior, but without a change in the culture of contact sports, conditions such as recurrent concussion and its related psychiatric symptoms will continue to be seen in those presently competing in sport as well as those who have retired.

Sports can impact the collective psyche of an entire city or county [1]. This phenomenon helps psychiatrists understand why individuals may become dysphoric when their team is defeated. It is much more than merely losing the game or match; it becomes personal. In such situations, people's identity becomes a reflection of their team's successes and failures. The thrill of victory and agony of defeat extend far beyond the players. This process of identifying with one's team has become so pervasive that one is often chastised for "missing the big game." Apart from whether or not someone's favorite team or athlete wins a given contest, whether or not it is someone's favorite sports season often impacts her mood. For example, patients with major depressive disorder may find themselves less depressed during the Olympics or during football season if they find enjoyment in watching the contests on television or in person.

To be successful in their work with athletes, sports psychiatrists must be knowledgeable about the prevailing sports cultures and subcultures that influence their patients. Just as an appropriate diagnosis would never ignore demographic information such as age and sex, when diagnosing and treating athletes, psychiatrists must also avail themselves of all relevant cultural factors regarding sports participation. Dating back to the birth of the Olympic movement, sport and society have been intertwined within the many cultures of the world. At the risk of overstating the obvious, the player is first a by-product of the culture in which he grows. Culture, often described as "the blueprint for living," provides the environmental forces that shape the morals, values, thoughts, feelings, and behaviors of the world's athletes. Such factors must be considered when considering the psychiatric ramifications of sport participation.

MULTICULTURALISM

In 1978, Engels introduced us to the biopsychosocial model. Since publication of the model, we have seen the underlying philosophy permeate many areas of psychiatry. Psychiatry training programs around the world teach their trainees about cross-cultural issues. Over the past half century, the world has become a smaller place. Prior to the mid-1950s, it was very unlikely that a clinician's practice would include patients outside of the clinician's local community. This is no longer the case. Today, the "social" aspect of the biopsychosocial model is perhaps even more relevant than was described in the late 1970s. A lack of appreciation and understanding regarding a patient's culture will clearly diminish the therapeutic outcomes. To ignore the folkways and morals embedded in one's culture is to increase the chance of an improper diagnosis and to decrease the chances for productive and effective treatment. This is even more likely in the world of sport.

SPECIFIC EXAMPLES OF IMPORTANT CULTURAL ISSUES IN SPORT

Violence

Violence associated with sports is a cultural issue of great importance. Regretfully, acts of violence are not necessarily seen as an anomaly in the world of sports. As sports psychologists and sports sociologists study such events, the underlying causes become all too clear. For some, the "rage" exhibited on the "field of battle" cannot be turned on and off. Thus, such criminal acts of violence become off-field displays of what is culturally accepted on the field.

Examples of sport-associated violence are many. In 2010, an up and coming elite goalie committed suicide. His decision to end his own life appeared to be the result of his recent poor performances as a member of his country's national team. In 1994, a Columbian soccer player named Escobar was murdered weeks after the 1994 World Cup. Columbia was a pre-tournament favorite, and Escobar had become a national hero expected to help the country win the World Cup. The players openly acknowledged that their desire to win went well beyond the athletic achievement; they wanted to win to help change a growing negative view of their country. As such, the pressure to win was great. After a poor performance, highlighted by Escobar scoring an "own goal" against the United States, the team returned to a disappointed, and in some cases hostile, country. Eventually the anger led to violence, and Escobar was shot and killed. In the Basque region of Spain, the emergence of soccer teams Real Madrid F.C. and F.C. Barcelona led to a geopolitical split. Although the supporters were from the same region, the fans were so devout in their support that the region literally split. In the 1990s, a professional hockey player was brought up on charges after throwing his pregnant wife from a moving car.

Though the sport may be played on the same surface with the same rules around the world, there are massively important cultural factors that must be considered when it comes to the lives of those who participate. You are less likely to find a soccer goalie in the United States committing suicide due to a few poor performances, nor are you likely to find a player murdered for a world cup loss in Canada. It is also unlikely that you will find fan violence outside a professional basketball game in Israel.

Collectivism versus individualism

Important issues such as whether or not a given society is collectivist or individualistic must be considered. Such differences can be understood within the movie *Rocky V*. The character "Drago" is portrayed as somewhat of a puppet of the state and is proud to serve in such a role. As the fight between he and Rocky (a very stereotypic American from Philadelphia, Pennsylvania) continues, the proud Russian audience begins to be swayed by Rocky's efforts. As Rocky begins to exert himself, the Russian head of state finds his way to the ring to threaten their national hero. Drago responds, "I fight for me," in what is a wonderful Hollywood portrayal of a shift from collectivism to individualism. Such differences can also be seen with regard to the ultimate goals of young soccer players. Do they dream of representing their national team or a club team? Are they driven to "wear the jersey" or make a lot of money? Such cultural forces have clear mental health ramifications. Had the previously mentioned goalie not grown up placing state above self, his demise by suicide would have been very unlikely.

Movement away from home

In some countries and for specific sports, it is common for children who show promising physical talent to move away from their homes, families, and friends to engage in rigorous training regimens in hopes of becoming Olympic greats. The process of "developing" Olympic athletes differs across countries. In the United States, the rather unique system of college sports is the primary source of Olympic athletes. Importantly, though, American colleges not only provide a home for American athletes, but also for athletes from around the world who come to the United States to participate in college athletics and academics. In other parts of the world, Olympians are often created via centralized plans administered by state-run sports ministries, a network of sports clubs across the country, or a combination of the two.

There have been no systematic, long-term studies of the impact of these different models of athletic development on athletes' psychiatric trajectories as they grow older. The media sometimes speculate that there may be long-term problems with children who move away from home at a young age for the purposes of sport, but this is largely speculative and anecdotal. Intuitively, the concern makes sense. Though the young athletes have impressive physical attributes, mentally they are still children or adolescents. Their brains are still developing, and they are vulnerable in many ways. Whether or not athletes do well after a childhood of international travel and upbringing away from home may also have to do with the extent to which they were allowed to develop an identity outside of sport and the extent to which primary attachments were maintained.

STIGMA AND ACCESS TO PSYCHIATRIC TREATMENT AROUND THE WORLD

Around the world, stigma toward mental illness is quite common. In most places, this stigma is compounded if it involves mental illness in athletes. In fact, it often does not occur to coaches, parents, fans, the media, physicians, and even athletes themselves that athletes could suffer from mental illness. Appearing physically robust on the outside suggests to the world that inner mental struggles are impossible. Moreover, athletes themselves often feel that "admitting" to psychiatric suffering is an admission of weakness, which they worry may translate into weakness on the field [2]. The stigma against mental illness in athletes is likely even stronger in those countries with more baseline stigma against mental illness in the general population.

At the broader level, stigma against mental illness in athletes truly is representative of stigma against anything that makes an athlete appear weak. Nowhere has this "culture of toughness" in sport, as discussed earlier, raised more concerns as of late than in the realm of concussion in athletes. Athletes are socialized to "shake it off" rather than come out of the game if they experience signs or symptoms of concussion. This cultural attitude transcends geography, and in recent years has come to affect not only traditional male sports but also women athletes (see following section).

Countries with more stigma against mental illness may have fewer psychiatrists in practice. Thus, in such countries, even if athletes were to acknowledge their psychiatric symptoms, they may not have access to psychiatric care. Even apart from the stigma issue, athletes in relatively resource-rich countries simply have fewer logistical (including financial) barriers to seeing physicians of any specialty, including psychiatrists. For example, an athlete in a relatively wealthy country who has attention deficit/hyperactivity disorder may wish to obtain a therapeutic use exemption so as to be allowed to continue taking his stimulant during elite-level competition (see Chapter 15). That may well prove much more feasible in a resource-rich country.

The flip-side of athletes in wealthier countries having access to higher-quality psychiatric and medical care is that they may also have more access to performance-enhancing drugs. Whether these drugs are surreptitiously provided by unethical physicians, obtained through the internet, or otherwise, they provide an unfair advantage to athletes in a manner that clearly is not proportionately spread out among all countries and cultures.

EPIDEMIOLOGY OF MENTAL ILLNESS IN ATHLETES ACROSS DIFFERENT CULTURES

Risk factors for mental illness in athletes differ depending on culture. Rates of many mental illnesses in athletes probably approximate rates in nonathletes [2]. Furthermore, rates of different psychiatric conditions are presumed to be fairly equivalent in countries around the world, and the between-country equivalence of these rates presumably extends to athletes as well. Of note, though, some studies do show that higher rates of mental illness are found in some countries than others, with, for example, lower prevalence rates sometimes found in Asian countries in general [3]. However, poor diagnosis in countries without affordable access to mental health services, low reporting rates, and the predominant use of self-report data rather than semi-structured instruments are widely felt to be important confounding factors. Importantly, athletes in some parts of the world may be more or less likely to develop mental illness depending on cultural circumstances. Eating disorders, mood disorders, and substance use disorders are examples of this as played out in sport.

Eating disorders have traditionally afflicted athletes from Western countries with widespread exposure to idealized media images of girls and women. However, with much of the world now having access to media, and with the realization that media do not by themselves cause eating disorders, there has been a realization that athletes from around the globe can and do suffer from eating disorders. Recent reports attest that women in North Korea, Seoul, Hong Kong, Singapore, the Philippines, India, and Pakistan are increasingly suffering from the "self-starvation syndrome," and this extends to athletes in those and other countries as well [4]. Moreover, men athletes from around the world are increasingly reported to suffer from eating disorders [2].

Retirement from elite sport and serious injuries are significant risks for development of mood disorders in athletes [2]. This is particularly the case if athletes have not developed an identity outside of sport. In those countries and sports, then, in which the athlete identity is all-consuming, transition to retirement and sidelining by injury are going to be even greater risks.

Beyond retirement and injury, other factors that are differentially present in various cultures may contribute to the risk of mood, as well as anxiety, disorders in athletes. Increasingly chief among these is the prevalence of media, especially the internet and social media, in a given culture. Athletes almost universally feel pressure to succeed in sport, and such pressure can be magnified when every loss or poor performance is met with critical comments on various sources of social media. An athlete who already is feeling badly about a poor outing may be tipped over the edge into depression or crippling anxiety when overwhelmed with critical Tweets, Facebook posts, or internet message board threads.

Likewise, risk for substance use disorders varies depending on the drinking and drug use culture within a given country. An athlete living in a country or as part of a group that has a culture of no alcohol consumption will be relatively protected from alcohol use disorders. However, if and when such an athlete moves to train in another country, for example in parts of Europe or the United States where alcohol use is quite acceptable and in fact even encouraged in the sporting world, alcohol use disorders will become more of a risk. Furthermore, in some countries in which alcohol use is disapproved, other substance use disorders may be relatively more common among athletes who are looking for some outlet for the stress of the world of elite sport.

WOMEN, SPORT, AND CULTURE

Recent years have brought increased participation of women in sport around the globe. This has cultural implications for the way women are perceived in terms of physicality, sexuality, power, and dominance. In many ways, women's increased sports participation has been a positive thing. Within the realm of psychiatry and mental health, exercise and sports participation are known to confer benefits to participants, for example, in the form of decreased rates of depression and anxiety. However, sport certainly does not bring universal protection from these conditions, and in fact can itself increase the risk for certain psychiatric conditions. Women in particular may be *more* likely to suffer from certain psychiatric conditions such as eating disorders if participating in particular sports (see Chapter 5). Moreover, as women's sports take on male standards of success, women athletes are increasingly likely to suffer from the same mental illness stigma as do male athletes. Thus, for women athletes to "admit" to symptoms of mental illness is seen as a sign of weakness, much as it is for men athletes. This makes it less likely that women athletes, like their men counterparts, will be able to get psychiatric treatment for conditions from which they may be suffering.

As women around the world have become more likely to participate in all types of sport, cultural clashes with religion have arisen. Citizens of some countries comment on the uniforms of women athletes, including swimmers and runners, and suggest that they should wear more "suitable" costumes for women in accordance with rules of the religion. Thus, tension exists between what is functionally optimal for these women athletes to be wearing and what is culturally deemed acceptable.

Several other issues impact women athletes in unique ways. Such issues include gender stereotyping in the media and homophobia. These issues impact the way that women athletes see themselves and are important to consider in understanding the athlete's world and the biopsychosocial underpinnings to any mental illness they may manifest.

Gender stereotyping in televised sports

Television and other media reflect the attitudes of a given society and culture. The manner in which media cover, or fail to cover, women in sport conveys something about the status of women in a given culture. Not surprisingly, research has found that women's sports are underreported, and when reported, coverage is of inferior quality and quantity as compared to men's sports coverage [5]. Other findings have included the following:

- Commentators are more likely to refer to women athletes only by their first names and to men athletes by both first and last names or simply last names.
- Women in nonathletic roles are often included in broadcasts of both men's and women's sporting events. For example, women appear in the role of comical object of the newscaster's joke or as a sexual object. Women are also shown as scantily clad spectators.
- Announcers more often refer to women athletes as "girls" than they refer to men athletes as "boys."
- Women's sports events are much more often gender marked than are men's events. Thus, for example, women's basketball coverage includes continual reminders to viewers that they are watching the "Women's Final Four" or the "NCAA Women's National Championship Game," whereas men's games are not as often marked in this way.
- Announcers' descriptions of athletes vary greatly depending on if they are discussing men or women athletes. For example, men athletes are more often described with such words as powerful, confident, smart, big and strong, brilliant, gutsy, leader, dominant, and aggressive. On the other hand, women athletes are relatively more frequently referred to with attributions of weakness such as weary, fatigued, frustrated, jittery, not comfortable, panicked, indecisive, vulnerable, shaky, worried, dejected, and choking [5].

Homophobia in women's sports

Of course, there are gay and lesbian people in every population such that it is not surprising that there are lesbian athletes in the world of women's sports. The presence or absence of lesbian athletes is not the issue. Rather, the problem arises when "lesbian" is applied as a label to stereotype members of a group, as is often done with women athletes. This stereotype seems to be applied in order to keep women from playing sports, sometimes certain sports more than others, or from playing for certain coaches or with certain teams. Use of many cultures' fear of homosexuality is one of the remaining ways that society attempts to keep women from participating in sport.

Ways that this manifests may include the following [6]:

- Women who play on varsity or elite teams are labeled as "lesbians."
- Prospective college athletes are deterred from choosing a particular college because of the suggestion that there are lesbians on the team.
- A candidate for a coaching position is asked whether she is married, and if not, she is assumed to be lesbian and not hired for the position.

These factors certainly influence many women in their choices about sports involvement. Girls and women may be discouraged from pursuing traditionally "masculine" activities such as contact sports and team sports. One study has shown that 51% of women coaches and 46% of women athletes felt that their involvement in sports led others to assume they were lesbian [7]. Parents sometimes worry that their daughters' involvement in sports may lead them to become lesbian. Elite women athletes sometimes fear that going public with their sexuality, if lesbian, will cause them to lose corporate sponsorships.

Case Study

Samantha was a 23-year-old woman who had recently completed a successful collegiate career as a cross-country and track and field runner. She signed a contract for a corporate sponsorship with a shoe company upon graduation so as to be able to continue her running career with financial support. During her first season as a professional runner, she decided to cut her hair to chin-length. She was dismayed to get a call from her agent, who reported that her sponsoring shoe company was upset that she had cut her hair and wanted her to grow it long again. The implication was that she would no longer be as "marketable" and thus not worth as much to the shoe company with short hair. Though not explicitly stated, it was also strongly implied that her salary from the shoe company would be markedly decreased if she did not comply with their request.

Beyond the issue regarding her hair length, Samantha was also bothered by the types of racing uniforms she was expected to wear. Her sponsor sent her bikini briefs and racing tops that she felt very uncomfortable wearing. In college, she had always felt more comfortable wearing racing shorts rather than briefs, and while some of her teammates made fun of her for her uniform choices, she was not forced as a college athlete to wear the bikini-style uniform. However, as a professional athlete, if she wanted to retain her corporate sponsorship, she was not being given a choice.

Because Samantha needed to keep the sponsorship in order to be able to train full time without getting another job, she chose to wear the required uniform and to grow her hair long again. However, she continued to feel uncomfortable in the selected racing uniform. She also could not help but wonder if her male professional running colleagues received mandates from their sponsors about types of hairstyle they needed to adopt.

Over the ensuing 2 years, Samantha developed an eating disorder. She would not necessarily say that the shoe company was to blame. However, when her psychiatrist explored with her the psychosocial factors potentially contributing to her disorder, cultural expectations of femininity did seem to be likely issues of importance.

CONCLUSIONS

A thorough biopsychosocial formulation is a part of any good psychiatric evaluation of a patient. Consideration of the psychosocial and cultural contributors to a patient's psychiatric symptoms may be particularly important in athlete-patients, given the numerous cultural facets of a life that substantially involves sports participation. It is not feasible for all psychiatrists to be experts on all cultures, but at the very least, we should know the questions to ask to ascertain the role that culture may be playing in our patients' lives and in their psychiatric symptoms and disorders.

REFERENCES

1. Arehart-Treichel J (2012). Why sports evoke passion, for better or worse. *Psychiatric News* **47** (9), 13.
2. Reardon CL, Factor RM (2010) Sport psychiatry: a systematic review of diagnosis and medical treatment of mental illness in athletes. *Sports Medicine* 40 (11), 1–20.
3. Demyttenaere K, Bruffaerts R, Posada-Villa J, *et al.* (2004) Prevalence, severity, and unmet need for treatment of mental disorders in the World Health Organization World Mental Health Surveys. *The Journal of the American Medical Association* 291 (21), 2581–2590.
4. Efron S (1997) Women's eating disorders go global. *The Los Angeles Times*, October 18. http://www.hartford-hwp.com/archives/50/103.html. Accessed on 16 September 2012.
5. Birrell S, Cole CL (eds.) (1994) *Women, Sport, and Culture*. Human Kinetics, Champaign, IL.
6. Feminist Majority Foundation (1995) *Empowering Women in Sports. The Empowering Women Series, No. 4*. Feminist Majority Foundation, Arlington, VA.
7. Women's Sports Foundation (2012) Homophobia in Women's Sports. http://www.divinecaroline.com/31/29668-homophobia-women-s-sports. Accessed on 16 September 2012.

18 Ethical Issues in Sports Psychiatry

David A. Baron,[1,2,3] Joshua Tompkins,[1]
Sally Mohamed,[4] and Samir Abolmagd[5]

[1] International Relations and Department of Psychiatry, Keck School of Medicine at the University of Southern California, USA
[2] Keck Medical Center at the University of Southern California, USA
[3] Global Center for Exercise, Psychiatry, and Sports at USC, Health Sciences Campus, USA
[4] Kasr El Maadi Hospital, korniche El Maadi, Egypt
[5] Addiction Medicine Unit, Cairo University, Egypt

KEY POINTS

- Medical ethics serve as a guide for what is considered the proper and humane practice of medical care. In the United States, the United Kingdom, and many other Western cultures, modern medical ethics reside on four key principles: beneficence, nonmaleficence, patient autonomy, and justice.
- Sports psychiatry, while governed by these principles, presents unique ethical challenges and potential conflicts of interest concerning performance enhancement, physician accountability, and other considerations.
- Successful navigation of these ethical challenges requires both a sound understanding of ethical principles as well as the capacity to identify the principles, stakeholders, and potential consequences in the real-life ethical problems that can arise in sports psychiatry.

INTRODUCTION: THE EVOLUTION OF MEDICAL ETHICS

The story of medical ethics starts with a colossal irony: Hippocrates of Cos (460–370 BCE), the Greek physician considered to be the founder of Western medicine, probably did not write the Hippocratic Oath. Though many modern scholars say the real author remains unknown, the deontologic nature of the Oath – binding physicians to their solemn vow to do no harm, to perform no abortions, and to attempt no surgery, among other stipulations – proves that *someone* in Ancient Greece was starting to reflect on the virtues that doctors should possess and the guidelines that should shape the humane practice of medicine. It should come as no surprise, then, that the Oath, which placed the power of healing squarely in the hands of human physicians, not vengeful gods, appeared during one of the greatest medico-cultural enlightenments in medical history, when forward-thinking Greek doctors began to view diseases in a framework based on science, not superstition. Whether a person was stricken with seizures, poisoned blood, chest pain, or a hopelessly nasty disposition, no medical condition was the product of a divine curse; instead, disease stemmed from an

Clinical Sports Psychiatry: An International Perspective, First Edition. Edited by David A. Baron,
Claudia L. Reardon and Steven H. Baron.
© 2013 John Wiley & Sons, Ltd. Published 2013 by John Wiley & Sons, Ltd.

imbalance of the four body humors – blood, phlegm, yellow bile, and black bile. Laugh as we may at the relative naiveté of this physiologic model in comparison to the modern biopsychosocial version, we should stand in of the Greek medical writers' ethical prescience. For example, more than 2000 years before the Health Insurance Portability and Accountability Act (HIPAA) became U.S. law in 1996, creating the nation's first rules protecting the confidentiality of personal medical records, Greek writers were instructing physicians to safeguard the privacy of their patients [1].

After the decline of Greece, the nascent flame of medical ethics was taken up by the Roman physician Galen (129–200 CE), who felt that physicians should be educated in philosophy and live modest, virtuous lives. In Medieval Europe, medical care came under the purview of the Christian church, which viewed healing the sick as a profound act of charity and compassion and thus a natural extension of the Church's spiritual function. Early Christian physicians adapted the Hippocratic Oath to suit their worldview, removing references to the Greek gods but upholding the Hippocratic prohibition on performing abortions. At the same time, far to the east, Persian physicians in intellectual centers such as Bagdad were recording ethical tracts of their own. Drawing upon Arabic translations of Hippocrates, Galen, and countless other classical thinkers, Islamic physicians agreed with the Christian medical ethic of treating the poor by necessity and, like Christians, saw their work as a form of devotion to God. Jewish life also flourished in Mesopotamia under Islamic rule, and Jewish physicians earned a reputation for being highly gifted. Jewish writers cautioned doctors to be prudent and not to covet wealth, and the celebrated writer and physician Maimonides felt the saving of life superseded religious doctrine, such as the observance of the Sabbath [1].

As medical science progressed rapidly during the Renaissance, physicians struggled with ethical issues such as the duty to put patients' welfare above their own (e.g., by treating victims of the Black Plague and thereby exposing themselves to a deadly infection). By recognizing their obligations not just to individual patients but to society as a whole, physicians endeavored to become a bona fide profession in the eyes of the public [1].

Internecine bickering hindered this effort until 1803, when an English physician named Thomas Percival coined the term "medical ethics" and published a book by the same title. *Medical Ethics* was a code that spelled out practitioners' duties to their patients, their colleagues, and the society in which they practiced, and it forever changed the way British and American physicians saw themselves and regarded the sick. It was quickly translated into other languages as its influence spread across Europe and beyond. The era of modern medical ethics had begun [2].

MODERN MEDICAL ETHICS

The continuing revision of medical ethics since the publication of Percival's *Medical Ethics* is a nuanced and engaging narrative whose details lie beyond the scope of this chapter. Suffice to say that medical ethics, which in recent decades has been folded into a broader category called bioethics, is not a musty old quarto but a living document subject to constant reexamination – and interminable dispute. In recent decades, events such as the Nuremberg trials, the discovery of DNA, the advent of organ transplantation, the Tuskegee experiments, and the AIDS epidemic have only further complicated the effort to weigh the needs of all parties and chart the fairest course through the turbid waters of medical morality.

Putting specific issues aside for a moment, we can appreciate the four cornerstone tenets of Western medical ethics as established by Beauchamp and Childress [3] as the following:

- *Beneficence* – the duty to act in the best interest of the patient. This requires physicians to possess the necessary education and experience to select beneficial therapies for patients while taking every effort to minimize adverse consequences.
- *Nonmaleficence* – the duty to avoid harming the patient. Practically synonymous with the principle of beneficence, the principle of nonmaleficence, for example, is generally interpreted as forbidding physicians from assisting in the execution of condemned prisoners or aiding a patient's suicide.
- *Justice* – the duty to treat all patients fairly and equally. This principle pervades issues such as the allocation of donated organs and other scarce resources and the limited availability of sophisticated and costly measures such as genetic testing and MRI scans.
- *Patient autonomy* – the duty to allow patients to choose or refuse treatment. Not only is a physician required to get a patient's permission to provide medical care, but the patient's wishes supersede the physician's expert opinion even in cases where the patient's choice will result in certain death. The principle of autonomy is dependent on the concept of informed consent, that is, that a patient's decision is supported by his or her complete understanding of the risks, benefits, and alternatives to any proposed medical action, or inaction.

MEDICAL ETHICS AROUND THE WORLD

Though our discussion has focused on Western medical ethics, a brief global perspective is warranted, given that (i) virtually all peoples of the Earth engage in sports and (ii) psychiatry's role in sports is already entrenched in some non-Western cultures and will become even more involved in the future. In Africa, where traditional medicine shares an awkward coexistence with the Western style of medical education and practice established during the colonial period, the Hippocratic Oath is the chief source of ethical guidelines for practitioners of Western medicine, but medical schools offer little instruction in ethics. Doctors of both the Western and traditional paradigms emphasize patient privacy and confidentiality, but the HIV/AIDS epidemic has forced officials to revisit the concept of privacy in the face of a dire public health threat. In Kenya, for instance, the rules of disclosure have been revised to permit physicians to reveal a patient's HIV-positive status to the patient's spouse or sexual partners [4].

In India, as in Africa, tension exists between Western medicine and traditional medicine (namely, the Hindu-based Āyurveda). The Hindu *Carka-samhitā*, written in the third century BCE, described the ideal physician as "truthful," "peace-loving," and "vigilant" as well as charitable and devoted to "spiritual power." Ancient Indian physicians were instructed not to treat patients who had no chance of recovery for fear of preserving the profession's image of competence. Āyurveda incorporated many features of Western medicine (e.g., vitamins, antibiotics, and chemotherapy) in the late twentieth century and, conversely, has gained a following in Western societies as patients have turned to alternative and complimentary therapies [5].

China, a nation beset – and perhaps defined – by political and cultural revolutions during the twentieth century, has witnessed a revolution of its medical ethics as a result. Traditional Chinese medicine, which traces its roots back to the early teachings of Confucianism, Buddhism, and Daoism, has been heavily supplanted by Western medicine, and the ethical code of the American Medical Association was first translated into Chinese in 1912. The Communist Revolution abandoned traditional ethical concepts such as humaneness, righteousness, and justice and infused Chinese health care with a new socialist outlook – "revolutionary humanitarianism," in the words of Mao Zedong. In 1981 the nation's Ministry of Health issued the first official code of medical ethics, which exhorted physicians to "respect the patient's dignity, will, and rights." Informed consent was emphasized also, and when confronted with gravely ill patients, doctors were instructed "to make one-hundred-percent effort to save lives even though the hope is only one percent" [6].

ETHICAL ISSUES IN PSYCHIATRY

Psychiatrists are physicians tasked with diagnosing and treating mental illness [7]. Like other physicians, they observe the fundamental ethical principles of patient autonomy, beneficence, nonmaleficence, and justice, and like all professionals they employ special knowledge and training to serve others. Among all physicians, psychiatrists occupy the most intimate place in the lives of their patients and bear the added responsibility of safeguarding their patient as well as the public.

The clinically intimate nature of the relationship between psychiatrist and patient evokes a skein of ethical issues that are unique to the profession. Yet despite the formidable and intricate nature of many areas of psychiatric ethics, relatively scarce attention has been paid to the subject.

Lubit [8] elucidated most of the major ethical issues that weigh specifically on psychiatrists, starting with the necessity of committing – and sometimes medicating – patients with serious mental illness against their will out of concern for their well-being and the safety of others. While clearly warranted in many cases, such curtailment of patients' personal liberty violates the ethical principle of patient autonomy, jeopardizes the therapeutic alliance, and may disincline the same patients to seek mental health care in the future [8].

Following the most ethical course becomes even more treacherous when a patient is not psychotic or a danger to others – for example, a suicidal patient with severe major depressive disorder. Can such a patient be justifiably medicated or given electroconvulsive therapy (ECT) against his or her will within the four-part framework of modern medical ethics described earlier in this chapter? Answering this question on a case-by-case basis requires careful circumspection into the likely risks, benefits, and alternatives; the potential degree of infringement on the patient's freedom; the possible need for collateral information from the patient's family and friends; and the potential impact on society of not administering the treatment. The patient has legal recourse through the court system, but the process is slow and judges often side with psychiatrists, placing the doctor in the virtually omnipotent position of having both the first and last word on the patient's therapy and civil rights [8].

The issue of boundary violations is no less critical to ethical psychiatric practice. Sexual relations with current patients is a professional anathema (for it violates the core tenets of beneficence, nonmaleficence, and autonomy), and intimate involvement with former patients is also prohibited by American Psychiatric Association (APA) guidelines, as any possibility of a future relationship might engender harmful fantasies on the part of the psychiatrist and therefore bias the course of therapy in a manner not beneficial to the patient. (It is worth noting that the prohibition on romantic relationships with current and former patients violates a patient's autonomy as an individual who should otherwise be free to choose his or her sexual partners, but on this matter, beneficence – the duty to safeguard a patient's well-being – outweighs autonomy.) [8]

Modern psychiatrists have a responsibility to uphold other ethical principles, many of which take on special significance in the psychiatric realm. Confidentiality – the duty to safeguard each patient's personal information and medical records – is vital both to facilitating the therapeutic alliance and to protecting the patient's reputation from a society in which mental health care is still widely stigmatized. Conversely, confidentially has become superseded in recent years by the duty to report, whether it be informing law enforcement authorities of an abusive parent of a young patient or warning the potential victim of a patient who has expressed a desire to harm others. Other tenets of psychiatric ethics govern areas such as double agentry (when psychiatrists have a responsibility both to the patient and to the agency that hired them, such as the military), cooperating with outside evaluators, and treating a child who is at the center of a parental custody battle. The point here is not to explicate every single concept but to mention the most pertinent ones in brief as a way of describing the gestalt of psychiatric ethics [8].

Psychiatry, like the entire medical profession, must continually revisit and revise its ethical guidelines to suit and serve the culture in which psychiatrists practice. These exigencies will vary widely from one nation to the next as each culture imposes its own moral values on the basic framework of psychiatric ethics. In the United States, for example, the compromising relationships between some psychiatrists and the pharmaceutical industry have been the subject of much attention. New issues will emerge as the fields of genomics and advanced brain imaging propel psychiatry toward a more biologically based model of diagnosis and treatment.

Case Study

An elite college soccer player is sent by his coach for a neuropsychiatric evaluation. The athlete has been missing practices, complaining of forgetfulness, poor concentration, and dizziness to his coach. There is no report of recent head trauma. On psychiatric examination, the player denies suffering from the aforementioned symptoms but no longer wants to play organized soccer. "It's just not fun anymore. They've made it into a high-pressure job," he professes. The player asks the psychiatrist to tell the coach he is suffering from an injury and is not cleared to play. "I just need some time off to decide what to do," he remarks. "I don't want to let my teammates down – or my coach. You could really help me by doing this."

Comment: From an ethical perspective, this case raises a number of issues. Going along with the athlete's request might be interpreted as beneficence, the duty to act in the best interest of the patient. Similarly, nonmaleficence, the duty to avoid harming the patient, might justify telling the coach the player must sit out for psychiatric reasons. Honesty can never be disregarded when considering an ethical interpretation. Discussing the athlete's moral dilemma and offering him advice on how to address his feelings and concerns with his coach, possibly with the psychiatrist in the meeting to offer emotional support, would be an ethical approach.

MENTAL HEALTH IN THE ATHLETIC ARENA

The world of athletics functions as a cultural entity, complete with its own language, norms, and values. Similar to the professional arena, team uniforms and other university-identified apparel worn by athletes are one example of the outward expression of an athletic department's culture. Likewise, team members are expected to conform to norms of behavior established and enforced by the coaches and administrators [9].

Mental health professionals who provide treatment to athletes must be knowledgeable about the stressors unique to this population. Athletes tend to underutilize available counseling resources despite data suggesting that the levels of psychological distress they may experience approximates the levels found in the nonathlete population [10, 11].

Researchers have explored the barriers to help-seeking behavior faced by the athlete and have identified internal factors, such as a need to be "strong" and "self-sufficient," as well as external factors, such as the lack of available counselors knowledgeable about athletes, time limitations, and some discouragement from seeking help outside the athletics system [11–13]. Their data indicated relative constancy over a 13-year period in the frequency of less severe presenting concerns (e.g., developmental issues, situational emotional concerns, and academic skill difficulties). However, during the same time period, frequency rates of more serious concerns (e.g., relationships, stress/anxiety, family issues, physical problems, personality disorders, suicidal thoughts, and sexual assault) significantly increased by approximately twofold [14].

SPORTS PSYCHIATRY: A NEWCOMER TO THE FIELD

In the intricate realm of athlete mental health, sports psychiatry is an endeavor in its infancy. It is not believed to be an officially recognized subspecialty of psychiatry in any country, and an internet search revealed no evidence of any medical or psychiatric governing bodies offering board certification in sports psychiatry. There is no English-language medical journal dedicated to the field of sports psychiatry. A recent search on amazon.com found only two English-language textbooks on the subject of sports psychiatry, the older one published in 2000 [15]. The International Society for Sports Psychiatry (ISSP) was founded in 1994 and has no code of ethics (E-mail correspondence with ISSP member Eric Morse, MD) [16].

It is partly for these reasons that medical literature on the ethics of sports psychiatry is virtually nonexistent. A recent PubMed search using Medical Subject Headings (MeSH) of "sports" plus "psychiatry" plus "ethics" yielded only 11 results dating back to 1986, and most of those held no actual relevance. Clearly, this poverty of information does not stem from any shortage of medical literature on sports (97 690 MeSH citations), psychiatry (82 919 MeSH citations), or ethics (132 933 MeSH citations). Unlike the psychiatric subspecialties such as forensic, child, adolescent, geriatric, and military, sports psychiatry does not have a separate MeSH subject heading, further highlighting the field's novel status.

ETHICS OF OTHER SPORTS HEALTH-CARE PROFESSIONS

We can compare the ethics of sports psychiatry, in its current inchoate form, to those of the field of sports psychology, which is already supported by a national association in several countries, including the United States [17], England [18], Spain [19], and Germany [20]. (Whereas sports psychiatry is concerned with mental illness suffered by athletes, sports psychology focuses on performance enhancement and the achievement of optimum mental functioning in the athletic environment.)

Sports psychology's ethics are quite explicitly formalized. The Association for Applied Sport Psychology (AASP), which was founded in 1986 and whose members hail from "38 different countries outside of North America," has produced a code of six general principles (competence, integrity, professional and scientific responsibility, respect for people's rights and dignity, concern for others' welfare, and social responsibility) plus 26 general ethical standards covering an extensive range of subjects including harassment, misuse of influence, bartering, fees, and informed consent. The AASP website instructs visitors to address concerns about "the ethical behavior of any AASP member" to the Chair of the Ethics Committee and refers questions regarding research ethics to the Editor of the *Journal of Applied Sport Psychology* [21]. The International Society of Sport Psychology, whose members hail from 73 nations and territories, uses a Code of Ethics based largely on the AASP's six general principles [22].

Conversely, it is also useful to examine the development of ethical standards of sports medicine, a much older field whose goals align with those of sports psychiatry and whose patient population is essentially the same. The International Federation of Sports Medicine (IFSM), which was founded (albeit under a different name) in 1920, has a detailed 13-part Code of Ethics that places the work of sports medicine physicians squarely under the umbrella of general medical ethics but also touches upon the concerns most likely to arise in the athletic context. "The same ethical principles that apply to the practice of medicine shall apply to sports medicine," the Code begins before continuing to explicate the ethical issues that bear specifically on sports medicine, such as the physician–athlete relationship ("that of absolute confidence and mutual respect"), the question of clearing a patient to play after injury ("the outcome of the competition or the coaches should not influence the decision"), and the use of performance-enhancing substances ("it is contrary to medical ethics to condone doping in any form") [23].

Prima fascia, these principles seem logical and self-evident, but the evolution of sports medicine ethics has threaded its own separate course within the theater of medical history and ethics as the role of physicians in athletic contests has grown in stature. The earliest evidence of sports medicine as a practice dates back (like the history of medical ethics) to ancient Greece, when the staggering prizes awarded at some of the early contests made the professional training and conditioning of athletes a profitable endeavor. Yet many Greek and Roman physicians derided the lack of adequate medical education of many trainers and felt the goal of winning at any cost stood in contrast to the fundamental health principle of balance (homeostasis, in modern terms). Athletes were overworked, under-rested, and some were compelled to eat 10 pounds of lamb per day [24]. The celebrated physician Galen, mentioned earlier, began his career as a doctor for gladiators and was an ardent critic of what he perceived as the abuse of competitors for the sake of victory:

> The athletes each day labor at their exercises beyond what is suitable: and they take their food under force, often extending their eating until midnight.... For when those who live according to nature have come home from work, needing food, then these athletes are getting up from sleep – so that their lives are like that of pigs – except for the fact that the pigs do not work beyond measure or eat under force [24, Part II, p. 21].

Medicine's disdain for the perceived harmful excesses of athletic training persisted well into the twentieth century, when the growth of the modern Olympiad, the burgeoning popularity of professional sports, and the emergence of medicine as a respected and capable profession spurred the rapid specialization of sports medicine physicians. This only served to heighten concerns on the part of some observers over the potential conflict of interest, that is, that such physicians could place the goal of victory above the well-being of their patients, many of whom were more than happy to sacrifice their long-term health for the sake of championship. These persisting fears spurred the establishment of the IFSM's aforementioned Code of Ethics, which made the health of the athlete paramount above all other considerations. The IFSM Code arose, by no coincidence, as a new concern for patient autonomy pervaded medicine and supplanted the outmoded ethos of physicians as paternalistic caretakers whose judgment was not to be questioned [24].

Case Study

An athlete makes an appointment for a consultation with a sports psychiatrist who is an expert in treating the mental health issues surrounding doping. The athlete admits he is considering using a drug recommended by a trainer to help him recover from a sports-related injury. He is not seeking performance enhancement as he believes such behavior would constitute cheating, but he wants to continue competing nonetheless. He does not want to take a banned substance or something that has potential adverse long-term health effects. How should the sports psychiatrist respond to the athlete's request?
Comment: The ethical concept of autonomy addresses a physician's duty to allow patients to choose or refuse treatment. Since the athlete is seeking a private consult and the behavior is not illegal, the patient holds the confidence. The psychiatrist can make a personal decision on how to proceed.

ETHICAL CHALLENGES FOR THE SPORTS PSYCHIATRIST

A handful of writers have touched upon ethical issues that are germane, if not always specific, to the sports psychiatry world. In their overview of sports psychiatry, Glick and Horsfall [25] enumerated six "principles of treatment," the fifth of which was entitled "Do the Right Thing," defined as "delivering appropriate and adequate treatment"[25].

Patient autonomy

Psychiatrists must maintain control of the patient–physician relationship and not "acquiesce to an athlete's inappropriate requests" while at the same respecting the patient's input in the interest of fostering compliance. Likewise, patient autonomy must be firmly respected whenever the best interests of the patient misalign with the goals of the team. "That the patient comes before the sport is a principle worth reiterating," Glick and Horsfall wrote. This is true regardless of the source of payment (i.e., the team itself, the school the team represents, or a third party such as a health insurer) [25].

Yet, due to the inherently competitive and intense nature of both scholastic and professional sports, a patient's medical autonomy is more likely to conflict with the ethical principles of beneficence and nonmaleficence in the sporting milieu than in the normal clinical setting. Such a situation will arise whenever the athlete values individual or team victory over his or her welfare. The same patient is more likely to attempt to conceal or deny his mental health issue in an effort to keep playing. Per the accepted bioethical hierarchy, autonomy trumps both beneficence and nonmaleficence in sports psychiatry, just as it does in all other fields of medicine, with the same caveats: the patient must be a legal adult and must be mentally competent to make decisions. Declaring an athletic patient mentally incompetent would represent an extreme measure that would rarely be warranted in most sporting situations and would almost always require obtaining a second opinion before proceeding with actions that could potentially end the patient's athletic career.

Doctor–patient confidentiality

Brown and Cogan [26], in discussing the ethics of sport psychology, touch upon several issues that apply equally to sports psychiatry. The most important is confidentiality, a matter that can become complicated when an athlete is referred to the psychiatrist by a third party (usually a coach, teammate, or parent) who expects to be kept apprised of the patient's condition by the psychiatrist. One effective approach in such a situation is to refer the third party back to the patient for an update (albeit with appropriate vigilance regarding patient autonomy if the patient has demonstrated unusual susceptibility to the third party's influence and/or the third party is known to be overzealous in the pursuit of victory). If the athlete's playing status depends on receiving treatment, it may be necessary to educate the athlete on the need for disclosure and then ask his or her written permission to discuss his or her condition with the coach or other officials [26].

Case Study

A team handball player is referred to a sports psychiatrist by the team's trainer for evaluation of self-reported poor sleep and increasing anxiety. During the initial intake, the athlete reports seeing an assistant coach touch another player inappropriately on several occasions. The athlete claims the increasing anxiety and lack of sleep are related to worrying about what to do in this situation. The team is having a successful season, and the athlete does not want to risk creating a distraction from the negative publicity going public would create. Despite encouragement from the psychiatrist, the athlete feels unable to discuss the situation with anyone else and demands the psychiatrist not divulge the story or, "I'll deny it".

Comment: From an ethical perspective, this is a challenging case. Confidentiality in the established doctor–patient relationship does not apply if child abuse is suspected. A minor cannot consent to sexual contact. To help determine the ethical, moral, and legal responsibility of the psychiatrist, the age of the potential victim would need to be determined, along with the type of contact observed. Any intimate touching could require immediate reporting for further investigation, depending on the ages involved. From a clinical perspective, the psychiatrist should address the anxiety symptoms and inform the athlete of the legal and ethic obligation of all physicians regarding potential sexual abuse of a minor.

Ethics and patient diversity

Ethical issues confronting the consultants working with athletes take on added importance when paired with the demands of practicing with individuals from diverse backgrounds and the issues they often face [27]. Counseling professionals need to equip themselves with the proper tools to deal effectively with the changing composition of various world populations. For example, according to the 2000 Census, 25% of the U.S. population is classified as "minority," and some experts have calculated that this percentage appears to be growing exponentially [28].

One ethical issue confronting consultants working with male and female athletes is the mandate that practitioners be knowledgeable about gender oppression issues and their impact upon the work they do with their clients. It is safe to say that this may be challenging to the consultant in light of the athletic culture's strong valuing of stereotypically male-identified characteristics of strength and domination over more female stereotypes of emotionality and caretaking [29].

Illicit drug use by athletes

Both public opinion and medical wisdom hold that use of banned substances is both unhealthy and contrary to the ethics of sport. It is necessary to protect the physical and spiritual health of athletes, the values of fair play and of competition, the integrity and the unity of sport, and the rights of those who take part in it at whatever level [30]. Not only does drug use constitute cheating and present an ethical dilemma for coaches, doctors, and officials, but it also jeopardizes the health of the athlete. Despite the potential danger of using a performance-enhancing substance, modern athletes may feel compelled to self-medicate due to many compounding factors, including: his or her psychological need for athletic success; external pressure applied by third parties such as coaches, teammates, parents, and the media; considerable financial incentive to win; the tacit acceptance of doping by authorities in some sports; and the athlete's belief that victory is impossible without doping [31].

Clearly, sports psychiatrists must not aid or abet the use of banned substances by athletes, and this holds true even if the substance in question can otherwise be legally prescribed, as is the case in many jurisdictions with anabolic steroids, stimulants, or narcotic analgesics. Sports psychiatrists must likewise be vigilant for signs of covert substance use by their patients and stand ready to intervene for the sake of the patient's well-being. Yet the tangle of interlaced motivations mentioned in the previous paragraph can make a sports psychiatrist's task quite difficult when treating an athlete who is using banned or potentially dangerous substances and has no intention of ceasing. In such a case, does patient autonomy still supersede beneficence and nonmaleficence? This apparent paradox highlights the need for teams and athletic governing bodies to craft explicit policies regarding the situations in which a psychiatrist would be obligated to inform officials of a player's health issue (e.g., doping) without the player's permission. Players should be required to sign waivers attesting to their understanding of such a policy [32, 33].

CONCLUSION

Sports psychiatry is a novel field endeavoring to define itself. Because the perpetual and virtually universal popularity of professional and scholastic sports makes increasing demand for sports psychiatry likely, the pioneers of the nascent subspecialty will be pressed to define and maintain the standards of practice for the growing ranks of care providers, and it will be necessary to codify a code of ethics that specifically addresses all issues of concern. Such a code should be considered a prerequisite for sports psychiatry's eventual elevation to a full-fledged, boarded subspecialty of psychiatry, and ethics education should be an explicit and mandatory component of all graduate medical education programs (e.g., fellowships) that lead to licensure in sports psychiatric practice. In the interim, sports psychiatry should be considered as beholden to the same general ethical principles that underlie all medical practice (i.e., benevolence, nonmaleficence, patient autonomy, and justice) as well as the established ethical standards of psychiatry, with special emphasis on confidentiality. We look forward to sports psychiatry's positive impact on athlete health and to the formal implementation of ethical standards that champion patient welfare above all other considerations.

REFERENCES

1. Jonsen AR (2000) *A Short History of Medical Ethics*. New York: Oxford University Press.
2. Baker RB (2009) The discourses of practitioners in nineteenth- and twentieth-century Britain and the United States. In RB Baker, LB McCullough (eds.), *The Cambridge World History of Medical Ethics*. New York: Cambridge University Press.
3. Beauchamp TL, Childress JF (2001) *Principles of Biomedical Ethics*. New York: Oxford University Press.
4. Wasunna AA (2009) The discourses of practitioners in Africa. In RB Baker, LB McCullough (eds.), *The Cambridge World History of Medical Ethics*. New York: Cambridge University Press.
5. Young KK (2009) The discourses of practitioners in India. In RB Baker, LB McCullough (eds.), *The Cambridge World History of Medical Ethics*. New York: Cambridge University Press.
6. Nie JB (2009) The discourses of practitioners in China. In RB Baker, LB McCullough (eds.), *The Cambridge World History of Medical Ethics*. New York: Cambridge University Press.
7. Proposed Changes to APA Guidelines. http://www.stanford.edu/group/psylawseminar/Ethics.htm. Accessed on 23 July 2012.
8. Lubit RH (2009) Ethics in psychiatry. In BJ Sadock, VA Sadock, P Ruiz (eds.), *Kaplan & Sadock's Comprehensive Textbook of Psychiatry* (9th edn). New York: Lippincott Williams & Wilkins.
9. Loughran MJ (in press) Counseling the gay, lesbian, bisexual, transgendered, and questioning (GLBTQ) student athlete: issues and intervention strategies. In EF Etzel (ed.), *Counseling College Student-Athletes: Issues and Interventions* (3rd edn). Morgantown, WV: Fitness Information Technologies, Inc.
10. Broughton E (2001) Counseling and support services for college student athletes. Paper presented at the Annual Conference of the American College Personnel Association, March 3–7, Boston, MA.
11. Watson JC (2006) Student-athletes and counseling: factors influencing the decision to seek counseling services. *College Student Journal* 40(1), 35–42.
12. Brooks DD, Etzel EF, Ostrow AC (1987) Job responsibilities and backgrounds of NCAA Division I athletic advisors and counselors. *The Sport Psychologist* 1, 201–207.
13. Ferrante A, Etzel EF, Lantz C (1996) Counseling college student-athletes: the problem, the need. In EF Etzel, A Ferrante, J Pinkney (eds.), *Counseling College Student-Athletes: Issues and Interventions (2nd edn)*. Morgantown, WV: Fitness Information Technology.
14. Kadison R, DiGeronimo T (2004) *College of the Overwhelmed*. San Francisco, CA: Jossey-Bass.
15. Amazon.com. http://www.amazon.com/s/ref=nb_sb_noss_1?url=search-alias%3Dstripbooks&field-keywords=sports+psychiatry. Accessed on 23 July 2012.
16. International Society for Sport Psychiatry. http://sportspsychiatry.org/. Accessed on 23 July 2012.
17. American Board of Sport Psychology. http://www.americanboardofsportpsychology.org/. Accessed on 23 July 2012.
18. The British Association of Sport and Exercise Sciences. http://www.bases.org.uk/Psychology. Accessed on 23 July 2012.
19. Spanish Federation of Sport Psychology. http://www.psicologiadeporte.org/indexingles.htm. Accessed on 23 July 2012.
20. German Association of Sport Psychology. http://www.iupsys.net/index.php/iupsysresources/84-germany-articles/1057-german-association-of-sport-psychology. Accessed on 23 July 2012.
21. Association for Applied Sports Psychology. http://www.appliedsportpsych.org/about/ethics/code. Accessed on 23 July 2012.
22. International Society of Sport Psychology. http://www.issponline.org/p_codeofethics.asp?ms=3. Accessed on 23 July 2012.

23. International Federation of Sports Medicine Code of Ethics. http://www.fims.org/en/general/code-of-ethics/. Accessed on 23 July 2012.

24. Mathias MB (2004) The competing demands of sport and health: an essay on the history of ethics in sports medicine. *Clinics in Sports Medicine* 23, 195–214.

25. Glick ID, Horsfall JL (2005) Diagnosis and psychiatric treatment of athletes. *Clinics in Sports Medicine* 24, 771–781.

26. Brown JL, Cogan KD (2010) Ethical clinical practice and sport psychology: when two worlds collide. *Ethics & Behavior* 16(1), 15–23.

27. Berg-Cross L, Pak V (2006) Diversity issues. In P Grayson, P Meilman (eds.), *College Mental Health Practice*. New York: Routledge.

28. LaRoche MJ, Maxie A (2003) Ten considerations in addressing cultural differences in psychotherapy. *Professional Psychology: Research and Practice* 34, 180–186.

29. Benton SA *et al.* (2003) Changes in counseling center client problems across 13 years. *Professional Psychology: Research and Practice* 34, 66–72.

30. Steven U (2006) Steroids are dangerous. Opposing Viewpoints Resource Center. Gale Group. San Joaquin Delta College Library, Stockton, CA, 28 November 2007. http://galenet.galegroup.com. Accessed on 18 January 2013.

31. Doug W (2007) Steroids are harmful. Opposing Viewpoints Resource Center. Gale Group, 2006. San Joaquin Delta College Library, December 5, Stockton, CA. http://galenet.galegroup.com. Accessed on 18 January 2013.

32. Collins GB (2000) Substance abuse and athletes. In D Begel, RW Burton (eds.), *Sport Psychiatry: Theory and Practice*. New York: W. W. Norton & Company.

33. Hendrickson TP, Burton RW (2000) Athletes' use of performance-enhancing drugs. In D Begel, RW Burton (eds.), *Sport Psychiatry: Theory and Practice*. New York: W. W. Norton & Company.

Part Four

The Field of Sports Psychiatry

19 Sports Psychiatrists Working in College Athletic Departments

Eric D. Morse

Carolina Performance, North Carolina State University, USA

KEY POINTS

- Discussion around whom the sports psychiatrist is serving, confidentiality, medical record keeping, and design of a Team Assistance Program (TAP) should be made prior to seeing college athletes.
- Performance enhancement/psychology is an important part of why most college athletes might be willing to see a sports psychiatrist initially. Sports psychiatrists need to seek additional education, training, and supervision in performance enhancement/psychology.
- Location of the service is essential. Sports psychiatrists should be working in the training room just like other members of the sports medicine team.
- Sports psychiatrists must be able to discuss budget and funding issues with the athletic department as utilization of TAP services will likely increase.

BACKGROUND

Few, if any, psychiatry residency training programs teach psychiatrists how to market their skill sets. It may seem foreign to psychiatrists who want to work with athletes to describe what they do and suggest that they can assist athletic departments with problems they may have. How, then, does a sports psychiatrist get his foot in the door? Cold calls or emails to athletic directors, athletic trainers, academic support, and sports medicine physicians may not be effective and go unanswered. Working at the university's counseling center may help. Having a good working relationship and pairing with a sports psychologist who has experience with marketing her skills to an athletic department may add to success. Walking in and sitting down with the decision makers may be the most effective method. When walking in, a sports psychiatrist needs a brief, polished sales pitch with a list of common difficulties or disorders that he can help manage. Substance use, attention deficit/ hyperactivity disorder (ADHD), depression, anxiety, eating disorders, suicidality, performance psychology, and anger issues are what most athletic departments feel they need assistance with. A good sports psychiatrist must be able to say with confidence that she can

Clinical Sports Psychiatry: An International Perspective, First Edition. Edited by David A. Baron,
Claudia L. Reardon and Steven H. Baron.
© 2013 John Wiley & Sons, Ltd. Published 2013 by John Wiley & Sons, Ltd.

help with all of these concerns. Sadly, it sometimes takes a critical incident, such as a death or criminal activity that has been made public, to lead to a turning point for an athletic department. A knee-jerk reaction of hiring a sports psychiatrist can lead to an opportunity. Coming in with the idea of taking existing resources and helping to manage them with a Team Assistance Program (TAP) approach usually seems more cost effective than other potential proposals to the athletic department's decision makers.

DESIGN

When a sports psychiatrist has the opportunity to work with a college athletic department, some thought into the design of the relationship should be made before consulting. While just coming in to see student athletes when called upon and leaving thereafter may seem like the easiest approach, establishing a TAP model might be more impactful and increase utilization [1]. Will the sports psychiatrist come to the training room or another department office, or will he remain in his office off campus? Who gets the medical records? Who pays, and how much, for the sports psychiatrist's time? The sports psychiatrist may decide to act as the point person for a TAP or as one of the consultants within the TAP. It is important to ask who is already consulting with the athletic department and from there to try to be inclusive. Taking the time to gather existing campus resources and assemble an interprofessional staff for the TAP will facilitate referrals. TAP professionals may include a sports psychologist, an eating disorders counselor, and a substance abuse counselor, all of whom may already be at the college's counseling center, a career counselor at the college's career counseling center, an eating disorder nurse at the women's center or at student health, a sports nutrition expert in the nutrition department or student health, a health promotion counselor at the health education office, a domestic violence counselor on campus, and counselors or educational experts within the academic support program. It is not unusual for most athletic administrators or trainers to be frustrated with a lack of communication from the campus counseling center prior to the establishment of a TAP. The sports psychiatrist may need to find some of these resources off campus and bring them into the TAP model.

BUDGET

The funding for the TAP may come from different departments. Some of the professionals may be willing to use their professional time or volunteer some time. Grant writers may be used for local, state, or conference monies for substance use prevention, eating disorder prevention, and other professional programs. A decision of an hourly rate, a rate per appointment, or a yearly stipend for the sports psychiatrist should be made with the overall budget in mind. A sports psychiatrist should not price himself or herself out of a job. However, as the TAP and the sports psychiatrist's time is utilized more with each passing year, there needs to be an understanding that the costs may rise. It is important to ask what the budget is and to pace the sports psychiatrist's time appropriately. One way to decrease costs is to create a sports psychiatry elective and supervise a psychiatry resident physician. There are few electives available for residents to gain valuable experience. Many sports psychiatrists would like to start a sports psychiatry fellowship, but funding such a fellowship is a significant challenge.

WHO IS BEING SERVED

The ethical question of who is the sports psychiatrist's identified client must be addressed in the beginning. Is the sports psychiatrist working for the university, the athletic department, the sports medicine department, academic support, the coaches, or the student athletes? Can the sports psychiatrist truly work for all equally? When an athletic director asks the sports psychiatrist to evaluate a coach to help decide on the coach's future, or when a coach asks the sports psychiatrist for a prognosis on an athlete to decide whether or not the athlete should have their scholarship renewed, that is not the time to decide for whom the sports psychiatrist is really working. Thought and discussion needs to transpire prior to these types of scenarios occurring. Certain professionals within the TAP might be bound by different rules and expectations.

CONFIDENTIALITY

Everyone needs to know what type of personal, confidential information can be released to whom and when. At the beginning of the first appointment with a student athlete, the topic of confidentiality and signing releases of information must be discussed. Choices of more confidential, off-campus resources should be given. Who pays for these resources must be decided ahead of time. Another challenge may be that certain professionals within the TAP may have different understandings about who needs to know what. For example, the nutritionist and trainers may need to know about a student athlete's disordered eating behaviors, but does the career counselor need to know this?

BOUNDARIES

Sports psychiatrists may have internal and external pressures to treat college athletes differently. Other TAP professionals may have different standards in professional boundaries. Maintaining proper professional boundaries can safeguard against ethical dilemmas.

A common boundary challenge may lie in diagnosing and treating ADHD in student athletes. The athlete may recognize and seek the performance-enhancing effects of stimulants, which are first-line treatment for ADHD. It is very easy to research and memorize the diagnostic criteria for ADHD in hopes of being prescribed stimulants for performance enhancement. When prescribed for well-documented ADHD, stimulants may be viewed as performance-enabling, not performance-enhancing. The prescription of stimulants strictly for performance enhancement must be considered a doping violation and unethical and the sports psychiatrist should be reprimanded. Some of the external pressures to diagnose and aggressively treat ADHD may come from coaches, trainers, academic support, and/or athletic directors. The sports psychiatrist may want to feel like a team player and treat the athlete before proper testing is performed. The athlete may border on academic ineligibility and feel pressured by his support system to initiate stimulants as soon as possible. He may fear the loss of his scholarship or college career. The sports psychiatrist might feel that her position may be in jeopardy if she refuses to prescribe without a proper evaluation.

Sports psychiatrists may be asked by athletes, coaches, and trainers about the half-lives of performance-enhancing (stimulants, anabolic steroids, etc.) or recreational drugs (marijuana, cocaine, etc.) in urine drug testing, about masking agents, and about other methods of doping. Some sports psychiatrists may be asked by a trainer to prescribe anabolic steroids to athletes, "since they are going to use them anyway," in a request that may be framed as "a harm reduction." Besides the 1990 Anabolic Steroid Act making such a practice illegal, such behavior is unethical, immoral, and violates the purpose of sport. A sports psychiatrist's special knowledge unfortunately can be misused for doping purposes, and educational information must be given with the proper ethical considerations.

Without proper professional boundaries, sports psychiatrists may feel beholden to certain athletes, athletic directors, trainers, and others if gifts are accepted. Common gifts include game tickets, gear, or personal jerseys. They may have no, or very low, monetary value to the person giving and/or accepting the gift. However, the gift must be fully examined and processed by the sports psychiatrist. Is this ticket to this game solely for the purpose of evaluating this athlete or team, or is it a form of thanks or compensation? The answer must be made clear to all parties involved. Athletes may be very respectful of their work with the sports psychiatrist and view giving their jersey (and expecting it to be framed and prominently displayed in the sports psychiatrist's office) as a way of thanking, or providing a testimonial for, the sports psychiatrist. Ethically, this would take advantage of the therapeutic relationship.

Another professional boundary that sports psychiatrists must consider is time. College athletes have busy schedules. Sports psychiatrists have busy schedules. There may be pressures to "fit" an athlete in and spend less time than necessary to make a clinical decision, to prescribe a refill without fully evaluating the athlete, or to provide phone appointments. In the training room, other sports medicine providers have a list of athletes who may be seen on a first come, first served basis. It may be easy to just "drop in and be seen." Sports psychiatry may be very different from other sports medicine disciplines, but we may be expected to function like any other sports medicine clinic. Sports psychiatrists may be expected to work evenings or nights like other sports medicine disciplines and provide round-the-clock access. Sports psychiatrists must remain aware of the professional boundary of time and examine transference and countertransference reactions to limit-setting on this front.

One question that sports psychiatrists should ask themselves in dealing with professional boundaries is: How is my treatment of this athlete different from any other nonathlete in my private practice? Significant differences should prompt further examination. Are the reasons for the differences justifiable? Are the athletes' needs being met, or are the sports psychiatrists' needs being met? Am I bending the standard rules of my practice for my convenience or the athlete's convenience? What is that saying about my athlete or me?

Lastly, when a sports psychiatrist is not certain about maintaining proper professional boundaries, supervision must be sought. Other TAP professionals may or may not be able to assist with supervision. Off-site supervision with colleagues may be required.

IMPROVING UTILIZATION WITH A TEAM
ASSISTANCE PROGRAM MODEL

Bringing together on-campus resources into a TAP model can improve utilization of and communication between all TAP professionals. Improving utilization may appear to increase costs, but an ounce of prevention is often worth more than a pound of cure. McDuff, Morse, and White have made 10 recommendations when establishing a TAP [1].

Provide services on-site

If the sports psychiatrist is out of sight, he or she will be out of mind. Attending practices and games, and interacting with athletes, coaches, and sports medicine personnel help to develop relationships, referrals, and trust. Being seen as part of the team is important. Having a consistent presence in the training room, even on days when the sports psychiatrist does not have anyone scheduled, creates a feeling of caring. Brief interactions and curbside advice on life stressors or performance issues can lead to more involved discussions. Trainers will refer more athletes to the sports psychiatrist the more the sports psychiatrist is seen.

Hire a diverse staff

A diverse staff by gender, ethnicity, professional discipline, and competencies allows for athletes and staff to have a choice. Some athletes relate better to males or females, younger or older, a particular race, or a particular look. Introduce all of the TAP staff at orientation or early in the season and step back and watch which athletes naturally gravitate to which TAP professional.

Connect with preparticipation physicals and injured athletes

The preseason physical evaluation is a good time to ask about past or current concerns with any mental health or performance issues. A review by Joy *et al.* [2] recommends that these questions become standard practice. Forms are sent out in advance of coming to campus and they should include these questions and be reviewed by trainers. Any affirmative responses should be referred to the TAP for at least a short interview early on. Supportive interactions with injured athletes are also important. Severe athletic injuries, especially those requiring surgery or prolonged rehabilitation, often produce emotional distress and lowered self-esteem [3]. Return to play and career termination decisions relating to injury, especially head injury, are now more clinically complicated [4]. An expert panel of Sport Medicine professionals recommended that psychosocial issues be included in the return-to-play processes [5] and TAP professionals can be useful in that process.

Give prevention talks

Giving brief talks to athletes, coaches, and trainers is a good way to remind them that you are present and to catch small difficulties before they become larger problems. Tying the topic to athletic performance and winning is essential to getting participants' attention and to stimulating discussion. For example, along with having the TAP nutritionists and strength and conditioning coaches discuss supplements, mixing in some substance use prevention material can not only stimulate discussion but also create opportunity for funding as part of a substance prevention grant. Most prevention talks lead to more referrals.

Offer tobacco cessation services

The adverse health effects, the increasing cost of using, and the resulting drop in conditioning and performance make athletes and coaches interested in tobacco cessation. There may be state or university resources for smoking cessation programs. The preparticipation physical forms and sports medicine physicians routinely screen for use and support quitting by referring to TAP professionals. Studies have shown that brief interventions can reduce spit tobacco use in athletes [6]. Besides nicotine replacement and FDA-approved medications for nicotine dependence, using substitutions such as sugar-free gum, aromatic hardwood branches, herbal dips, toothpicks, or drinking straws cut to the size of a cigarette can be helpful in the handling of oral fixation.

Offer performance enhancement services

Having a sports psychologist with a lot of performance psychology experience working with the sports psychiatrist is ideal. If not, some TAPS have modeled these services after the approaches recommended by Dorfman and Kuehl in *The Mental Game of Baseball* [7]. Identifying major barriers to performance (i.e., divided attention, negative self-talk, poor emotional control, pregame arousal, inability to let go of mistakes) in individual or team sessions is important. Athletes should record information about thoughts and emotions (positive and negative) during competition using a mental training log as recommended by Porter [8]. Well-trained TAP professionals should regularly review the records while updating short-, medium-, and long-term goals in an improvement plan with the assistance of the coaching staff.

Provide critical incident stress management services

Athletic departments occasionally experience traumatic events or unexpected tragic losses. Deaths of coaches or athletes can obviously disrupt individual and/or team functioning. TAP professionals would be expected to respond to such challenges by offering comprehensive support services for the athletic department. Already having a good working relationship with the athletic department makes the critical incident response seem seamless. It is important to respond quickly and in person. It is also recommended to collaborate with a chaplain and give extra support to the medical and conditioning staff.

Know something about fitness and supplements

Supplement use by college athletes has increased. While most athletes are looking to gain a competitive advantage, they are still concerned about false claims, cost, long-term side effects, and contamination. Sports psychiatrists need to know the athletic department's drug policy. Current, factual information about the policy and about the risks and benefits of various supplements is most helpful. Whether presented in prevention talks or in printed materials that are posted in the training room, coaches and players are interested. Collaboration with the team physicians, trainers, strength staff, and nutritionists is necessary to ensure a consistent message. The more the knowledge about exercise physiology, cardiovascular fitness, speed, strength, and flexibility training, the more credibility sports psychiatrists will have with their athletes.

Think about sleep, jet lag, chronic fatigue, and burnout

College athletic training and competition are now year-round endeavors. Most college athletes do not truly get an off-season. It is therefore critical to monitor athletes for sleep and stress recovery. Long seasons can bring on chronic mental and physical fatigue and poor sleep because of chronic injuries and performance pressure. Travel adds to the demands of studies and competition, especially if across two or more time zones or if circadian rhythms are disrupted [9]. When asked for sleeping medication, sports psychiatrists should screen for poor sleep hygiene, excessive stimulant or alcohol use, high stress levels, or sleep, mood, or anxiety disorders that might explain the insomnia. They are good prevention talk topics. Chapter 15 contains more information on the use of sleep aids in this population.

Reach out to family members

Many college athletes have prolonged family separations. Some degree of homesickness is normal. In severe cases, reaching out to family can be helpful. Sometimes helping athletes and trainers with limit-setting for over-involved or enmeshed parents can be challenging but essential work. It is difficult to be fully present in college if the athlete is constantly calling home or texting her parents. Setting limits on the number of calls, texts, or time spent per week can be of great assistance to the athlete and the family. When evaluating a college athlete for a mental illness, the family may have important collateral information about the athlete or family history. Some college athletes already have children and miss seeing them. Helping to arrange regularly scheduled Internet visits can be very helpful for the college athlete and child.

TREATMENT ISSUES

What do most sports psychiatrists do when working with the college athletic department? Besides providing mental health services to student athletes through sports medicine, sports psychiatrists serve as the education, prevention, and intervention arms of their athletic department's substance abuse or drug testing policies on an individual or team level, assist in team building and improving group dynamics, and evaluate and treat learning disorders in their academic support services. It is difficult to do it all alone, so establishing a TAP is recommended, as already emphasized.

In college athletics, ADHD is probably the most common mental illness that sports psychiatrists will treat. Stimulants are still first-line treatment, but are on the prohibited list at the college level in most countries. Since stimulants can be performance-enhancing, standardized testing and clinical interviews by possibly more than one TAP clinician to make a certain diagnosis, rule out other issues and diagnoses, and provide documentation for applying for special accommodations is recommended. Sports psychiatrists should make certain that proper documentation makes its way to the sports medicine chart, so that any urine testing positive for stimulants is not considered a violation of policy. Any college athlete competing at an Olympic level would need to apply for a therapeutic use exemption (TUE) from their country's Olympic governing body. In the United States, the governing body is the United States Anti-Doping Agency, and the TUE forms can be downloaded from www.usada.org. The sports psychiatrist needs to complete a TUE depending on the country for which the athlete is competing.

Treating depression or anxiety is probably the next most frequent referral to a college sports psychiatrist. The stress of being a student athlete can be immense. Often, the athlete's exercise and nutrition are healthier than nonathletes. Thus, when they meet DSM-IV criteria for a mood or anxiety disorder, medication management is often required, as lifestyle factors may already have been optimized. Sports psychiatrists can provide psychotherapy and medication (or can provide split treatment with another TAP clinician). Accustomed to being coached and taking instructions, college athletes do well with cognitive behavioral therapy (CBT) by completing their homework assignments (thought records), as discussed in Chapter 11. College athletes may tend to be more reluctant but more compliant with medications than are nonathlete patients. Because there is pressure to get better faster, so they can compete at a higher level and remain eligible academically, using psychotherapy in conjunction with medication is quite common.

Sports psychiatrists working in athletic departments should remain current in the latest treatments of addictions. They should assist in updating the athletic department's substance abuse or drug testing policy to encourage prevention and treatment of addictions and not just sanctions for positive urine drug tests. The use of motivational interviewing techniques in college athletes is essential in addiction work because so many athletes are in the precontemplation stage. Twelve-step facilitations, such as Alcoholics Anonymous or Narcotics Anonymous groups, may be a challenge due to some athletes' high profiles and concerns about confidentiality. CBT for relapse prevention is helpful. Because college athletes have so much to lose by testing positive again, they tend to be willing to try pharmacologic interventions (disulfiram, acamprosate, naltrexone, etc.). Co-occurring illness (an addiction together with another mental illness) is the rule, not the exception. The co-occurring mental illness must also be treated. This is why most sports medicine physicians have learned to refer college athletes suffering with addiction to sports psychiatrists over substance abuse counselors, although split treatment with another TAP clinician may be more cost effective.

For team substance use prevention work, it is best for sports psychiatrists to work with other TAP clinicians. Substance use problems on a team can be part of the team's culture. Teammates tend to use together. Substance use can be a negative part of team-building rituals or hazing. Since current players have a pivotal role in recruiting, players tend to select recruits that will go along with the existing team culture. The TAP should work on these aspects with team-building exercises or leadership training and then relate them to substance use. The use of role play can be helpful.

Eating disorders are more prevalent in college athletes than in the general college population [10]. Many athletes fall into the category of "Anorexia Athletica," which is not a DSM-IV diagnosis but meets criteria for Eating Disorder NOS [11]. Anorexia Athletica often includes a fear of gaining weight despite being lean, but muscular development maintains weight above the anorexic threshold (85% or less of expected per DSM-IV), and there is excessive or compulsive exercise. Sports psychiatrists need to be aware of "The Female Athlete Triad" which refers to the interrelationships among energy availability, menstrual function, and bone mineral density, which may have clinical manifestations including eating disorders, functional hypothalamic amenorrhea, and osteoporosis [12]. CBT and motivational interviewing techniques are helpful in treating disordered eating [13, 14]. Female athletes may feel more comfortable working with a female TAP clinician, which may necessitate split treatment in some cases. Proper and frequent communication within the treatment team is essential. Many athletic departments use eating disorder treatment contracts that involve input from coaches, parents, athletic trainers, sports medicine physicians, nutritionists, and mental health providers. Disordered eating is a good prevention talk topic. The TAP may need to provide support to the team or affected teammates and do some educational programs and address the team culture. College athletes may have "The Over-Doers Triad," consisting of symptoms of eating disorders, obsessive-compulsive disorder, and exercise dependence [15]. They overthink and overdo. They can be so obsessional that when the sports psychiatrist asks them to estimate what percent of their waking hours they think about their weight, nutrition, calories, exercise, or body issues, it is not unusual to get answers above 90%. They would like to have new thoughts. Selective serotonin reuptake inhibitors (SSRIs) can be extremely helpful in reducing this percentage of obsessional thinking and in helping the athlete to do better in psychotherapy [16].

PART OF THE SPORTS MEDICINE TEAM

It is essential for sports psychiatrists working in college athletic departments to be part of the sports medicine team. Sports psychiatrists need to communicate and use the same language as the rest of the sports medicine team. When the sports medicine team gives the sports psychiatrists a sports medicine shirt, jacket, cap, etc., the sports psychiatrist should wear it. It gives the athletes a sense that the psychiatrist is just another sports medicine physician who comes into the training room on the same assigned day. It reduces stigma for the athletes and the staff.

LOCATION

Sports psychiatrists should work in the training room along with the rest of sports medicine. As discussed, this is the first recommendation in establishing a TAP. If the sports psychiatrist decides not to create a TAP, being in the training room will still give the sports psychiatrist more access to engage college athletes and staff, reduce stigma, and gain more referrals.

Case Study

A sports psychiatrist consulted for a Division I National Collegiate Athletic Association university from 2002 to 2004 and created a TAP. A brochure was designed and presented to sports medicine physicians and trainers that included every TAP professional's phone number and email. It was posted in the training room for college athletes to see. The TAP was presented annually at a monthly compliance meeting to remind the coaches and administrators to use the TAP. At the beginning of the 2002 season, a letter attached to a screening questionnaire introduced the TAP to every college athlete. The TAP sports psychiatrist also met each incoming freshmen and transfer college athlete while giving lectures in a required health and human behaviors course. The TAP included a sports psychiatrist, a sports psychologist, a nutritionist, two substance abuse counselors, two career counselors, a domestic violence counselor, and an eating disorder specialist. The sports psychiatrist was the point person for the TAP, so if the referral source was not certain as to which TAP professional should get the referral, the sports psychiatrist was called first.

The sports psychiatrist came to the training room every Wednesday afternoon. Appointments were scheduled in 1-h sessions for intakes and half-hour sessions for follow-ups. College athletes, trainers, sports medicine physicians, the chiropractor,

Table 19.1 Utilization data for a college Team Assistance Program.

Year	No. of intakes	No. of visits	No. of athletes[a]	Utilization %[b]
2002 (3 months)	6	10	354	1.7
2002–2003	43	224	328	13.1
2003–2004	47	201	322	14.6

[a]No. of Athletes = number of athletes who were in the athletic department that academic year.
[b]Utilization % = percentage of athletes in the athletic department who used the sports psychiatrist formally with an appointment in that academic year. It does not include work by other TAP professionals, or informal discussions in the training room or after prevention talks.

coaches, and academic support staff all had access to the sports psychiatrist's schedule kept by the sports medicine director. No shows were limited by training staff reminder calls on Wednesday mornings. There were no "wrong doors" for referrals. Referrals came from any TAP professional, the sports medicine team, college athletes themselves, coaches, or administrators. The sports psychiatrist gave prevention talks and worked with teams on performance enhancement, mental skills, positive self- and team talk, and communication skills and conflict resolution between teammates and coaches in early morning, evening, and weekend time slots.

Records were kept in separate folders double-locked in the sports medicine director's office. TAP notes were written with as much discretion as possible. The sports psychiatrist only documented prescribed medications and dosages in the general sports medicine charts. Only one athlete refused treatment because of this arrangement, and she was given a referral to a preferred provider in her insurance network.

College athletes were reluctant to seek treatment unless initially asking for performance enhancement. The one notable exception was the self-referrals that come in after the "Disordered Eating" prevention talk given in the health education class for athletes by the sports psychiatrist each semester. Athletes usually walked in the following Wednesday afternoon with a chief complaint of "I think I have an eating disorder." All walk-ins were seen.

Table 19.1 shows utilization data for 3 years kept by the sports psychiatrist in this real-life case study. Only individual sessions with the sports psychiatrist in the training room are included in the utilization data. Neither formal sessions with other TAP members nor informal advice by the sports psychiatrist are included. The prevention talks and team consultations are not included.

Most referrals were self-referrals, with a minority of referrals made by trainers, team physicians, and coaches. Some athletes were seen repeatedly. In fact, 22 athletes initially seen in 2002–2003 were seen again in 2003–2004. A total of 69 different student athletes were seen over 3 years. Visits averaged five per intake, although some athletes were seen once or twice and others more frequently. No significant gender utilization rate differences were noted. Few college athletes were seen in 2002 as the sport psychiatrist's time was used primarily for staff recruitment presentations and coaches meetings.

Identifying a primary problem for individual athletes was not always possible. Therefore, if athletes had two or more significant problems, each was included in

Table 19.2 Common problems faced by college athletes during appointments with the sports psychiatrist in the Team Assistance Program.

Performance enhancement (23)[a]	Domestic violence (3)
Stress reaction to injury/rehab (9)	Learning disorder (2)
Depression (9)	Exercise dependence (3)
Attention deficit disorder (8)	Insomnia (2)
Substance use (7)	Panic disorder (2)
Eating disorders (7)	Bipolar disorder (2)
Post-concussive syndrome (4)	Anger management (2)
Obsessive-compulsive disorders (4)	Dysthymia (1)
Stress reaction to breakups (3)	Social phobia (1)
Generalized anxiety (3)	Specific phobia (1)
Grief (3)	

[a]Actual numbers of athletes facing a given problem during 27 months of tracking are listed in parenthesis. The prevalence data do not include problems discussed occurring informally in the training room or after prevention talks. TAP professionals other than the sport psychiatrist did not collect data.

Table 19.2, which highlights the common problems with which athletes presented. Interestingly, two athletes had three problems – "The Over-Doer Triad," which includes an eating disorder, obsessive-compulsive disorder, and exercise dependence, as described earlier.

As more college athletes were being assisted, they referred their teammates. The program continued even after the sports psychiatrist left for another university. The sports psychologist took over as the TAP point person. Budget and funding problems led the sports psychiatrist to find another Division I school to start another TAP. It was an excellent learning experience for the sports psychiatrist, both in how to establish a TAP and in how important it is to discuss the budget and funding on a more regular basis.

CONCLUSION

Before a sports psychiatrist begins working in a college athletic department, decisions must be made about design, budget, who is being served, confidentiality, boundaries, and location of services. Gathering on-campus resources and creating a TAP is a significant way to improve referrals, utilization, and outcomes, while hopefully reducing costs to stay on budget. The sports psychiatrist needs to stay current on the treatment of the common problems that are sometimes unique to college athletes. If following these guidelines, sports psychiatrists will hopefully become an essential part of sports medicine teams.

REFERENCES

1. McDuff DR, Morse ED, White RK (2005). Professional and collegiate team assistance programs: services and utilization patterns. *Clinics in Sports Medicine* 24, 943–958.
2. Joy EA, Paisley TS, Price R, *et al.* (2004). Optimizing the collegiate preparticipation physical evaluation. *Clinical Journal of Sports Medicine* 14, 183–187.

3. Smith AM, Scott SG, Wiese DM (1990). The psychological effects of sports injuries. Coping. *Sports Medicine* 9, 352–369.

4. Cantu RC (2003). Recurrent head injury: risks and when to retire. *Clinics in Sports Medicine* 22, 593–603.

5. McFarland EG (2004). Return to play. *Clinics in Sports Medicine* 23, xv–xxiii.

6. Walsh MM, Hilton JF, Ellison JA, *et al.* (2003). Spit (smokeless) intervention of high school athletes results after 1 year. *Addictive Behavior* 28, 1095–1113.

7. Dorfman HA, Kuehl K (1995). *The Mental Game of Baseball*, 2nd Edition. South Bend, IN: Diamonds Communications, Inc..

8. Porter K. (2004). *The Mental Athlete*. Champaign, IL: Human Kinetics, pp. 26–27.

9. Waterhouse J, Edwards B, Nevil A, *et al.* (2002). Identifying some determinants of jet lag and its symptoms: a study of athletes and other travelers. *British Journal of Sports Medicine* 36, 54–60.

10. Johnson C, Powers PS, Dick R (1999). Athletes and eating disorders: the National Collegiate Athletic Association study. *International Journal of Eating Disorders* 26(2), 179–188.

11. Currie A, Morse ED (2004). Eating disorders in athletes: managing the risks. *Clinics in Sports Medicine* 24, 871–883.

12. American College of Sports Medicine (2007). The female athlete triad. *Medicine and Science in Sports and Exercise* 39(10), 1867–1882.

13. Williamson DA, White MA, York-Crowe E, Stewart TM (2004). Cognitive-behavioral theories of eating disorders. *Behavior Modification* 28(6), 711–738.

14. Wilson GT, Schlam TR (2004). The transtheoretical model of motivational interviewing in the treatment of eating and weight disorders. *Clinical Psychology Review* 24(3), 361–378.

15. Morse ED (2004). Eating disorders in athletes. Presentation given at the International Society for Sports Psychiatry's scientific session at the American Psychiatric Association's annual meeting, May 2, New York.

16. Power PS, Santana C (2004). Available pharmacological treatments for anorexia nervosa. *Expert Opinion on Pharmacotherapy* 5(11), 2287–2292.

20 Sports Psychiatry: Current Status and Challenges

Ira D. Glick,[1] Thomas Newmark,[2]
and Claudia L. Reardon[3]

[1] Psychiatry and Behavioral Sciences, Stanford University School of Medicine, USA
[2] Department of Psychiatry, Robert Wood Johnson Medical School, Cooper University Hospital, USA
[3] Department of Psychiatry, University of Wisconsin School of Medicine and Public Health, USA

KEY POINTS

- The aims of the field of sports psychiatry are to: optimize health of athletes, ethically improve athletic performance, and manage psychiatric symptoms or disorders of athletes.
- Sports psychiatry as a field faces many challenges, including: stigma, difficulties breaking into the field, negative publicity about physicians who work with athletes, an underdeveloped research base, and the need for elevation of the status of the field.
- Professional sports psychiatry organizations are important to provide networking, research, and educational opportunities.

BACKGROUND

The field of sports psychiatry had its origin in 1990, when Dan Begel, M.D., carved out a new subspecialty within psychiatry, which he defined as "the application of the principles of and practice of psychiatry to the world of sports" [1]. Sports psychiatrists are physician-psychiatrists who diagnose and treat problems, symptoms, and disorders associated with an athlete, the athlete's family or significant others, the team, or the sport. Primary aims of the specialty are to:

1. optimize health,
2. ethically improve athletic performance, and
3. manage psychiatric symptoms or disorders [2].

Factors that illustrate the necessity of sports psychiatry as a subspecialty include:

1. an athlete's state of mind has a significant impact on performance,
2. participation in sports affects the mood, thinking, personality, and health of the participant, and
3. the psychiatric care of the athlete must be adapted to the athletic context in order to be effective [3].

Clinical Sports Psychiatry: An International Perspective, First Edition. Edited by David A. Baron,
Claudia L. Reardon and Steven H. Baron.
© 2013 John Wiley & Sons, Ltd. Published 2013 by John Wiley & Sons, Ltd.

Education and training to practice as a sports psychiatrist include medical education to impart knowledge and skills unique to physicians, psychiatric training to provide knowledge and skills unique to that specialty, and training or experience in sports psychiatry to provide knowledge and skills unique to psychiatric aspects of sports [2].

The work of the sports psychiatrist usually consists of:

1. making an individual and family-systems diagnosis of the clinical situation, as appropriate,
2. setting goals for the athlete and any significant other parties involved, and
3. delivering treatment based on the psychiatric disorder or problem using a combination of medications, psychotherapy, and strategies targeted to specific sport performance issues [2].

EVOLUTION OF THE FIELD

Historically, athletes and teams have readily consulted with large medical and nonmedical staff (sometimes including psychologists) to improve performance. However, they have not typically involved psychiatrists, as professionals who can diagnose and treat psychiatric problems and disorders. This has started to change over the past two decades, as mental health professionals have become more incorporated into college and professional team sports [4]. Reasons for this change include competitive pressures to win, fallout from bizarre behavior on and off the field, inappropriate aggressive tactics or overt cheating, steroid scandals, concussions, gambling, and substance abuse. Sports psychiatrists increasingly are especially involved in management of substance abuse problems [2].

CHALLENGES FOR THE FIELD

Despite the positive evolution of the field in recent years, working within sports psychiatry presents many challenges [2]. Stigma is a primary one, and this manifests in many ways. Athletes have a tendency to minimize apparent signs of weakness, including symptoms of mental illness. As a result, they do not seek out psychiatric treatment, even when psychiatric symptoms are interfering with athletic performance. Athletes may fear that they will be labeled as "crazy" or not be allowed to participate. Moreover, the tendency to idealize athletes leads coaches, teammates, family members, and health-care professionals to deny the existence or significance of psychiatric symptoms in athletes [5]. As a result, teams, coaches, and agents are reluctant to hire and pay psychiatrists to deal with behavioral problems of athletes, and they more commonly discuss behavioral issues "off the record" [2].

In the absence of a perceived need, then, it is difficult for psychiatrists to break into the field. It often takes many years to establish the connections needed to enter this subspecialty. Chapter 19 addresses some of these difficulties, many of which apply regardless of the setting in which a sports psychiatrist would like to work.

A third challenge relates to negative publicity about physicians unethically providing treatments to enhance performance [2]. This most prominently involves prescription of banned substances, such as anabolic steroids and stimulants. It can also involve use of unproven procedures [6].

An important challenge is the underdeveloped research base in the field. This too likely relates to the tendency to deny the existence of mental illness in athletes. Sports psychiatrists will be better positioned to provide evidence-based treatment to their athlete-patients as the research base continues to grow. Areas in which the field desperately needs more epidemiologic study include the relationship between major depressive disorder and over-training syndrome, given the prevalence of the latter in athletes and its potential implications for performance and quality of life; diagnosis of psychiatric symptoms during times of transition (e.g., post-injury and retirement), given the increased risk of psychological distress during these times; eating disorders, given that these probably represent one of the few areas in which the disorders are actually perpetuated by sports participation itself; ADHD, since treatment involves using potentially performance-enhancing stimulants; and addictive disorders, since athletes appear to use substances of abuse more than the general population does [5]. Additionally, little research attention has been placed on the most complex patient within this group: the elite athlete [7]. Elite athletes are at increased risk for injuries, psychological abuse by coaches and parents, and self-abuse. Beyond epidemiologic research, much more study of *treatment* of mental illness in athletes is needed. In particular, researchers need to further examine the use of psychiatric medications in athletes, as described in Chapter 15.

A final challenge involves the need for elevation of the status of the field by development of a code of ethics and a curriculum of subspecialty training for those who wish to specialize in this area [2].

THE ROLE OF PROFESSIONAL SPORTS PSYCHIATRY ORGANIZATIONS

Given the challenges facing the field, psychiatrists wishing to establish a career within this subspecialty must have local as well as larger-scale support. National and international organizations are particularly important as sports psychiatry continues to establish recognition within the medical field and among athletes and teams.

The International Society for Sports Psychiatry (ISSP) was incorporated in 1997 and is the premier professional organization devoted to promoting the field. It provides networking opportunities and education for psychiatrists around the world interested in the field. Members are invited to present their work at the annual ISSP Scientific Session, which is held in conjunction with the American Psychiatric Association Annual Meeting. The ISSP also provides a website on which members' clinical contact information, publications, and media appearances are featured. Goals for the ISSP include: increasing global membership, developing standards of clinical practice, and developing linkages to other stakeholders in the field, including psychologists and athletic trainers [2].

In addition to the ISSP, the World Psychiatric Association (WPA), which includes several sections devoted to specific professional interests, has a Section on Exercise and Sports Psychiatry. The purpose of this section is to collect, analyze, present, and disseminate information concerning clinical service, research, and training and to advance scientific knowledge within the field. The section endeavors to establish working relations with national and international organizations sharing similar goals, organize scientific meetings and symposia on sports psychiatry for presentation at the World Congresses of Psychiatry and other meetings organized under the auspices of the WPA, and establish proposals for adoption as WPA consensus and position statements [8].

REFERENCES

1. Begel D (1992) An overview of sport psychiatry. *American Journal of Psychiatry* 49: 606–614.
2. Glick ID, Morse E, Reardon CL, Newmark T (2010) Sport psychiatry – a new frontier in a challenging world. *Die Psychiatrie* 7: 249–253.
3. Glick ID, Kamm R, Morse E (2009) The evolution of sport psychiatry, circa 2009. *Sports Medicine* 39(8): 607–613.
4. Nicholi A (1996) Psychiatric consultation in professional football. *The New England Journal of Medicine* 31: 1095–1100.
5. Reardon CL, Factor RM (2010) Sport psychiatry: a systematic review of diagnosis and medical treatment of mental illness in athletes. *Sports Medicine* 40(11): 1–20.
6. As sports medicine surges, hope and hype outpace proven treatments. *New York Times*, September 5, 2011. http://www.nytimes.com/2011/09/05/health/05treatment.html?pagewanted=all. Accessed on 1 April 2012.
7. Glick ID, Stillman MA, Reardon CL, Ritvo EC (2012) Managing psychiatric issues in elite athletes. *Journal of Clinical Psychiatry* 73(5): 640–644.
8. World Psychiatric Association (2012) Purpose of the sections, March 29. http://www.wpanet.org/detail.php?section_id=11&content_id=539. Accessed on 1 April 2012.

Index

Clinical Sports Psychiatry: An International Perspective, First Edition. Edited by David A. Baron,
Claudia L. Reardon and Steven H. Baron.
© 2013 John Wiley & Sons, Ltd. Published 2013 by John Wiley & Sons, Ltd.

.

Printed and bound by CPI Group (UK) Ltd, Croydon, CR0 4YY

29/07/2024

14533712-0003